A New Approach to
Women and Therapy
2nd Edition

A New Approach to
Women
&
Therapy

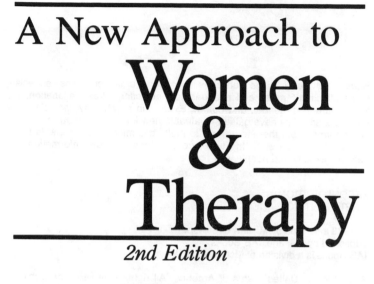

2nd Edition

MIRIAM GREENSPAN

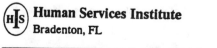

Human Services Institute
Blradenton, FL

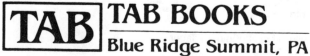

TAB BOOKS
Blue Ridge Summit, PA

Human Services Institute publishes books on human problems, especially those affecting families and relationships: addiction, stress, alienation, violence, parenting, gender, and health. Experts in psychology, medicine, and the social sciences have gained invaluable new knowledge about prevention and treatment, but there is a need to make this information available to the public. Human Services Institute books help bridge the information gap between experts and people with problems.

SECOND EDITION
FIRST PRINTING

© 1993 and 1983 by **Miriam Greenspan**.
Published by HSI and TAB Books.
TAB Books is a division of McGraw-Hill, Inc.

Library of Congress Cataloging-in-Publication Data

Greenspan, Miriam.
    A new approach to women and therapy / Miriam Greenspan. — 2nd ed.
      p. cm.
    Includes bibliographical references and index.
    ISBN 0-8306-4167-X   ISBN 0-8306-4168-8 (pbk.)
    1. Feminist therapy. 2. Women—Mental health. I. Title.
RC489.F45G73 1993
616.89′14′088042—dc20   92-34036
                                                         CIP

Questions regarding the content of this book should be addressed to:

Human Services Institute, Inc.
P.O. Box 14610
Bradenton, FL 34280

Acquisitions Editor: Kimberly Tabor
Cover by Holberg Design, York, Pa.

Contents

Preface to the Second Edition

In the past decade, I have received many letters from women thanking me for *A New Approach to Women & Therapy*. Most of these women spoke of the validating and empowering experience of reading this book. Some said they had given the book as an offering or challenging opportunity to their therapists or as a gift to their friends. Many women talked about how their emotional and social problems had gone unrecognized or were worsened in therapy. Too many told stories of emotional and sexual abuse that they suffered in the privacy of their psychotherapists' offices. Some women declared that the book helped them gather the courage to leave abusive therapists.

I thank all of you who have corresponded with me. The honesty and courage reflected in your letters have filled me with gratitude for being able, in some small way, to contribute to your journeys out of traditional psychotherapeutic straightjackets and toward emotional and social freedom.

Preface to the First Edition

This book is about women, therapy, and society. In particular, it is about therapists and female patients, and the relationship between them. Its specific focus is on individual therapy, which, despite the growth of group, couples, and family therapy, remains the most widely practiced mode of therapy today.

In ever increasing numbers, people today are putting their psyches on the line in the hope of finding someone who will help them find themselves. Most of these therapy patients have been, and remain, women. Therapists are supposed to be psychological healers, but how often they fall short of this ideal is all too evident in the research on the outcome of psychotherapy and in the countless stories of therapy patients and ex-patients who feel cheated. Patients too often find themselves paying enormous fees for "cures" or fulfillments that never come. Therapy too often becomes an instrument of constraint rather than an instrument of liberation—at best ineffectual, at worst psychically damaging.

I have tried to explore some rather complex themes relating to both women and therapy in language that is accessible to a lay reader. I hope that therapists, students and teachers of female psychology, and people generally interested in women and therapy will find the book useful. But it is addressed primarily to the people therapists treat—especially women who have been, are, or would be patients in individual psychotherapy. My goals are to expose the myths upon which currently accepted therapies are based, to show how these therapies fail women, and to present a new basis for understanding female psychology and for working with women in therapy. In offering a woman-oriented model of therapy, I have tried to incorporate the best elements of past therapies while avoiding those aspects which are inadequate or destructive, particularly to women. Most of all, my aim is to help the female reader gain a greater sense of herself as a person, and of her power to choose and demand the kind of therapy that will best serve her.

In my approach to women and therapy, I have tried to take account of the ways that the class of the therapist and patient affects the therapy, as well as of how class affects the psychology of women. But, for the most part, in my discussions of the latter, I have stressed what is generally true for women of *all* classes. I have tried to develop a psychology of women that acknowledges what we all share as a result of being part of a common "sex class."

A word about the use of pronouns in this book is necessary. In my discussion of traditional therapy, I have consistently used the pronouns "he" for the therapist and "she" for the patient. This is because most traditional therapists are men and most therapy patients are women; and also because, even when the therapist is a "she" and the patient a "he," the model of therapy itself is a male model. In presenting my own approach to therapy, I have used "she" for the therapist and "she" for the client because it is a female therapist and client I have in mind in this new model of therapy. I have also substituted the word "client" for "patient" in this new model in order to avoid the medical connotation of the latter, which is inappropriate to the kind of therapy I am proposing.

When referring to women as a whole, I have used the pronoun "we" rather than "they." This is because I consider myself part of the subject I am writing about, rather than a professional outsider researching a particular population.

Throughout this book, I have described the stories of women with whom I have worked in therapy. To protect their privacy, I have changed names and identifying characteristics. Within the limits of these modifications, I have tried to be true to these women's accounts of their own lives.

Acknowledgments

Many people shared in the making of this book, both directly and indirectly, and I am indebted to all of them. My first thank-you must go to the women's movement itself, for the book grew out of the movement and is inspired by a commitment to it. I am particularly grateful to the many women whom I have had the good fortune to work with in therapy, and who have taught me so much. A special thanks must go to those clients who gave their support and encouragement when it was necessary to take a therapy sabbatical in order to finish the book.

For reading and commenting on portions of early drafts of the manuscript, I thank Janet Kahn, Susan Galvin, Bronwen Murphy, Aidla Greenspan, Naomi Bock, and Carol Hymowitz. I was lucky to have the benefit of Carol's always astute writer's tips, as well as her continual support as a friend.

I am especially thankful for the detailed suggestions and criticisms of portions of earlier drafts which I received from Rochelle Ruthchild, Lou Ferleger, Barbara Ehrenreich, and Jean Baker Miller. Barbara provided some important criticisms of Part I. Jean's page-by-page suggestions were invaluable, as was her early encouragement regarding the importance of the book.

For their encouragement and faithful friendship over the years of writing, I am grateful to Susan Kaplan, Debbie Taylor, Myra Hindus, and Betsy Abrams. Betsy was always there when I needed a reader or a listener, a critical or a friendly ear. For their help and support, I also thank Ellen Keniston and Susie Dickler. For the generous loan of his typewriter, I thank Mordechai Leibling.

For their work in helping to create a theory and practice of feminist therapy, I am indebted to many, many women throughout the country. In particular, I would like to thank the members of the Brookline Women's Counseling Group and the Women's Mental Health Collective in Somerville. My association with both of these groups at different times helped in the development of my ideas about female psychology and feminist therapy. I also thank my colleagues in mutual supervision of therapy cases, especially Julie Schneider, Susan Calvin, and Bonnie Engelhardt.

The ideas about psychology and therapy developed in this book would not be possible without the work of certain people to whom I am intellectually indebted. These include Phyllis Chesler, Jean Baker Miller, R. D. Laing, Thomas Szasz, Frantz Fanon, Dorothy E. Smith, Naomi Weisstein, Sheila Rowbotham, and the radical therapy and mental patients' liberation movements.

For their excellent and efficient typing, I thank Ellen Holzman and Jeanne LeClare.

For her diligence, intelligence, ceaseless support and devotion to this book, I thank the best all around literary agent and mensch anyone could hope to know—Frances Goldin.

I had two editors at McGraw-Hill and I am grateful to them both. For her incisive organizational and editorial assistance, especially in the initial stages, I thank Peggy Tsukahira. My second editor, Gail Greene, contributed helpful suggestions to every chapter of the book. No author could fail to appreciate the encouragement and sense of excitement about one's work which both Peggy and Gail provided. But I owe Gail much more than an author's thank-you. The final stages of the book's completion coincided with the birth of my first child, Aaron, and his death two months later. For her compassion as a human being at this time, I will always be grateful.

For teaching me to trust myself and to have the courage of my convictions, for their love and support and for their consistent confidence in me, I thank my parents, Aidla and Jacob Greenspan.

Most of all, for being my constant supporter, unflinching critic, emotional counselor, astute editor, loving companion and overall "wife" during the years of making this book, I am grateful to my husband, Roger Gottlieb. There is not a single page of the many drafts of manuscript that did not benefit from his careful editorial and conceptual assistance. He was always there even when we both couldn't stand it anymore and wanted to throw the book out the window. I could not have written it without him. For his humor, warmth, and love, for having faith in me when I couldn't muster it myself, for his remarkable intelligence, and last, but most certainly not least, for all the years that he did the housework, I cannot thank him enough.

Miriam Greenspan
Boston, Mass.
May 1982

Introduction to the Second Edition*

This book is ten years old. The seeds of its creation were planted some twenty-five years ago when across America small groups of women sat in their living rooms and committed one of the great radical acts of our time: telling our stories in our own voices and honoring our common experience. Whether we were suburban housewives suffering from "the problem with no name" or radical women tired of serving male leaders in the civil rights or new-left student movements, we had one thing in common—we wanted to find our own truths about ourselves and our world. We listened to each others' stories about relationships with husbands, children, and friends; about sex, love, work, and depression; about housework and thwarted aspirations; about the joys and agonies of motherhood; and about the hidden violence in our lives. We found the place where being a woman in a man's world felt like an unnamed, unvoiced rage. We "heard one another into speech."[1]

Some spontaneous social combustion occurred. In hearing one another's seemingly individual stories, we found out who we really were—not who we were told we were or thought we should be. In finding ourselves in one another, we were *empowered*—a concept that was not in the social vocabulary of the time but that we discovered in action. In breaking the isolation and silence surrounding women's authentic experience we came to know ourselves and our power, changing ourselves and our world in the process. This was consciousness-raising.

* A special thanks to Jan Surrey for her help in thinking through the overall scope of this introduction and for her sisterly support and laughter, and to Roger Gottlieb for his painstaking editorial assistance and love.

In consciousness-raising, women broke through some unspoken codes of conventional psychological thinking: first, the notion that women's problems and dilemmas are strictly personal, having to do with individual flaws and inadequacies; and second, the cherished, professional idea that to really understand who we are we must submit ourselves to an expert who knows us better than we do. We broke through the pervasive male bias of our culture that defines women's experience through a masculine lens masquerading as "objective truth." We found out that the truth about the oppression of women in our society could be searched for and known *subjectively*—and that this truth had the power to transform not only individual women, but also society as a whole. Consciousness-raising was the best kind of therapy—the kind that changes self and world together.

A New Approach to Women and Therapy is rooted in and reflects this process of healing called consciousness-raising (c-r). It has been a small part of the major shift from patriarchal to women-centered ways of re-visioning and transforming self and world that has been happening in the past quarter of a century. In writing this book, I had two basic intentions. First, I wanted to show how traditional psychology and psychotherapy reflect a culture that denies the social origins of women's emotional problems and how institutionalized psychology and psychiatry thus tend to silence, devalue, and misunderstand women and perpetuate women's emotional suffering. Second, I wanted to present a model of woman-centered psychotherapy that is grounded in the recognition of women's subordination in patriarchal society, a psychotherapy that is committed to women's individual and social empowerment.

The deepest and best intention of feminist therapy has been to be part of the personal, social, and global changes that are needed if we are to heal the psychic wounds of patriarchy.* This intention is certainly as important now as it was a decade ago.

The good news of the past decade is that feminist therapy has come of age. Variations of the general approach to women and therapy put forward in these pages are being practiced throughout the United States and Europe, as I learned in my travels as a workshop leader and public speaker after this book's publication. The feminist movement

---

* By *patriarchy*, I mean a system of male domination of economic, political, religious, cultural, and family life in which women's experience, authority, and powers are systematically denied, distorted and subjugated.

has had a broad impact on psychological theories and practices, from conferences on psychiatric diagnosis to television portrayals of battered women, rape victims, and incest survivors.

The bad news is that the status quo of male-biased theories and practices in the world of psychotherapy has not changed enough. And we are already seeing signs of how feminist advances are being co-opted into the tired old Father-Knows-Best system of therapy that I explore in Part I of this book.

This has been an eventful decade in the world of women and healing. Women of courage have broken the silence surrounding patriarchy's longest-held, best-kept secret: incest is out in the open. The enormous trauma of childhood sexual violence visited on at least a full third of the female population has been disclosed. Hundreds of thousands of women have begun the healing process that was by and large not possible for them in psychiatric treatment. This same decade has seen the flowering of Goddess-centered, feminist spirituality and the ecofeminist movement—which holds that the healing of the planet is irrevocably connected to the liberation of the world's women. We have also seen the phenomenal growth of the New Age, self-help, and 12-step recovery movements that have claimed the minds, hearts, spirits, and pocketbooks of millions of people—many of them women—who are searching to heal the "inner child."

Coexisting with these various movements toward healing has been the ongoing drift toward global destruction—the ecocide of earth that we are committing as a species. This process has cast its shadow over all of us—men, women, children, plants, animals, and all life forms.

In looking back at this book ten years later, I am glad to ponder these astonishing events and the possible threads that connect them:

● How feminist therapy has contributed to the healing of women in our society.

● The significance of the sexual abuse survivor movement and its impact on psychiatric practices and views of women.

● The contributions and drawbacks of the co-dependence recovery movement for women's psychological healing.

● The flowering of Goddess-centered feminist spirituality as a source of women's healing in therapy and out.

● How feminist therapy might enlarge its vision to contribute to the urgent need for planetary healing.

1. Feminist Therapy Comes of Age

There was a time, less than twenty years ago, when women were routinely pathologized and devalued in the traditional system of psychotherapy. Unfortunately, many women are still undergoing this brand of "therapy" today. However, with the growth of feminist therapy, women now have choices that did not exist two decades ago. Traditional theories of female psychology and psychotherapy are still with us, but their male-centered thinking has been radically challenged. Theories of female psychology that start from an authentic understanding of women's experience in sexist society are replacing theories that blame the victim. Feminist therapies aimed at healing the psychic wounds women suffer in patriarchy and honoring women's strengths are an available alternative to "treatments" that perpetuate female adaptation to the gender hierarchy. We have places of refuge for victims of patriarchal violence, including battered and abused women and children, and survivors of rape and sexual abuse. Hundreds of thousands of women have been helped to transform the energies of self-hatred, self-destruction, and shame into self-renewal, self-love, and individual and social empowerment. These gains of feminist therapy are cause for celebration.

When I began this book, feminist therapy had not yet penetrated the male-dominated institutions of professional psychology and psychiatry. The feminist therapy challenge began with a rejection of the notion that having a fancy credential from a prestigious academic institution made a therapist an "expert" in understanding or healing women's psyches. (More likely it meant that the therapist was trained in a system of thought in which the cultural male-bias was enshrined as truth.) Feminist therapists created their own institutions for training, education, and sharing knowledge. Some of these organizations, such as the Association for Women in Psychology and the national Feminist Therapy Institute are still going strong. Women's collective therapy and training enterprises exist in cities throughout the country. The American Psychiatric Association and the American Psychological Association both have women's divisions. Departments of psychiatry, psychology, social work, and counselling have been affected by the analysis of gender in the understanding and treatment of women. Family therapy (itself a maverick offshoot that rejected traditional psychiatry) has been profoundly rocked by a feminist contingent that has exposed the inherent sexism of viewing the family system without a social analysis of the position of women in the family and in the larger society as a whole. Jungian theory has also had its feminist revisionists.[2]

During the same period, feminist theories of female psychology have found a national audience. The entire field owes a debt of gratitude to the two books that started it all off. Twenty years ago, Phyllis Chesler's *Women and Madness* exploded psychiatry's pretensions to scientific objectivity, showing how women were systematically misunderstood and mistreated in sexist psychotherapy and in psychiatric institutions. Then, in *Toward A New Psychology of Women*, Jean Baker Miller began her feminist re-formulations of psychoanalytic theory, starting from the premise that female psychological development occurs in a context of the social subordination of women as a group.[3] When *A New Approach to Women and Therapy* first came out, there were, in addition to these two works, only two or three slender volumes on the subject of women and therapy. Since then, the body of literature in feminist psychology and therapy has grown substantially.[4]

For a creative, feminist theory of women's psychological development, it is worth noting the ongoing work of five women at the Stone Center for Developmental Studies and Services at Wellesley College: Judith Jordan, Alexandra Kaplan, Jean Baker Miller, Irene Stiver, and Janet Surrey.[5] Their work challenges the male-biased psychoanalytic idea that human development proceeds by separation from the primary caretaker (mother) toward an ideal stage of "autonomy" characterized by a rigidly separate, self-sufficient self. This model of selfhood is not accurate for men, much less women. The Stone Center model sees the growth of women's sense of self as embedded in relationships. The healthy "self-in-relation" develops in relationships that are characterized by a search for mutuality, empathy, and empowerment. This core idea of women's growth toward connection replaces that of the male journey of separation toward autonomy.

A woman-centered model of therapy presented in Part III of this book was developed during the same period as the Stone Center writings. Both models focus on a mutually empathic and empowering therapeutic relationship rather than a powerful, neutral expert in a hierarchical relationship with a disempowered patient. The Stone Center has had substantial (though still limited) impact in bringing this feminist model of development and therapy to mainstream psychoanalytic psychotherapy.

In short, feminism in some form has become a feature of the "mainstream" in all the various helping professions. Though feminism might not have changed the landscape of psychotherapy altogether, it is finding an institutional place for itself that is a welcome relief and shelter for women in thousands of therapy offices throughout the country.

Psychiatry, the dominant institution in the hierarchy of the helping professions, has had to contend with this call for change in what therapists see and do when they "treat" women in therapy. The radical challenge that feminist therapy poses is embodied in a new kind of empowered patient: one who insists that her therapist be, at the very least, willing to learn about women's social and emotional realities in male-dominated society or risk losing the patient. The passive, victimized "patient identity" that I write about in Chapter 10 of this book has been undergoing a massive transformation through the feminist therapeutic process of individual and social empowerment. The increasing willingness of women to hold psychotherapists morally and legally responsible for power abuses in psychotherapy has been the tip of this iceberg.

An important aspect of feminist approaches to psychology and therapy that has been emphasized in recent years is the necessity of learning from the diversity of women's experience. This emphasis warns us against seeing any one theory as monolithically applicable to the varied lives of women of different races, classes, sexual affiliations, and ethnic and religious identifications. While there is some value in developing a unified theory of women's psychology, this enterprise poses thorny problems when considering the racism and class biases that tend to pervade psychological theory in general. The voices of women of color, lesbians, and women of different ethnic and religious affiliations tend to be "ghettoized" in occasional courses or training in "multicultural" approaches to mainstream psychology and/or psychotherapy. Feminist psychologists have been reflecting on the ways that feminist theory also overgeneralizes the perspective of white, middle-class, Protestant Western women.[6]

Looking back at the history of feminist therapy, it is clear that the progression is from the women's movement to theory, not vice versa. The authentic voices of the social movement for women's liberation tend to be incorporated into psychological theory about a decade later. As feminist psychology develops, it is important not to lose sight of this history. The original insights of feminist therapy about the effects of patriarchy on the psyches of individual women were indeed "radical" in the sense of "going to the root." The mainstreaming of feminist psychology and therapy is of a double nature, as is always the case when a radical movement is absorbed by dominant cultural institutions—there are both gains and losses from this sort of progress. On the one hand, bringing a feminist perspective into the mainstream brings immediate benefits to women in therapy. On the other hand, when radical ideas are adapted by the dominant culture, something of the original vision of basic social change is often lost in the bargain. My hope is that feminist therapy at the grass-roots level, will continue to be a vital force for *both* individual and social change.

2. Women Break the Silence about Incest and Childhood Sexual Abuse

Violence against women has noticeably escalated in the past decade—precisely in the period when women are more and more breaking the silence about it. The statistics we now have in all likelihood underestimate the actual extent of this violence, since so many women never report abuse by their husbands, boyfriends, fathers, and other intimate male figures. We know that at least one in four women are battered by boyfriends or spouses (some estimates are much higher, citing one-third to one-half of all women). "Domestic abuse" (a euphemism for violence against women by men they know intimately) has been declared a national epidemic by the Surgeon General of the United States—it is the number one cause of injury to women in this country. A woman is battered every 18 seconds. Approximately 4,000 battered women die each year in this country, and more than 40 percent of all women who are killed die at the hands of their spouses. One woman is raped every three minutes, and approximately one in three will be raped in their lifetimes. (This doesn't count the instances of marital and date rape that go undocumented). The statistics emerging on childhood sexual abuse vary, but it is clear that as many as one in three girls are sexually abused, often by a close relative, before the age of eighteen.[7]

These statistics begin to paint the picture of the routine physical and sexual violation of women and female children in our society, including the social secret of incest as a common feature of family life. Twenty years ago radical feminists were saying that the social and psychological domination of women is kept in place through the threat and perpetuation of violence directed at women as a group. Pick up a newspaper nowadays, and it is hard to deny that this is true. The violent men who are raping, battering, sexually assaulting, and murdering little girls and women at alarming rates are not all pathological deviants. Many of them are "respectable" men who would fit a "normal" profile in the battery of psychological tests that are used to assess normality and pathology. What these tests do not tell us is that *the social system itself is pathological.* There is an epidemic of violence against women because it is "normal" in patriarchal society for men to learn that they have power over women and children, especially female children, and that they are entitled to take what is rightfully theirs and to lash out when threatened. As feminism begins to alter patriarchal society, there is the inevitable masculine backlash.[8] Under the threat of economic decline and social chaos that we are experiencing today, this backlash is strengthened, and violence against women escalates.

We now can see more clearly that latent and actual violence against women is the underpinning of patriarchy, as much as psychiatry and the self-help movement might say otherwise. While psychiatry continues to individualize violence without bothering to look at the systemic causes of it, much of the self-help literature continues to hold women responsible for the violence against them. We see this blame-the-victim mythology in best-sellers about women who "love too much" or make "foolish choices." We see it again in men's movement literature in which there is, for the most part, a resounding silence about men's violence towards women. The work of Robert Bly and other men's movement heroes glorifies masculinity and celebrates male bonding while pointing the finger of blame at shrewish mothers and wives who have undermined male authority.

It is astonishing to think that a little more then ten years ago, the term "sexual abuse survivor" was barely in the vocabulary of women or therapists.[9] The sexual abuse survivor movement has become in the past decade a national and international phenomenon. It has changed the lives of hundreds of thousands of women who have been able, for the first time (often not until they are in their forties, fifties, or sixties), to consciously know the truth of their violation and begin the healing process. It has also forced psychiatry, for the first time, to admit that the trauma of sexual violence against female children is real and not imagined—as Freud posited in his Oedipal theory.[10]

Because women have had the courage to remember and tell their stories of incest and childhood sexual abuse, we have discovered the truth: that the "haven" of family life has been built on the widespread physical, sexual, emotional, and spiritual violation of female children. Any form of violence that occurs routinely to at least one-third of the female population cannot be accurately called a deviation from the norm. The violence itself—and its threat—*is* the norm. This has been perhaps the most earth-shattering revelation of the twentieth century since the "secrets" of Auschwitz were told following World War II.

It is not, in short, incest that has been taboo, but speaking about it. Women in the past decade have broken this taboo—hopefully, for all time.

This world-historical change has been encouraged by the existence of feminist therapy. The hallmark of feminist therapy has been the simple tool of consciousness-raising in which women's stories are told, heard, and honored rather than diagnosed, pathologized, or reduced to pseudo-medical categories. After a decade or more of women's consciousness-raising and public speak-outs about rape and battering, breaking the silence about incest and the sexual abuse of children had to follow. In many cases, the disclosure came in the form of women telling their stories to feminist therapists who refused to collude in the massive social cover-up.[11]

Some of the problems that women typically bring to psychotherapists and that I specifically address in this book include: low self-esteem, including feelings of worthlessness, inadequacy, and powerlessness; poor body image; chronic anxiety and depression; sexual "dysfunction"; psychosomatic disorders; marital or relationship problems; the fear of being or going "crazy." I call these "symptoms of female subservience in a man's world." Looking at them ten years later, I am struck by the fact that almost all of them are signs of possible physical or childhood sexual abuse. (Although you don't have to be a sexual abuse survivor to suffer these symptoms.)

In this book you will find stories about rape (Andrea's story), emotional abuse (Susan's story), and sexual harassment (Polly's story), but no story of physical or sexual abuse or incest. Perhaps when I first began writing this book I was not ready myself to see the awful truth about the pervasiveness of incest and what this says about our society. A little more than a decade ago, most therapists, including myself, didn't inquire much about sexual abuse because we did not suspect how widespread it was. In my training there was not a single mention of the sexual or physical abuse of women in families. This professional denial not only mirrored the overall social denial, but actively contributed to it. Freudian dogmatists for 50 years have re-traumatized the victims by labelling their ordeals Oedipal "fantasies."

The fact that incest is no longer a secret reaffirms that the true understanding of women cannot come from an aloof elite of experts but must come from women themselves. We *are* the experts in our own experience. The world—including many professionals—needs to hear what women know about the violation and fear of violence in women's lives. If it is truly grasped by society and not reabsorbed and imprisoned once again in the narrow confines of a strictly intrapsychic psychology, this knowledge must have widely felt consequences for how we see our world and what must be changed if women, children, men, and the planet itself are to be truly safe, free, and healthy.

3. Psychiatry Diagnoses Women's Voices

As the secrets of the patriarchal family system have been un-earthed, how has the dominant system of psychological theory and practice responded? Psychiatry has been forced to make some accommodations to the reality of violence against women because both patients and clinicians have struggled (in therapy rooms, case conferences, conventions, professional associations, and committee rooms) for the recognition of women's realities. In these struggles, psychiatry has been held accountable for the sexist double standard of mental health in general and the sex bias in some of psychiatry's most prized theories and diagnoses.

The 1980s was a decade of much internal struggle within the psychiatric establishment around the issue of diagnosis and misdiagnosis. In the spirit of masculine backlash, the old-guard psychoanalysts in the American Psychiatric Association resorted to pushing several new reactionary diagnoses with names like Masochistic Personality Disorder and Premenstrual Dysphoric Disorder. The Masochist or Self-

Defeating Personality is known for her display of "symptoms" such as engaging in excessive self-sacrifice and failing to accomplish tasks crucial to personal objectives while helping others with their tasks. In a parody of so-called "objective social science," this diagnosis blames the victim and ignores the patriarchal context of women's socially conditioned "symptomatology." The diagnosis of Premenstrual Dysphoric Disorder cites women's emotionality around the menstrual period as "symptomatic." This is the contemporary equivalent of the ancient Greek medical diagnosis of "wandering womb" for "overly emotional" women. In this case the diagnosis makes all menstruating women eligible for the diagnosis of a personality disorder.

The Coalition Against Misdiagnosis (a working group of feminist professionals) and the fathers of psychiatric nomenclature battled over the terms in which women's emotional suffering would be catalogued in the *Diagnostic and Statistical Manual*—the bible of psychiatric fundamentalism. Feminists won some partial victories.[12] However, while individual battles over diagnoses might have been won, the war itself will go on as long as diagnoses are considered to bear the truth about women's psychic pain. For this war is, ultimately, about who has the power to name and define women's psychological realities.

The current *Diagnostic and Statistical Manual-III-R* lists several diagnoses that reflect its own failure to understand the inherent sexism of many of its diagnostic labels. For example, Borderline Personality Disorder and Histrionic Personality Disorder are both widely used for female patients and are two of the most male-biased and demeaning categories in the entire psychiatric lexicon. A Borderline Personality is easy to spot—she exhibits intense and frequent displays of anger. (Angry women beware—you are easy prey for this diagnosis.) The Histrionic Personality is also a breeze to diagnose—she is characterized by rapidly shifting emotions (which she displays to male therapists who are characterized by the conspicuous lack of any display of any emotions whatsoever). No amount of feminist agitation has erased these and other equally sexist diagnoses from the *DSMIII-R*. (See Chapter 2, "How to Diagnose Patients.")

There is one new diagnosis, however, that has appeared in recent years and is the product of a partial feminist victory—Post-traumatic Stress Disorder (PTSD). Before this diagnosis, a woman battered by her spouse or boyfriend was likely to be diagnosed as a Borderline Personality. A female victim of sexual abuse or incest was out of luck—her trauma would go unrecognized and remain a festering psychic wound. Worse still, if she was a victim of father-daughter incest, and if she had the courage to remember her story and tell it to an orthodox psychoanalytic psychotherapist, she might very well be told that her father's actions were her "wish" or that she was making it up.

Because of the pioneering work of feminists like Lenore Walker who worked with battered women and who wrote about the "Battered Woman Syndrome,"[13] the physically and emotionally abused woman's loss of self-esteem, intense psychological distress, daytime and nighttime terror, difficulty sleeping and concentrating, and "outbursts of anger" can now be diagnosed as symptoms of PTSD. Her suffering is seen as the domestic equivalent of being a prisoner of war. The survivor of sexual violence, especially the survivor of severe and recurrent instances of incest, can also be diagnosed as someone who is suffering the real effects of extreme physical and emotional trauma. Psychiatry has finally admitted that psychological suffering is inflicted on women as a result of victimization by others, often men intimately known to the victim, and that such suffering is not a manifestation of some inner mental disorder!

The baring of women's hidden injuries contains a potentially explosive energy for social transformation that is quite lost, however, when psychiatry, like a giant amoeba, incorporates women's secrets into the system of psychiatric diagnosis. The diagnosis of PTSD is described in the DSM-III-R as a *"disorder"* that occurs when "the person has experienced an event that is *outside the range of usual human experience* and that would be markedly distressing to almost anyone . . . "[14] What the APA seems at a loss to recognize is that physical and sexual violence is very much *inside* the range of human experience when the humans are female children or adults. (The readily available statistics, daily newspaper accounts of battered and raped women, and hundreds of thousands of women telling their sexual abuse stories don't seem to have registered as "scientific" evidence!) This conspicuous oversight allows psychiatry to continue to ignore the sexual oppression of women as a whole in its way of thinking about and treating them.

Thus, even in this partial victory of feminist diagnosticians, we can see that the entire pseudo-medical system that relies on diagnosis is as misguided today as it ever was. Diagnoses have always arisen with certain specific socioeconomic contexts—and are changed within a social context too, as the struggle over these and other diagnoses within the APA illustrates. Diagnosis is ultimately a social act with social uses masquerading as a medical act with medical uses. What's at stake here is how people look at reality and understand suffering, especially the suffering of socially induced violence. The truth of the normative violence and threat of violence against women and its individual effects on women's minds, bodies, and spirits is being tamed by the psychiatric establishment—primarily through the use of diagnosis.

Psychiatry is the religion of contemporary society. Like the shamans and priests of the past, psychiatrists define the holy and profane; but in our society, those terms are secular: the healthy and the sick. In psychologizing reality, psychiatry reduces a complex set of social, economic, emotional, and spiritual dimensions to the terms of a single diagnosis. The diagnosis then converts the plethora of emotional problems under patriarchy into diseases or disorders that are treated by a professional elite in a totally individual way. Ultimately, what gets denied in all this is the pathology of the social structure itself. The locus of attention and the responsibility shifts from society to the individual. If a society is sick, we need to change it. If a person is sick, she needs to go to a psychiatrist. Certainly, psychiatry as an institution has a vested interest in helping people adapt to a belief in the latter, not the former. Women as Patient is what keeps psychiatry in business as usual.

In short, despite some feminist victories, the psychiatric system as a whole continues to be a regressive force in the lives of most women. Women who tell their incest stories to most orthodox psychoanalytic psychiatrists and psychologists nowadays are being heard by the same folks who still believe in the Freudian dogma that sees female sexual abuse as female fantasy. There has been no public admission of psychiatric error in the American Psychiatric Association or anywhere else. There has been no public repudiation of Freud's denial of and contribution to female victimization in the form of the Oedipal theory.[15]

Despite the appreciable successes of feminism, psychiatry as a whole continues to operate out of and perpetuate the three myths that I write about in the first part of this book. They are:

● Myth 1. *It's "all in your head"*—the myth that the psyche can be understood by separating it from the social system in which it takes its shape.

● Myth 2. The *medical model of psychopathology*—the idea that emotional suffering is essentially a matter of individual illness or disease and can be treated in a medical model of practice.

● Myth 3. The idea that there is a father-like *Expert* who can cure this suffering through his superior knowledge and power.

These myths continue to be widely and deeply held by helping professionals today. They are inimical to genuine healing, not only for individual women in therapy, but for anyone of any age or sex. Psychiatry, mirroring the culture from which it springs, has yet to recognize the psychopathology of our social system and its destructive effects on individual psyches, bodies, spirits, and the planet as a whole. Until psychiatry understands this, the "cure" it offers is often an unwitting contribution to the psychopathology itself.

4. The Co-dependence Recovery Movement: Is it Good for Women?

Healing has become big business in the past decade. The bookshelves are overflowing with books about recovering from every kind of "addiction" and "disease"—from drinking too much to loving too much, from substance abuse to co-dependence.

Psychiatry, the once unchallenged authority on psychological illness and cure, is being given a run for its money by the new self-help/recovery movement. The power of psychiatry is being eroded by the astounding popularity, increasing respectability, and sheer economic clout of the recovery movement. This movement has considerable implications for the healing of women.

The foundation of the recovery movement is, of course, the original 12-step program of Alcoholics Anonymous. This program—which was totally repudiated by psychiatry when I was a trainee—has clearly proved to have a greater success rate in the treatment of alcoholism than psychiatry could ever claim. The form of the 12-step programs of AA, Al Anon, etc., is a distinct counterpoint to the traditional form of therapy. People meet in leaderless groups that conduct themselves on the basis of principles of egalitarianism and peer support. No exchange of money takes place. The model emphasizes personal honesty in the context of a non-authoritarian, mutually supportive peer community. It puts forth a spiritual as well as a communal basis for the process of healing.

There is no doubt that this form has been a literal lifesaver for millions of alcoholics, drug abusers, and their friends and families. The program has, however, also been problematic for many women. The 12-step emphasis on surrendering one's will to a "higher power" (in whatever way one understands that power) has often been all too easy for women who are socially conditioned to surrender their wills to the "higher power" of masculine authority. Of course, this is not what is meant by AA philosophy, but it points to the special needs of female alcoholics and addicts to recover their sense of self before they can surrender it.

This problem with the 12-step programs for women has increased with the rising popularity of the concept of "co-dependence" and the proliferation of co-dependence groups and treatment programs. Women are increasingly diagnosing themselves as co-dependent and seeking treatment for their "disease." Though the term co-dependent originally referred to those whose lives were significantly affected by living with someone who abused drugs or alcohol, it has now become an all-purpose category in the literature of "self-help" and recovery. For example, in one popular self-help book, co-dependence is defined as "any suffering and/or dysfunction that is associated with or results from focusing on the needs and behavior of others."[16] Symptoms of this "disease" include caretaking, low self-worth, external referencing for one's sense of self, weak "boundaries," anger, and sexual problems.

These "symptoms" sound startlingly similar to what I call in this book the symptoms of femininity in the victim psychology of women in a patriarchal social context. Diagnosing oneself as or being diagnosed by others as co-dependent, if you are a woman, ends up in yet another of the many double binds of female psychological adaptation—the normally socialized traits of femininity, such as focusing on the needs of others, are declared to be symptoms of a disease by a whole other group of (non-psychiatric) experts!

One of the major tenets of feminist therapy found in this book is the need to reexamine and re-vision what has been called female emotional "pathology" as a manifestation of women's adaptation to an oppressive social system. We need to see the core of strength in women's culturally devalued "weaknesses." This strength in weakness tends to be lost in the co-dependency movement. Here, in a context altogether different from psychiatry, there is still the same model of the healthy ego as a masculine-style bounded ego, a fortress with firm ego boundaries, self-sufficient, autonomous, and masterful. The socialized feminine characteristics of empathic connection and caretaking are not seen as a sign of compassion but of sickness. This is not to say that compulsive altruism or caretaking in women who are in abusive or unequal relationships is not a problem. However, the co-dependency approach once again removes the problem from its social context. This move inevitably, if inadvertently, ends in blaming the victim.

It is ironic that the co-dependency movement, which has scathingly attacked psychiatry for its ignorance and refusal to treat addictions of all kinds, should end up embodying the three myths of the traditional psychiatric system in new forms. Myth one, the myth that "it's all in your head" has here become myth 1a: *"it's all in your family."* The idea of the dysfunctional family as the bedrock of the "disease" of co-dependence once again ignores the social context of families within the social and cultural system of patriarchal capitalism. Recovery guru John Bradshaw declares that almost 100 percent of all families are dysfunctional, yet comes short of questioning: if this is the case, where does the basic pathology lie? Instead, myth 1a holds us to a view of a massive bunch of dysfunctional individuals all stepping forth from a massive array of dysfunctional families without coming to any understanding of the social sources of these ills. "Toxic" parents or toxic families or toxic people are blamed for all one's suffering. Parents who have not totally, superhumanly protected their children from all the emotional and spiritual ills that fester in an unnurturing and destructive social order are as likely to be diagnosed as "dysfunctional" as families in which fathers nightly rape their daughters. Something very important is lost here, and healing as an act of ritual whining is ushered in.

The co-dependency movement, despite its anti-psychiatry bent, has also retained the core of the medical model idea of "sickness" as the basis of all human suffering. The real life-threatening disease of alcoholism becomes trivialized by labelling almost any behavior of caretaking as a disease or addiction. We are all "sick sickos" according to Pia Mellody.[17] Myth 2—the idea of emotional suffering as "disease"—has never been stronger! The notion that a disease is essential to your identity as a self-enclosed individual might have some temporarily positive effects, largely because it entitles you to air your feelings in a supportive group atmosphere. However, in the long run, such an identification with disease entrenches the suffering it seeks to alleviate. It keeps one encapsulated in pain, grievance, and illness, and keeps one running to the bookshelves and workshops for yet another "fix" of self-help and recovery. (The only addiction book that's not on the recovery shelf is the one about addiction to books about addiction.)

This is what keeps myth 3—the myth of the expert—alive and well in the co-dependency movement, and makes the movement big business. The new expert is not the benign, fatherly doctor figure of the traditional medical system. He has been replaced by the charismatic TV talk show celebrity who offers simple fix-it solutions to the complex dilemmas and multifaceted emotional/social/spiritual problems of living in our world today. This was poignantly demonstrated in an evening speech given by one of the guiding lights of the co-dependency movement. Having presented her model of co-dependency, she was asked a question by a female member of the audience who said, in a very shaky, disempowered voice: "Now I can see what you are saying and I have come to believe that I am really very sick. But now that I know this, what can I do about it?" The answer from the co-dependency expert was: "Buy my book and then buy my workbook."

It is true that many thousands of women get much-needed day-to-day 12-step support by sharing their pain in co-dependence or Sex and Love Anonymous groups. However, without holding fast to a feminist analysis of women's pain, we are inevitably drawn back into blaming the victim. An alternative to the concept of women's co-dependence in relationships with men is found in this book in "Linda's Story: Depression as a Way of Life," in which "co-dependent" symptoms are viewed as aspects of male-identified femininity. Part II of this book, "Growth Therapy is Not Enough: The Failure of Humanist Therapy" is as relevant to the co-dependency movement as it is the various assortment of humanist therapies that I wrote about a decade ago.

Having said all this, it is important to acknowledge that the recovery movement's emphasis on healing the "inner child" has had some very positive effects on many thousands of men and women who have been removed from their inner emotional life, including survivors of physical and sexual abuse. What could be wrong with trying to teach people to love the child within? Nothing, per se. The problem comes when one separates the "inner child" from the world. Healing then comes to be seen as an "inner" process focused exclusively on the past and one's pain from the past, while ignoring the social context of both the past and the present. The world around us is not considered relevant to the process of healing. It comes to be seen as something from which to escape or to set up one's boundaries against. This emphasis on a closed and bounded inner child from the past is a way of trying to protect that child from continued violation and a way of fostering self-love. However, the kind of protection it offers is ultimately self-defeating, for healing happens in relationship—to others and to the world—not outside of it. Now, more than ever, our world demands not an embattled, separate self, but an empathic, open, boundless self that can feel and know the basic truth of our interconnectedness in the earth community and the necessity of bringing healing to the community as a whole.

5.   *The Goddess Empowered: Towards a Global Ecofeminist Psychology and Psychotherapy*

"To be conscious in our world today involves awareness of unprecedented peril . . . Until now, every generation throughout history lived with tacit certainty that other generations would follow . . . That certainty is now lost to us . . . That loss, unmeasured and immeasurable, is the pivotal psychological reality of our time." (Joanna Macy, *Despair and Personal Power in the Nuclear Age*)[18]

"I believe we are at a great watershed in history and that we hold in our hands a fragile thread, no more than that, that can lead us to our survival. I understand the rising up of women in this century to be the human race's response to the threat of its own self-annihilation and the destruction of the planet." (Sally Miller Gearhart, "The Future—If There Is One—Is Female")[19]

The social world of female oppression is as real today as it ever was. We live in an era in which the gains women have made are still in jeopardy—including the most basic right to reproductive and bodily freedom. Violence against women has increased. Patriarchal thinking on a global scale each day threatens to bring us closer to the edge of ecological disaster. Clearly, there can be no lasting or complete healing for women, men, or children until we make the planet safe and livable for all. Feminist therapy, grounded in this social reality, is still a necessity—despite the backlash ideology that says we live in a "post-feminist" era in which feminism is irrelevant.

In the past decade, there has been a grass-roots spiritual movement within feminism, within mainstream psychology, and in society as a whole. This movement seeks to integrate spirituality into the understanding and practice of healing. In the forefront of my own writing and work in psychotherapy during this period has been an effort to unify two realms that have long been seen as separate and antagonistic—the political and the spiritual. The guiding question in this work has been: can we create a holistic model of therapy that includes spirituality and builds upon (but does not constrict) the feminist social model presented in this book?[20]

My own spiritual awakening and its profound effects on the way I now work came not as an intellectual pursuit but as a result of the birth and death of my infant son just before the publication of this book. Aaron taught me that there was more to heaven and earth than is dreamed of in our psychological and political philosophies. Being touched by this child's spirit—loving him fully as he lived and died, letting him go when I had to, and seeing his spirit after his death— shattered my former spiritual agnosticism and opened me to undreamed possibilities of healing beyond the narrowly defined realm of psychology.

After Aaron, my work as a feminist therapist began to change gradually and intentionally to a practice in which I would no longer ignore or compartmentalize spirituality in my life and in the lives of my clients, but instead searched to find ways to welcome it directly into the process. For instance, in addition to the usual questions I asked clients, I began to ask questions like: What do you think of as the meaning or purpose of your life? What images do you have of divinity or the sacred? How do you feel about death? Have you had any experiences that you think of as spiritual, and how do you feel about them?

In so doing I experienced myself going through the palpable sense of "taboo" by which spiritual concerns are considered to be outside the proper domain of psychotherapy, indicative of inappropriateness on the part of the therapist or pathology on the part of the patient. This is hardly surprising, considering that when I was a psychology trainee in the early 1970s, I learned that a preoccupation with religious matters was a symptom of schizophrenia! No one in their right mind was supposed to think or talk about God-related experiences, concerns, or questions in psychotherapy. The current *DSM-III-R* still lists a number of transpersonal experiences as evidence of a "Schizotypal Personality Disorder!" For example, "odd beliefs or magical thinking . . . e.g., belief in clairvoyance, telepathy or "sixth sense" . . . unusual perceptual experiences, e.g., illusions, sensing the presence of a force or person not actually present . . . "[21]

Nowadays, "transpersonal" and mystical psychologies and various spiritually oriented therapies enjoy widespread popular and professional interest.[22] Feminist therapy also has begun to close the split between politics and spirituality. (Three years ago, when I gave a workshop on Spirituality in Clinical Practice at a Conference on Women sponsored by Harvard University, I knew that spirituality was beginning to be a little less taboo in psychiatric circles.)

As my own work changed, I discovered a door opening into a much deeper kind of healing that can take place when the therapy context is freed of the constraint of having to keep religious or spiritual experience out of the room. This is particularly striking in working with survivors of sexual abuse, many of whom carry spiritual gifts that sometimes come from profoundly traumatic experiences, gifts that have often been denied or pathologized by those around them. I didn't really have to "go after" spirituality in psychotherapy—I just had to stop keeping it out! My clients—as all of us do—had their own spiritual questions and challenges, especially the usual ones occasioned by loss, illness, disability, or death.

This initial period of integrating spirituality into feminist therapy came simply from my desire to be true to what my life was teaching me, to refuse to fragment the various parts of myself and to maintain my authenticity as a therapist. The model of therapy put forth in these pages emphasizes the authenticity of the therapist-client relationship and compassion as the cornerstone of feminist therapy. These foundations of feminist therapy were only deepened after my spiritual awakening.

I had two more children after Aaron died. Through my experience of mothering my two daughters, I am continually affirmed in the spiritual nature of women's gifts in bringing forth and nurturing life, how much these gifts are trivialized, demeaned, and disempowered in patriarchal culture, and the urgency of bringing the gifts of women to the world at this time. By and large, my spiritual path has been the path of motherhood, and my spiritual teachers have been my children. Anna, a feisty girl with ideas of her own, keeps me humble. Esther has a mysterious neuro-motor disability that diminishes her muscle tone throughout her body and challenges her capacity to perceive her body in space and to coordinate her movements. She is my daily teacher in the courage to overcome obstacles and meet unexpected challenges.

The experiences in my life that would be conventionally perceived as most "tragic" have been the doorways to spiritual opening, renewal, and healing. In my brokenness, I found a sense of wholeness; in my vulnerability, I found a place of spiritual empowerment. The "dark" emotions of grief, fear, anger, and despair have been my guides on this journey. The more I have befriended them and allowed them to take their course in a state of awareness, the more I have found them to be a source of healing and creativity. I describe this journey as the emotional alchemy of the dark emotions—a journey through grief to gratitude, through fear to joy, through anger to trust, and through despair to faith.

I was moved to use my personal experience as the basis of what might be possible for others. My therapy work shifted its focus from a practice dominated by individual therapy to a more group-work orientation. I began leading women's groups focused around working with the emotions of grief, fear, anger, and despair. These groups are designed to provide a supportive and empowering context for experiencing dark emotions and opening to their transformational possibilities. The groups include some re-education about emotions, to undo the patriarchal conditioning that tells us that painful emotions indicate psychological, moral, or spiritual inadequacy or dysfunction.

Dark emotions have been totally devalued in our emotion-fearing culture. They tend to be viewed psychiatrically as symptomatic of pathology. Seen as "negative" by traditional psychologists and New Agers alike, dark emotions are repudiated by a patriarchal culture that separates reason and emotion and associates dark emotions with weakness, irrationality, and women. Dark emotions are often seen as inimical to healing and are rarely experienced fully and with awareness. Yet, they are also the very emotions that I believe it is essential that we fully experience if we are to heal ourselves personally and globally.

My own experience has taught me that it is not transcendence but the fullness of living consciously that is healing. Healing for me has been journeying *through,* not above. What makes these emotions so difficult to go through (and often makes them destructive) is the apparently universal human aversion to anything unpleasant, the wish to deny or avoid the "darker" side of life. We disavow, deny, numb out, and addictively avoid feelings that are uncomfortable. We do this not only with feelings about individual experience such as childhood pain, neglect, or trauma, and with current experiences of personal loss, but also with feelings that we have about the painful crisis of the planet. Many of the disastrous and destructive processes operating in the world today are related to this kind of denial.

In these groups, I try to provide some of the conditions for the alchemy of dark emotions to take place. The groups are, in a sense, initiations for women who wish to journey together through the labyrinth of their most frightening feelings, to find their authentic sources and the extraordinary knowledge, power, and energy that can emerge when these emotions are allowed to take their sacred course. Women's individual, collective, historical, and archetypal experiences of domination, sexual violence, and physical, emotional and spiritual violation tend to be the one of the central themes of these groups.

I now routinely use a number of methods that I did not use when I wrote this book. Meditation, for instance, provides a ritualized structure by which women can focus their attention and concentration; it is also a method by which to develop our capacities to be present with painful experience—in ourselves and in the world. Meditation provides the "anchor" for a grounded awareness that is not a flying away from reality but an ability to be with it.

Despite the somber sound of all this, these groups are often playful. A great deal of laughter and expressive creativity is released when we are no longer using so much energy to repress or avoid difficult feelings. I have felt free to creatively experiment with more collective meditation modes—rather than the usual solitary, single-body, closed eyes inward-looking forms common to meditative traditions. I have found that when meditation takes a more collective female form, the individual ability to be present is more often heightened than distracted, and from this awareness grows an enlarged sense of Self that is connected to others and to the earth.

Another aspect of my work has been the use of prayer—by which I mean a heartfelt communion with something beyond our autobiographical egos. Whether we call this a communion with God, Goddess, Higher Self, Deepest Resources, Sacred Ground of Being, or Whatever is not important. Prayer includes finding gratitude in the midst of pain, asking for and finding help or guidance beyond our usual sense of self or ego, and expressing our deepest intentions for ourselves and for the world. The use of other methods like yogic breathing, body work, visualization, and artwork accompany the more traditional group-work methods of sharing our stories and supporting one another by listening closely for the commonalities in women's experiences.[23]

I have worked with sexual abuse and incest survivors, victims of rape and assault, women with disabilities, women grieving a lifetime of losses, ex-addicts and ex-prostitutes, professional women, and women with no visible means of support. I have found in these groups that when the therapeutic experience is enlarged to include the social and spiritual dimensions of women's lives, the connections between women's individual suffering and the collective pain of the planet seem to be made automatically. Our emotions, when shared in this way, guide us on journeys in which individual pain, experienced alone or in isolation, opens out into the healing energy of compassion for self and world. We feel ourselves to be part of a larger whole. Also, as women, we find our wish and power to nurture, maintain, and protect that whole.

There is a magic that can happen when what I call the "free child" is allowed to be present in the psychotherapeutic journey. Who is this free child? As one client put it, "she knows all about the pain but is free of the hurt"—and she is also connected to the spirit of the world. She is not simply some inner childhood remnant from the past but a very present spiritual energy that lives in women, even in the psyche that has suffered the most unspeakable physical, emotional, and sexual tortures. She is not an encapsulated smaller self of the past, but a spirit connected to the earth itself; This "free child" finds its voice through women's discovery and liberation of our power within. I have come to believe that the courage and powers of women, despite thousands of years of patriarchy, are more and more emerging and guiding us toward the healing of our world.

From the ground of my own most personal experience, my work has taken a turn toward connecting the personal and the global in a socially conscious and spiritually aware context. The creative challenge to any psychology and psychotherapy that hopes to contribute to the amelioration of the planetary crisis we face today is how to enlarge the scope of its paradigm to include the connections between personal pain and the plight of the earth. Some psychologists today are beginning to work on this together. Many women throughout the world are working with more creative, women-centered approaches to healing. We are finding the courage to trust our own voices and visions and create new healing forms that break the patriarchal mold.[24]

In the past decade, it has become more obvious to most ordinary people— however much it might be denied by politicians and CEOs— that we are living in an age of imminent threat to the survival of the ecosystem of the earth. The crisis is not an abstract matter that we can afford to leave to elected officials that we no longer have much faith in. All that has always sustained and nurtured us has now become poisoned or poisonous, dangerous, or deadly: the air, the water, the food, the soil, the sun. This threat has "democratized" the world in one way: no one can completely escape into a safe haven of gender or racial privilege. The earth itself is the killing field, and we are both the victims and the victimizers in the ecocidal holocaust that we are leaving as a legacy to our children.

We face a choice as a species: to survive or to self-destruct. I believe that this is fundamentally a choice between letting the planet die and holding on to patriarchy, or letting go of patriarchy and healing the planet.

In the past decade, as feminism has begun to chip away at patriarchal culture, there has been an entrenched holding fast to patriarchal institutions (with a somewhat higher quota of women in high places), a fierce gender backlash, and the international capitalist defense of the rights of corporate greed to overshadow any and all considerations of life. The ecology and ecofeminist movements have advanced their efforts to head off planetary disaster and place some sanctions on unlimited corporate and governmental destructiveness. Women's exposure of the dark and violent underside of patriarchy has been "earth-shattering." The feminist movement has found new vitality and creativity in the re-awakening of Goddess-centered spirituality. The recovery movement too has provided a channel for healing many who have been devastated by the alienation, cruelty, and self-destructiveness of twentieth century post-modern life.

I believe these various movements are related. The connecting thread is found when we take a larger, aerial view of the world in which we live. These movements are different responses to what Joanna Macy calls "the pivotal psychological reality of our time": the

Introduction to the Second Edition

threat of planetary extinction.[25] The ecology and ecofeminist movements are clearly in the forefront of working on behalf of our ailing planet. However, we are all affected by the plight of the earth, whether we are consciously part of these movements or not. The earth itself cries out for healing, and in our seemingly private sufferings—if we are willing to abandon our archaic notions of individual selves separate from the world and begin to enlarge our sense of who we are—we can hear the voice of the earth calling for our help. It is the earth itself that is trying to heal, and we women are often her voices.

In the diseases of women and children—such as the epidemic of breast cancer, the diseases of the female reproductive system, the rising rates of infertility, miscarriage, stillbirth, birth defects, and the rise in childhood respiratory diseases and cancer—the cultural plague of patriarchy is made manifest. Often it is our diseases that call our attention, both to the cultural pathology and to the potential for spiritual healing.[26] Our bodies bring our attention to what is wrong, not only with our own individual psyches and bodies, but with the world. One startling example of this is the correlation feminist therapists are finding: that women who suffer from environmental illness are often also survivors of childhood incest and sexual abuse. Women, men, and, increasingly, children who are environmentally ill are the "carriers" of the knowledge we need to wake up. They are the "body prophets" who point to our fate as a species if we do not heal institutionally and globally as well as personally.

The voices of women speaking in grief and outrage about their abused bodies and psyches let us know not only of their own suffering but also of the need for healing of the whole. The emergence of incest survivors speaking their stories might well be part of the truth-telling, uncovering process that our patriarchal social order must go through before it is transformed.

The same cultural psychopathology that brings harm and death to the bodies of women, children, and men is also responsible for the pollution and desecration of the earth. The journey toward healing in our time can be seen as a journey through the Dark Goddess who opens our eyes and helps us see clearly the violation of women and the earth, the woundedness of men, women, children and other species, the fury of women in the face of this violation, and the sources of creativity, survival, and affirmation of life that arise as a response to our earthly crisis. The Dark Goddess speaks through women who tell us their stories of violation so that we can break through the massive social denial of the destructive force of patriarchy. To know the truth about patriarchy is to begin to change it.[27]

A sizable literature exists that brings us the riches of the flowering of the Goddess in our time.[28] Here, I will simply say that the feminist movement, which has been declared dead by the media, is still alive and functioning, and that much of its energy currently takes the form of the ecofeminist spirituality movement. This movement is growing in all areas of the globe and in all classes and races of women. Goddess-centered spirituality is in the forefront of connecting personal and global healing.

The recovery movement is, I believe, also an aspect of the response of a threatened population in desperate need of healing. The great power and promise of this grass-roots movement is that it brings to us, in popular form, important news about the pain of our "inner child." The inner child, however, is not just the child of individual, toxic parents. It is the wounded child of toxic patriarchy and of an ailing earth. This child must be recognized, seen, heard and loved. However, as long as we see the inner child as isolated and separate from the world, we fall back into the conceptual trap that is part of the wounding of patriarchy: the ethos of separation, autonomy, and competitive mastery that is also the ethos of war, aggression, rape, and domination.

The turning to the Goddess, or letting the Goddess come through us, is a way of experiencing healing of self and world in a woman-identified ethos that emphasizes connectedness, compassion, community, and cooperation. The primary search of the inner child for safety and protection in a heartless world is not just the search of the wounded child within who has been abused or neglected by "bad" parents. Inner safety, peace, and harmony are tenuous as long as we live in a world in which the radical unsafety we have created continues to pose a threat to all life. The healing we seek is both inner and outer, personal and transpersonal, individual and collective, social and spiritual, private and planetary. These distinctions fall away the more we are able to enlarge our awareness of our common suffering and the ties that bind us together as an earth family.

Healing is a movement into the wholeness of authentic connection in which we know ourselves to be interwoven strands of One Earth,

One Body, One Spirit—in its various manifestations. Enlarging our boundaries in this way, we find protection. Protection is not just in setting up "barriers" from others' potential to hurt us (though women, especially sexual abuse survivors, need to know how to do this). Protection is also in expanding our awareness and capacity for connection. Healing is healing of the whole through compassionate action for the whole. For we need to heal not just from the past but from the present and from the looming future. We are all suffering not from Post-Traumatic Stress Disorder but from Present Traumatic Stress Disorder and Pre-Traumatic Stress Disorder, traumatized by living on a dying planet. Certainly, we need to be strong to face this present and the possibilities of our future. Our "inner child" must face its own truths and sing its sad, angry songs out loud. So too must our adult citizen-self be strong—to imagine itself as more than a skin-encapsulated ego alternately flexing its own delusionary muscles of individual control and collapsing in a heap of powerlessness. What we need to develop is a sense of self that is larger and wider than this, and that can feel its connection to the larger whole, whether that whole is experienced as God, Goddess, Higher Power, Self, No-Self, Over-Soul, Buddha Nature, Eco-Self, or Gaia.

The connections between feminism, ecology, and psychology are vital. Liberating women, healing the wounds of patriarchy, and saving the planet are actually one and the same process. If we are to avoid a "spiritual bypass" of the suffering built into our social order, we must continue to be rooted in an unflinching understanding of the politics of patriarchy and its effects on the psyches of men and women and on the earth itself. We can no longer afford to keep psychology and therapy—feminist or otherwise—separate from spiritual growth and ecological awareness and activism. Psychology and psychotherapy have often functioned as forces for adaptation to a life-denying social structure. However, they nevertheless contain the potential to widen the horizons of what is known about self and world to help us meet the real healing challenges of our time.

May the Goddess be with us.

Miriam Greenspan
Boston, Mass.
August 1992

Introduction to the First Edition

My first experience of therapy was not as a therapist but as a patient. By the time I was twenty-four, I had already had three such experiences. As an undergraduate, I had learned from other female students that my daily anxiety about my worth as a student and the pain of my various romances was appropriate fare for therapy. (At the time, it never occurred to me to ask why my male fellow students and boyfriends seemed so oblivious to therapy while my female friends were so familiar with the campus counseling center.) In my first therapy session, the therapist asked me to tell him my earliest memories. I remembered myself at age three, wheeling my own baby carriage in play, and my father rescuing my kitten from the violent claws of a larger cat.

I learned from this therapist that these memories reflected a successful resolution of my Oedipus complex. The memory of my wheeling a baby carriage showed that I had adopted the proper identification with my feminine role as mother. The memory of my father's rescuing of my cat showed that I had the proper view of masculinity as a saving power. In short, I was a well-adjusted female.

My satisfaction at being declared a normal woman was dispelled, months later, when my therapist told me that I was an "obsessive-compulsive neurotic." Though I had no idea what this diagnosis meant, it struck me as undeniably accurate. Coming from his mouth, it had the ring of truth. Apparently, after divulging my diagnosis, there was nothing more that this therapist could do for me, for I was thereafter expelled from therapy.

By the time I got to my second therapist, my initial innocence was tinged with a bit of wariness. I was then a graduate student of English at Columbia University. In this male bastion of academia, I became a chronic female depressive. Neither my academic honors nor my professors' praise succeeded in convincing me that I was a "real" student. Like many women, I believed my success to be largely a sham. I was underweight, chronically sleepless, anxious, and depressed.

My second therapist took notes and listened attentively to my complaints for three sessions. He then told me that I had a chronic problem and that a university counseling center could do little for me: I needed long-term, intensive, individual psychotherapy. Assuming that I could afford the fee of a private psychiatrist, he was willing to recommend one. Being a poor student, I had no choice but to pass up this referral.

I left the university a year later, still plagued by insomnia, massive self-doubt, acute stomach pain, depression, and anxiety—symptoms that I later learned were quite typical for female therapy patients. Once again, I searched for a therapist. I was not alone. Most of my female friends from college—and hundreds of thousands of women throughout the country—sought in therapy the solution to the profound sense of being lost which we shared in those days of cultural upheaval. We had grown up in the fifties, the era of the Feminine Mystique; come of age in the sixties, the era of the sexual revolution and student politics; and were hitting the seventies with massive socially induced identity crises. Like many women in those days (and still today), I suffered from a numbing confusion about what I was supposed to "be" as a woman-person in 1969. A mother wheeling a baby carriage? A perpetual student? A career woman? A wife? A mistress? For reasons I did not yet understand, all of these options struck me with dread.

Finding Dr. B. provided a temporary answer to my dilemma about who to be. I was no man's mistress and no man's wife, but I was my therapist's patient. Psychotherapy gave my life a shape, the meaning it had been missing since I graduated from college. I embarked on what Phyllis Chesler has called the female "career" as therapy patient with all the enthusiasm and romantic idealism of a newly married bride.

In my first session, Dr. B. pointedly observed that I was wearing a low-cut sweater and that my pants were not completely zipped, and then waited for me to respond. I remember dimly feeling that this "meant something" terribly important that I would later learn from him. From that moment on, my "transference" (as I later learned it was called) was complete: my psyche belonged to the doctor.

With Dr. B. I explored the confusions, depression, and anger I felt as a woman trying to find my place in the world. Apart from an avid interest in my sex life and my feelings as a child, Dr. B.'s favorite psychic strategy was to get me to see how I fought my feminine identity. For instance, his response to my discontents in relationships with sexist men was that I evidently refused to allow myself to be taken care of by a man. While society shook with the initial blasts of the women's movement, I spent one hour each week getting psychologically groomed to be the kind of woman who would not make waves. When I rebelled against Dr. B.'s expertise and suggested that he had a sexist understanding of women, he lost his usual reserve and insisted that "women's lib" was not the subject of therapy. Indeed.

Getting a divorce from Dr. B. and reclaiming my psyche as my own was a difficult feat for me—as it is for many women in therapy who are dissatisfied with their therapists but cannot leave them. I could not have done so without the support of the women's movement which was surging through our society at the time. In my consciousness-raising group I learned that I could both understand and retrieve myself from my dilemmas as a woman without resorting to psycho-diagnosis or psycho-therapy. I began to see myself in relation to men, other women, and society from a woman's point of view. The very fact that there was a "woman's point of view," and that it was missing from psychiatry and male culture in general, was itself a profound, life-changing revelation. It became clear to me that the displeasure and anger I felt at Dr. B.'s approach to my problems were not the transference feelings of an obsessive-compulsive neurotic or the manifestations of failed femininity: they were the legitimate emotions of a woman who refused to adapt to her subordination in the way that both society and her therapist prescribed.

Two years after I gave up being a therapy patient, I became an intern in clinical and community psychology. It was only then that I began to see how typical my own experiences as a patient actually were. What I had taken to be the individual quirks of my first two therapists and the overt sexism of the third were essential aspects of the way in which traditional therapy functioned. The emphasis on diagnosis and its apparent irrelevance to helping patients in any concrete way, as well as the belief in a theory of women as feminine creatures whose normalcy rested on subordination to men, were all a part of the traditional theory and practice of therapy as taught to trainees in the field.

The initial ideas for this book were conceived during my apprenticeship as a therapist. The book reflects the personal/political/professional journey I have taken in these ten years: from learning how to perpetrate psychiatric injuries on patients to learning how to practice a kind of therapy that attempts to serve not only the personal interests of individual women but the social interests of women as a whole. The pain and anger that I felt in the years of my training, in seeing so many women (and men) come to harm in situations in which they expected help, fueled Part I's critical examination of the theories and practices of the traditional psychiatric system. Much of this analysis of psychiatry is told in the form of "inside stories" from my training. For the most part, I believe that these stories speak for themselves. Chapter 1 looks at the theory and Chapter 2 at the practices of psychiatry as a whole. Chapter 3 specifically focuses on the traditional theory of female psychology and the traditional practice of therapy with women.

In the eight years since my training ended, my private therapy practice has coincided with the emergence and growth of feminist therapy as a "movement." During this same period, the new growth therapies, based on a humanist model of psychology, have increasingly challenged the traditional modes of therapy and developed a large variety of alternative modes and techniques. Since the flowering of the counterculture in the late sixties and seventies, these therapies have become the most serious theoretical, practical—and economic—threat to mainstream psychology and psychotherapy in this country. They have deeply influenced the way many feminist therapists think about and treat women. They merit a close and critical analysis, which is the subject of Part II of the book. Chapter 6 looks at the limitations of the humanist or growth approach to psychology and therapy in general. Chapter 7 focuses on the limitations of this approach to understanding and treating women.

While borrowing ideas and techniques from the radical therapy and growth therapy camps, feminist therapy itself came about as a grass-roots uprising of women helping women, a part of the spread of feminist services in the seventies. Unlike other schools of therapy, it was not founded by one great personality. It evolved gradually from the thoughts and labors of countless women. Women's therapy collectives and associations sprang up in cities throughout the country. Many

of them offered therapy at fees that were negotiable on the basis of
what the patient could afford. These groups were often run collectively—each woman an equal partner, regardless of differences in
degree of professionalization or training. Feminist therapists saw
themselves as women working within a growing women's community,
rather than as members of a professional elite outside that community.
Therapists and patients together developed a definition of therapy for
women that deviated from the standard definition of therapy as treatment for pathology and the humanist definition of therapy as a means
of personal growth. Feminist therapy, by contrast, was considered a
process of both personal and political growth furthered by an egalitarian relationship between women struggling to challenge their subordination in our society.

I was fortunate to share in the emergence of feminist therapy ideas
and services. During the past eight years of working as a therapist and
speaking at universities, women's conferences, and women's centers
throughout the country, I have been one of the thousands of women
trying to develop a genuinely new approach to therapy for women.
Women in search of a nonsexist therapy now do have an alternative to
what has existed in the past.

But though feminist therapy services have proliferated throughout
the country, the need for a coherent theory of feminist therapy
remains. Indeed, as more and more people have come to call themselves feminist therapists, the term has come to mean less and less.
Phyllis Chesler's now classic book, *Women and Madness*, was the first
to express, clearly and forcefully, women's dissatisfactions with psychiatry and traditional therapy. This book owes a great deal to hers.
But conspicuously absent from *Women and Madness* is any suggestion
of what feminist therapy for women might be. In fact, Chesler leaves
an open question as to whether therapy of any kind can be useful to
anyone, Part III of this book is an attempt to find that gap. It starts
where *Women and Madness* left off. Its goal is to map out a therapy
specifically geared to the needs of women in our society, both theoretically and in practice.

Such a therapy requires, to start with, a theory of female psychology that doesn't suffer from the masculine bias of traditional theory.
Chapter 9 is a point of origin for the formulation of such a theory. It
grapples with the question of how the "outer" becomes "inner" in
women's lives—how not only cultural values and norms, but social

structures such as the family and the economy influence female psychology.

During the writing of this book, Jean Baker Miller published *Toward a New Psychology of Women*. It was invaluable in advancing my own thinking about women. The third section of Chapter 9, "Women and the Labor of Relatedness," builds on Miller's analysis of female ego-identity in male society, but with a more specific focus on how a woman's sense of self grows out of women's work in our society. Much of the analysis of female psychology in this chapter is told through stories of women with whom I have worked in therapy. Chapter 10 offers a woman-oriented model of therapy. It, too, is presented largely through stories from my practice.

To provide the reader with a concrete understanding of the three approaches to therapy examined in this book, each of the three parts ends with a chapter presenting a fictionalized account of a "typical" therapy session with a "typical" woman patient. Thus Chapters 5, 8, and 11 show what happens to Polly Patient (as I have affectionately named her) in traditional, growth, and feminist therapy, respectively.

Part of the difficulty of writing this book has been dealing with the apparently dizzying rate of social change in the condition of women over the years. I started writing in 1977, a time when women's anger at the enormity of our oppression coexisted with an unbounded optimism and exhilaration about the possibility of collectively overcoming it. I finished in 1982, a time when women's victories in the era of reproductive rights are under increasing attack, an era in which it is difficult not to despair about the future of women, men, children, and the planet.

Writing during these years about the emotional problems that women face as a result of the internalization of our oppression has often been perplexing. Certainly, one of the important achievements of the women's movement has been the collective redefinition of ourselves as women, from our own point of view. The dominant culture has no doubt been influenced by these efforts. The media image of the "liberated woman" has been incorporated into the way that society thinks about women. To the extent that feminism has succeeded in affecting the public image of femininity, it would appear that some of the more crippling emotional problems I write about (in Chapters 9 and 10) are a thing of the past, or at least apply to only a small number of women.

This conclusion, however tempting, is mistaken. In the first place, the dominant culture has a way of incorporating the ideology of feminism while pacifying its potentially revolutionary content. The "liberated" woman becomes yet another image on the TV screen of reality; her continued visibility in the culture depends upon her overall network ratings. For instance, at the midpoint of writing this book, I began to doubt whether the "Woman as Body" I was writing about in Chapter 9 still existed as a cultural ideal. Within a few months, fashion moguls came out with "hooker skirts" for women, a harbinger of the return in the last few years, to traditional femininity in fashion and social values. The "liberated" woman has become a chic combination of the Total Woman with her man and the ravishing career woman on the job: she is nothing short of Superwoman. Young women growing up today are internalizing this modified version of the pre-women's liberation norm of Woman as Body.

Furthermore, changes in the ideology of womanhood that occur over the span of a decade do not entirely negate the enormous weight of centuries of female social conditioning. To say this is not to minimize the extraordinary energy that women have devoted to the struggle to free ourselves from our psychological and social straitjackets. Nor is it to deny the success of these efforts in transforming women's lives for the better. On the contrary, my faith in the therapeutic effects of consciousness-raising informs my approach to women and therapy throughout this book.

Nevertheless, the female symptoms of oppression examined in Chapters 3, 9, and 10 continue to plague women. The conflicts that women experience in achieving a feminine identity are perhaps more puzzling in the era of post-women's liberation than before. They take some new forms, but they persist and are widespread.

Changes in the traditional "cure" that psychiatry offers for these symptoms and conflicts reflect similar ambiguities. During the course of writing this book, the academic and professional realms of psychology and psychotherapy have shown an increased tolerance of feminist scholarship, research, and teaching. Feminist therapy has arrived on the marketplace of available therapies. But, for the most part, this progress has not affected the traditional psychiatric treatments documented in Part I. These treatments—including the traditional method of individual therapy—continue to be taught and practiced with little modification. The male bias in this model of human psychology and therapy continues to affect millions of women *and* men in this country adversely. It is precisely because traditional treatments are still practiced as usual that Part I of this book will no doubt be controversial in psychiatric circles.

Because therapists work so intimately with the most deeply embedded layers of a person's consciousness, they are in a unique position to alter a woman's experience, awareness, and understanding of herself and her world. The potential for therapy to be a means of changing a woman's consciousness in a way that furthers the transformation of society to meet women's—and human—needs has yet to be fully explored. I hope that *A New Approach to Women and Therapy* will be a contribution to this task.

1

Father Knows Best:

THE FAILURE OF
TRADITIONAL THERAPY

1
CHAPTER

An Introduction to
Traditional Theory

1. What's the Problem?

If you are a woman in search of or in therapy, you may be suffering from one or more of the following typical problems. The most common, and the most serious of them, is depression —that familiar gray fog of emptiness and fatigue that numbs and envelops your life. Perhaps you sleep poorly, have little or no interest in sex or work or friendships or husband or family. Nothing seems to matter. If your depression is mild, you manage to function fairly well despite how you feel. But sometimes the depression becomes so intolerable that you may find yourself longing for the sweet oblivion of death.

For some women, the problem is recurrent aches and pains of unknown origins—headaches or migraines or stomach pain or back pain—which medical doctors ascribe to "nerves" and for which they prescribe Valium.

For other women, the problem is sexuality. Perhaps you think of yourself as sexually inadequate or frigid because you never or rarely have orgasms. Or perhaps you've been faking it in sex, disgusted with yourself and scared that your husband or lover will find out. He may be kind and considerate, yet nothing seems to work. Or he may never take the time or offer the tenderness that you need in sex. You may try to stifle the rage you feel because, deep down, you think that the bad sex is really your problem.

3

Sometimes it is your marriage or couple relationship that is the problem. You and your partner fight constantly but never resolve anything. Or you don't fight at all but feel more and more distant and unconnected. You find that "you can't live with him and you can't live without him." The thought of separation or divorce is terrifying, but so is staying in a relationship that feels like it's strangling you.

Or the problem may be that you are not involved with a man and would like to be—but just can't seem to make it work with anyone. You tell yourself that men are to blame: they are crass, insensitive, cruel, or inept. But deep down, you blame yourself: you are not worthy of being loved. You believe that you are too dependent, that your neediness chases men away. You feel that you are doomed to be alone, searching in every passing contact for the one man who will save you from your terrible fate. You blame yourself both for failing to hold a man and for needing one too much.

Or the problem may surface in any one of dozens of other typical female "symptoms": You may eat and diet compulsively and yet always hate your body. You may doubt your competence, constantly and addictively seeking the admiration and approval of others to confirm your sense of self-worth; yet when you get the approval, it leaves you cold. You may feel that you have no self at all—that you are a collection of other people's demands and desires. You may feel constantly anxious or lost. For some women, the problem is the terrifying fear that they are "going crazy," or even the profound longing to stop functioning so that they can be taken care of.

These are some of the leading forms of the problems that bring women to therapy. Psychiatrists call these "presenting problems." Whatever form it takes, the problem, you are convinced, is *you*. Something is wrong with you: you are sick, neurotic, crazy, or bad. Often enough your husband, your lover, your boss, your mother or father or children are telling you the same thing: *you* are the problem. You get to a point where you know that, whatever the problem is, you cannot possibly fix it yourself. You are afraid to burden your friends. You are convinced that the only possible solution to the problem is professional help: you need a psychotherapist, a shrink, a doctor, an expert.

The woman who can afford the going rate of approximately fifty to seventy dollars an hour arrives at the private office of a psychiatrist or psychologist. Otherwise, she is referred to a local mental health center or the outpatient clinic of a local hospital where she is introduced to a psychiatrist or psychologist (in most cases a trainee—but she is not usually informed of this). At some point, should her symptoms persist, she is likely to have tranquilizers or antidepressants prescribed for her. As a woman, she is more likely than her male counterpart eventually to be referred for inpatient hospitalization.

The mental health system in which she finds herself is a vast and growing system of interconnected institutions including psychiatric wards of general hospitals; state mental hospitals; private psychiatric hospitals; private and public outpatient clinics; community mental health centers; and private psychotherapy.

Women are *the majority of patients in all sectors of the psychiatric system* except for state and county mental hospitals.

- Women comprise almost two-thirds of the adult population of general psychiatric, community mental health, and outpatient psychiatric facilities.
- Of the approximately 3 million people admitted to private psychiatric hospitals, psychiatric wards of general hospitals, outpatient clinics, and community mental health centers, almost 2 million are women.
- Approximately 4 percent of all office visits to private doctors made by women each year are for symptoms that doctors ascribe to psychological or mental disorders. This amounts to more than 12 million women.
- An estimated 84 percent of all private psychotherapy patients are women.
- There are approximately 1.2 million new psychotherapy patients each year, 60 percent of whom are women.[1]

On the other hand:

- Approximately 73 percent of all medical doctors are men.
- Approximately 86 percent of all psychiatrists are men.
- Approximately 84 percent of all psychologists are men.

The clear picture that emerges from these statistics is that it is largely men who label the variety of psychological problems of those who seek therapeutic help and largely women who are seeking the help. It is a picture of a mental health system dominated by male practitioners who diagnose and treat female patients. It is a picture, in short, of Man as Expert and Woman as Patient.

Man as Expert and Woman as Patient are a complementary fit. Men, more than women, are both socialized to see themselves as authorities and institutionally encouraged to become them. Women, more than men, are socialized to see their problems as emotional in origin and to be willing to report these problems to such male authorities.

There is a world of difference between the posh Fifth Avenue office of the private psychiatrist and the back wards of the degenerating state hospital system. Yet, from psychotherapy to state hospitalization, the fate of Woman as Patient in the traditional system is the same: as helpless, passive patient, she is chaperoned into different parts of the system by various male Experts.

In the mental health field, as in most other arenas of social life, it is largely men who have the power to define reality—*to name the problem*. In this case, the typical male Expert is likely to construe the above statistics to mean that women are psychologically sicker than men. The numbers may be taken as evidence of the *problem of female mental illness*. But if we look closer, this way of defining the problem is itself a part of the problem. For statistics also show that male doctors will diagnose women as neurotic or psychotic *twice as frequently as they do men with the same symptoms:* Man as Expert simply sees women quite differently than he sees men.

In one research study, therapists were asked to describe the characteristics and behaviors of a healthy, mature *adult* (sex unspecified), and the characteristics and behaviors of a *man* and of a *woman*. The responses of these mental health professionals showed that behaviors and characteristics judged healthy for an *adult* and presumed to reflect an ideal standard of mental health correlated only with those behaviors and characteristics which they judged healthy for *men* and not with those judged healthy for *women*.[2] This study shows us that there is a double standard of mental health for men and women. More important, it is the male standard that is understood to be that of the healthy human being. Hence the double bind for Woman as Patient: to be seen as a woman by Man as Expert she must embody characteristics that are not seen as those of a healthy, normal adult. If she embodies those characteristics Man as Expert considers adult, she will not be seen as a woman.

The problem is not that of female mental illness. The symptoms of such "illness," as we shall see, are, for the most part, the systematically socially produced symptoms of sexual inequality. The problem is a matter of how women are seen and treated both inside the mental health system and in the surrounding society that it mirrors.

If you are a woman in traditional therapy with any one of the above presenting problems, you have found a new home. You probably initially feel a sense of great relief that you are finally getting some help. Your therapist seems competent, strong, authoritative—that is, male. You feel safe in the masculine protection that he seems to offer. For the first time in a long time, you feel hopeful. With his help, perhaps the problem that brought you to therapy will be solved. The problem—*you*—may be curable.

But after the initial honeymoon phase is over, you are often faced with another problem: that of being a female patient in traditional therapy. Perhaps you adore your therapist but you find that therapy has brought about no real change. You try not to blame him, but you feel increasingly frustrated and hopeless.

You blame yourself for your inability to change. Or perhaps you become suspicious or distrustful of your therapist. You feel acutely uncomfortable when you talk to him about yourself, more like a little girl than a grown woman. You may feel constantly scrutinized and evaluated and judged in his presence: as though he had one big Eye that was always open and glued to your every flaw. It becomes difficult just to be yourself with him, rather than to gear your words to what you think he would like to hear. You are afraid that if he knows the "real you" he will think that you are bad, mad, or crazy. Sometimes, you are secretly angry at him, even hate him—yet you are ashamed of these feelings. You believe that they prove how neurotic you really are. You blame yourself for being so unreasonable about someone who knows more about you than you do and has only your best interests at heart. You begin to question yourself habitually (in imitation of his way) about why you should feel these neurotic feelings toward him.

Despite your distrust, you may eventually come to feel very dependent on your therapist, even terrified of life beyond his all-seeing Eye. This dependency grows despite (perhaps because of) the fact that you walk away from most therapy sessions feeling that all your problems are your own fault.

In the end, you may be one of the millions of women who, after years of therapy, still feel lost and helpless. Despite your increased understanding of the childhood roots of your problems, they do not seem to go away. You believe, now more than ever, that *the problem is you.* You have become Woman as Patient, hooked on Man as Expert—with no cure in sight.

The problem is not you. The problem is that you feel trapped in your life and then further trapped in a system of therapy from which there is no way to emerge feeling powerful. The problem is how you are defined, seen, and treated in the mental health system as well as in society as a whole. The problem is how traditional psychotherapy works against you rather than for you.

To understand your problem, traditional therapy searches

your personal history. But for the real roots of the problem we must look beyond your personal history to your history as a woman in society and to the history of traditional psychotherapy itself.

2. The Traditional Approach to the Problem

Traditional psychotherapists believe that all the clues to your presenting problem(s) lie in the details of your past personal history. Therefore, the first thing that happens to you as a therapy patient is that your family, social, and sexual histories are taken in the initial or intake interview so that they can be evaluated against a hypothetical norm for human development. Any deviations from this norm are analyzed closely, for they are presumed to contain the causal explanations for your current problems.

All theoreticians and practitioners of psychology are concerned with the central question of how individuals psychologically develop from childhood to adulthood. As social scientists, psychologists and psychotherapists tend to frame this question in its absolute or universal forms: How does the individual develop in the normal developmental process? What are the stages of development through which *he* must pass? What factors determine individual development? This approach, which is largely unquestioned, poses several problems for women.

First, as we have seen, the "individual" is always presumed to be male. In patriarchal societies, there are, of course, bound to be profound differences in how women and men develop into human beings. For the most part, until recently, such differences were always ascribed to innate differences in the female and male "natures." Nevertheless, this did not stop traditional theorists of psychology from taking this "natural" difference between men and women as evidence of women's deviation from the human (male) norm. Because they did not follow the "normal" (male) course of development, women were not seen as normal. In this sense, by traditional standards, a close scrutiny of the past personal history of virtually *any* female would inevitably turn up some grist for the psychotherapist's mill. Women are simply born patients.

The problem, to start with, is in the way psychotherapists and social scientists in general frame their questions. Presumably it is scientific to ask "How does the individual develop?" The hidden assumption here is that such a question can be adequately answered without asking how specific individuals belonging to specific groups develop within a specific society. Women are simply one, and the largest, of such groups. In a society that is stratified by sex, race and class, as ours is, there are other groups of people who are essentially ignored by positing this general, presumably universal, question. For the model of the individual in this question is not only male but also white and middle-class. The hiddenness of women, blacks, and working-class people within this model is a reflection of the invisibility of these groups within the society as a whole.

Now indeed there may be common features in the development of male and female individuals or middle-class and working-class individuals or blacks and whites or men and women of *all* classes in *this* society and men and women of *all* classes in *every* society. But the unquestioned assumption in the social scientist's general query is that all of these common features can be understood while ignoring the specific differences in the individual's sex, race, and class. This is called the scientific approach, and it is based on the myth that there are no *essential* social divisions in our society—that the impact of social structure on the individual is the same for all. Were this the case, we might indeed be able to study the development of the individual divorced from his or her social, economic, historical contexts and assume that we are arriving at the "truth" currently enshrined by science. Until we create a totally egalitarian society, however, social scientists simply mystify the subject by affixing the label science to what is, at best, a partial and, at worst, an ideologically contaminated process of asking limited questions.

The problem lies in the way in which social science defines the problem.

Psychotherapy is a branch of psychology. Psychology, as one of the compartmentalized disciplines of the social sciences, isolates the individual from his or her social/historical/economic context and assumes that in so doing it can validly study the behavior of the individual in all societies for all times. This kind of compartmentalization and isolation is perhaps the distinctive feature of contemporary social science. The proliferation, in the last two decades, of all the multihyphenated disciplines—psycho-biology, neuro-psychiatry, physiological-psychology, psycho-history, etc.—is a manifestation of this tendency of social science to devolve into more and more "specialized" areas. In attempting to answer the broadest possible questions of human behavior, psychology paradoxically falls into asking increasingly narrow ones. The larger question of "What makes people depressed?" turns into "What happens to chemical x at the nerve synapse?" Or "What makes this particular woman so unhappy?" turns into "What is this woman's diagnosis?" These questions are not of the same order, yet they are mistakenly thought to be so. It is as though one could isolate one brain cell and in so doing understand the functioning of the entire brain. Or as though one could isolate the chemical functioning of the brain and in so doing understand the feelings and behavior of the whole human being. (The latter is, in fact, the aim of much of contemporary neuro-psychiatry.)

The western scientific mind thinks in dualities (mind versus body, the individual versus society, etc.). Reality becomes more and more subdivided. The social scientist must choose his "side": as environmentalist or geneticist, as psychoanalyst or behaviorist, as humanist or scientist. In the process, *the aim of social science, which is a totalistic account of the individual and his or her environment,* is irretrievably lost.

Instead of such an account, contemporary psychology offers us a choice between three equally limited ways of looking at the individual. The *traditionalists* (Freudians and neo-

Freudians) tell us that the person is a composite psychic mechanism whose behavior is determined by unconscious forces within. The *behaviorists* tell us that a person is a "black box" whose behavior is determined by "reinforcement" from the environment.* And the new *humanists* tell us that a person is a spiritual being whose behavior is totally determined by the self. All three of these theoretical orientations eclipse major portions of reality: the traditionalists and humanists (each in different ways) deny the impact of social reality, while the behaviorists deny the impact of consciousness.

For our purposes here, the "individual" is a woman, one of the millions whose problems lead them to psychotherapy. And our problem is how to understand and treat her problems. For this reason, it is the traditional orientation with which I am most concerned. For despite the existence of behaviorist and humanist psychology, most psychotherapy today, both private and public, inpatient and outpatient, is still of the traditionalist variety. It is called *psychodynamic therapy* and is derived from the original psychoanalytic practice of Sigmund Freud.

3. Grandfather Freud

Sigmund Freud is the undisputed grandfather of all modern psychotherapy. Before Freud, people were seen as self-

---

* Although there is much to be said about the impact of behaviorist psychology on psychotherapy today, I do not do so in this book. At the time of this writing, behaviorist principles of psychology have been applied more widely to prison "rehabilitation" programs than to individual psychotherapy, public or private. Such behavior modification programs are examples of the most overtly coercive and totalitarian use of psychology today, in many cases amounting to out-and-out torture. (Electroshocks applied to male genitalia to "cure" homosexual "deviants" is only one example.) Behaviorist psychology has entered the mental health arena mostly in the occasional use of behavior modification techniques in inpatient settings as well as in individual therapy, particularly in the cure of phobias. Nevertheless, the behaviorist approach to individual psychotherapy is still much more rare than the traditional (psychodynamic) approach to mental illness, which remains the reigning approach today. The humanist perspective is, more and more, coming to usurp some traditional therapy markets. In the form of pop psychology, literature, and media, the humanist approach to solving individual problems is one of the strongest ideological trends in the popular imagination of Americans today. It is a force to be reckoned with (and therefore occupies Part II of this book).

intentioned, conscious, and rational subjects whose mental disorders were a product of nervous degeneration. Freud tore the rug out from under this Victorian understanding (a leftover from the enlightenment era) of the individual as a fundamentally rational organism. He introduced instead the concept of the individual as a being ruled from within by forces largely beyond his comprehension or control. His major contribution was to name these forces as unconscious and to map their terrain, to expose the essential irrationalities that motivate much of human behavior.

The original ideas of psychoanalysis have by now become well-known even by those who have never read Freud:

1. that sexual drives and feeling starting in early childhood are at the core of human personality development, which proceeds by stages (from oral to anal to phallic to genital).

2. that the mind has an *unconscious,* which operates according to a logic very different from that of the conscious mind—a logic apparent in dreams.

3. that what Freud called the *psychic apparatus* of mind can be divided into three structures; id, ego, and superego. The id contains the libidinal drives—the unconscious instinctive desires and impulses. The superego is formed through the child's identification with his parents, through which he internalizes their wishes and demands in the form of conscience. The ego mediates between the demands of the id and those of the superego, helping the individual to adapt and mature.

4. that unconscious drives and feelings threatening to the ego or superego are repressed by *defense mechanisms*— thereby preserving inner conflicts in the attempt to stave off anxiety.

5. that there is much conscious and unconscious *resistance* to the surfacing of repressed *material.*

6. that—in a process Freud called *transference*—people transfer to others, especially therapists, feelings and atti-

tudes that were originally associated with important figures in their early life, particularly with their parents.

Freudian psychoanalysis was both a theory and a practice. It laid the groundwork for a truly sophisticated understanding of the workings of the unconscious mind and established a method of therapeutic work. The Freudian methods of psycho-analysis—including free association, dream analysis, interpretation of transference and of resistance—have remained indispensable tools of psychotherapy. Many of Freud's ideas have become deeply ingrained in our society. Without them, most forms of therapy as we know it would be virtually impossible.

As the original teachings of Christ were to the Church, so psychoanalysis was to modern psychiatry. Psychoanalysis became the foundation on which modern psychiatry built its theory and practice. The woman who ends up in the psychiatric outpatient clinic or in the private psychiatrist's office, or even in most inpatient wards, is both viewed and treated according to a system of thought rooted in Freudian theory.

But psychoanalysis, despite its indelible contributions, was mistaken in certain crucial ways. These mistaken ideas were taken up and perpetuated within the psychiatric context of practice.

Freud never abandoned the dualistic approach that is perhaps the hallmark of western thinking. On the contrary, psychoanalytic theory is deeply entrenched in these dualisms: conscious versus unconscious; id versus ego; eros (love) versus thanatos (death); pleasure principle versus reality principle; instinct versus culture; the individual versus society. What Freud tried to grasp was the presence of what appeared to him to be inescapable forms of *conflict* between incompatible elements both within the individual and between the individual and society. Freud saw a world in which the individual and society were at war, a world in which the most primitive or basic of human longings—for sexual love—was at odds with the dictates of civilization. In the face of the boundless Victorian faith in the inevitability of progress, Freud uncovered the reality of what seemed to be irreconcilable antagonisms. His effort was to understand these antagonisms *from the inside.*

In the end, however, Freud never fully escaped the constraints of Victorian ideology. In the Freudian world view, sexuality was still in some sense fundamentally evil, not by virtue of original sin, but because the free play of sexual drives was seen to be ultimately incompatible with the "highest" ends of humanity and culture. The instincts, seething in their unconscious cauldron, had to be repressed if society was to be maintained. For Freud, the most essential characteristics of the person—his or her innate instinctual life—were defeated by social organization. Harmony between the individul and society was impossible.

Freud's task was to elucidate the process of individuation —the process by which individual personality structure developed socially. He understood that even the most apparently biological aspects of the human being—the sexual instincts— were actually socialized through the mediation and intervention of society in the form of one's parents. However, in positing a permanent, inevitable, and universal antagonism between the instincts and civilization, between the individual and society, Freud abandoned his own understanding of individuation as a social process. In the end, his theory misunderstood the individual, society, and the relationship between them.

Freud's problem was that his conceptions of human nature and society were fundamentally ahistorical. The repressive demands of Victorian society, its need for the strict conformity of individuals to a rigid, sublimated style of heterosexual genital sexuality, and the concomitant social production of sexual neuroses in a vast number of people, all this was seen by Freud as a natural consequence of society—an inevitable process involving all individuals in all societies for all time. In fact, the "individual," in the sense that Freud talked about him, did not even exist before the advent of capitalism. Before this, the divisions between individual and society, private and public life, family and work that we now take for granted were fundamentally different. What Freud saw as society was actually a particular society; and what he saw as the individual was the particular kind of person demanded by that society.

Certainly, Freud was correct in his perception of an apparent war between people as individuals and the social order. But he misunderstood the nature of this war—its causes and the means by which to end it. Freud saw no end in sight; he had no vision of a society in which people could live in harmony with one another and with the demands of society as a whole. He started out as a sexual revolutionary and ended up as an apologist for current norms of sexuality and for the preservation of the social status quo.

The mistaken approach of psychoanalysis to the individual and society, along with its ingenious contributions to the study of the unconscious, was perpetuated by the psychologists and psychiatrists who succeeded Freud. The Freudian approach contained what then became the ruling myths of psychiatric theory and practice. Briefly, these myths can be stated as follows: first, the myth that the individual's psyche can be understood apart from the specific society in which s/he lives; second, that psychological symptoms can be understood apart from a person's social relationships; and third, that the patient's behavior in therapy can be understood apart from her relationship to her therapist. These myths continue to plague both those who practice therapy and those who receive it.

4. Three Myths of the Traditional System

MYTH 1: "IT'S ALL IN YOUR HEAD" ■ Myth 1 tells us that personal reality is essentially determined by unconscious forces within a person's mind. This is the myth of intrapsychic determinism or "It's all in your head." It views the private, personal realm of the individual as one polarity and the public, social realm of society as another. In isolating one polarity from

the other, it misses the interdependence of each on the other—
that is, the mutual impact of social structure and personality
structure. Instead, a person's emotional problems are divorced
from any current social, historical, or economic context. Causes
of emotional problems are ascribed to disorders or diseases of
internal psychic mechanisms. Such disorders or diseases are
said to be rooted in unconscious psychic conflicts engendered
in early childhood. The social environment considered relevant to a person's emotional problems and personality is defined, simply, as the family. The family—especially the mother
—is considered the only significant social context of human
personality development.

The picture, according to myth 1, is of individuals floating
in space with their families orbiting around them. There is no
particular relationship among the individuals or between the
families and other institutions in the social order. Emotional
pain is caused by unconscious forces within each individual.
And the sum total of all individuals taken together is "society."

As we have seen, this myth was deeply ingrained in Freudian thinking. The vicissitudes of the sexual and aggressive
drives and their mediation by ego and superego were considered to be the causes of human behavior. The warring and
integrating interreaction of id, ego, and superego were considered the driving mechanisms of personality development.
The individual, ultimately, was seen as an enclosed shell
whose behavior was determined by irrational forces from
within.

Abnormalities of behavior were ascribed to disorders in the
psychic apparatus of id-ego-superego. While Freud did acknowledge the importance of social environment in the development of this psychic apparatus, he saw this environment as
including only the child's immediate family: mother, father
and, to a lesser extent, siblings. The limitation of this thinking
was that he had no social conception of the family itself—of its
relation to institutions outside of itself. He had little or no understanding, for instance, of how the effect of the family on

individual development was also structured by the effect of socioeconomic organization on the family. The Oedipal scenario of mother, father, and son, so central to the Freudian view of human psychology, was possible only in a historically specific family: the family created by capitalism. Stripped of its former functions as an economic unit of production and reduced to the nuclear affective unit we now know, the family evolved into a crucible for intense emotion unparalleled in history. Only in this kind of crucible could the Oedipal drama unfold in the way Freud envisioned.* Had Freud been more aware of the historical nature of the family, he might have been able to make a more scientific study of the interdependence of social structure and personality structure in general, as well as of how the socioeconomic organization of the capitalist society of his day influenced the development of specific personality types.

Furthermore, Freud unquestioningly took for granted a crucial fact of family life which needed explanation—that mothers were the primary caretakers of growing children. The patriarchal nature of the family was assumed rather than explained by Freud; this resulted in a working definition of environment that, in effect, equated "environment" with "mother." By extension, both in Freud's practice and in the psychiatric practice which succeeded it, this led to one of the favorite abuses of contemporary psychology: the habit of blaming mothers for virtually every instance of human pain and distress in their offspring. Hence, for example, the common psychiatric practice of tracing the etiology (origins) of the mental illness schizophrenia to the "schizophrenogenic mother"— the mother who induces schizophrenia! Without an adequate conception of how motherhood is shaped by the patriarchal rule of the father in the family, the extent of a mother's power over her children is both wildly overestimated and severely misunderstood. The resulting contribution to women's oppres-

* With the advance of monopoly capitalism, the family unit of mother, father, and children is now being further eroded and, according to recent statistics, is increasingly less the norm in the United States today.

sion and therefore to women's psychic distress should not
be underestimated. (Some of the consequences of this particular Freudian mistake on the understanding and treatment
of women in traditional therapy are taken up in chapter
three.)

The myth that "It's all in your head" seriously misdefines
the relationship between the individual and society and between the family and other social institutions. It replaces the
complex interplay and interdependence of individual psychology and social structure with a dangerous simplification which
denies that social institutions create individuals as much as
individuals create social institutions.

Every society creates certain specific personality types
which will fit into, maintain, and reproduce the social order. In
order to perpetuate the sexual division of labor, patriarchal societies have historically structured the psyches of men and
women in very different ways. What psychologists have called
psychosocial "adaptation" is essentially the process by which
people unconsciously and consciously learn to accept and incorporate the social order, including the basic structural inequities upon which it rests—such as the inequality of men and
women. By ignoring or misunderstanding how and why our
society both requires and creates certain types of personalities
along sex/gender lines, myth 1 helps perpetuate a social status
quo that rests on the social subordination of women.

The most obvious (and therefore most neglected) fact about
theories locating all causality within the individual is that such
theories end up blaming the victim. If women are depressed or
sexually frigid, psychologists tell us, it is because they are
"masochistic" personalities. If the working man finds himself
feeling like a machine, he is suffering from a "somatic delu-
sion," a symptom of psychosis. The objective oppression that
women and working people suffer and which contributes to the
formation of such symptoms is thereby rendered invisible. Instead, the woman and the worker are labeled neurotic and
psychotic. Looked at from a social perspective, it is hardly surprising that a woman in a male-dominated culture may develop

certain symptoms of powerlessness such as depression and frigidity (see chapter three). Or that the working man (or woman) whose labor has been turned into another commodity on the marketplace, who must sell himself as an object for a wage, or whose labor has become completely mechanized, should end up feeling like a machine.

Myth 1's way of labeling such phenomena adds insult to injury. The oppression and exploitation of women and working people in our society is conveniently swept away and located *within*. It is not the social organization of the family or of the workplace that needs to be transformed—the individual woman or man needs to be fixed. The mental health professionals who subscribe to myth 1 form the army of experts who are there to do the fixing—to patch up the disorders and send the victims back to that which has broken them in the first place.

It is not that psychodynamic psychotherapy or prescriptions of Valium are never helpful to people. It is that, generally speaking, theories of individual determinism function largely to obfuscate the forces in people's lives that cause psychic distress, and thereby to defuse the energies that could be directed against these forces.

Since Freud, the belief that people's emotional problems (whatever their family roots) are ultimately of their own making has become widespread. It has caused countless men and women to blame themselves for problems that are social in origin. Freud did not say that *all* emotional problems originated in the unconscious, but he elaborated a system of thought and practice by which virtually any individual problem could be, and tended to be, viewed in this light. Whereas Freud thought that certain miseries were not amenable to psychoanalysis, his followers became more and more zealous in the application of psychoanalytic principles to all forms of human distress. Increasingly, the message of myth 1 became: "Your problems stem from unconscious psychological hangups which started in your early childhood. In overcoming these hangups (with professional help, of course) you can solve your problems and control your own reality." Because so many people in our society feel so out of control of their social reality, this message became extremely appealing. No wonder more than a million people each year join the swelling ranks of the millions of psychotherapy patients!

Women are especially vulnerable to this pervasive myth since women, more than men, tend to see their problems as emotionally based. This tendency is caused by female sex-role socialization and reinforced by a similar tendency of both the medical and psychiatric professions to diagnose women's physical ailments as psychological in origin. Myth 1 is all the more destructive to women, who are encouraged by it to see the socially produced symptoms of sexual inequality as their own solely individual pathology. This kind of self-condemning internalization is, in fact, a major aspect of the psychosocial oppression of women.

MYTH 2: THE MEDICAL MODEL OF PSYCHOPATHOLOGY ■ Closely related to the first, this myth tells us that human emotional pain in our society is a medical problem, that people in such pain are sick, and that their emotional problems can be cured in the same way that physical problems can: through medical means.

The psychiatric system that Freud helped shape, like the medical system in general, has a disease rather than health orientation. The "head" problems of myth 1 are presumed to be due to an illness or disorder which must be diagnosed and treated. Before Freud, psychiatry merely catalogued the symptoms of what were considered to be organically determined nervous disorders. Freud introduced the idea that many of these so-called nervous disorders were not derangements of the nervous system but had to do with profound psychological disturbances originating in the patient's early life. (By comparison to the psychiatrists of his day, Freud was, in this sense, an environmentalist.)

At the time, this was considered a highly controversial and speculative line of thought. Combined with the daring of Freud's original ideas about infantile sexuality, it made Freud a less than reputable figure in professional scientific circles. As a result, Freud had to work harder to prove his scientific credentials. He hovered dangerously on the brink of a rather revolutionary line of thinking about the social/political origins of human emotional pain. But he never crossed the threshold—possibly because he simply could not make the jump theoretically but also, in part, because he was simply too involved in making his own reputation as a scientist. In order to do so, he had to adhere to the basic disease-orientation of the science of his day. Not to do so would probably have gotten him laughed out of professional circles altogether.

Consequently, Freud originated a system of diagnosis, treatment, and prognosis in the psychological arena that imitated that of his colleagues in the medical arena. He categorized general types of mental disorders and then invented and catalogued the specific diagnoses that applied to people within each type. He named the diagnoses according to his system of fixed stages of psychosocial development: for example, obsessive-compulsives were fixated in the anal stage, hysterics in the oral stage, etc. But whereas Freud originated a limited number of diagnostic categories which he elaborately described and illustrated in his case studies, psychiatry added to and diluted this list to such an extent that the *Diagnostic and Statistical Manual of Mental Disorders* put out by the American Psychiatric Association in 1968 has no fewer than 304 psychiatric diagnoses, only one of which is "no mental disorder"! By the loose, subjective terms of many of these diagnoses, virtually anyone and everyone can be seen as psychiatrically ill.

As an example of how the medical model operates, let us take a typical outpatient: the working housewife and mother whose symptoms are constant headaches and depression. Typically, she has few or no available social resources to help her support herself and her family. Life is a constant economic struggle, even with the combined incomes of her husband and herself. There are no affordable day-care centers in her neighborhood. Her workplace does not offer flexible work hours for working mothers. Her spouse neither believes in nor practices egalitarianism in marriage. As a result, this woman works a double shift—one at the workplace and one at home.

She takes her problems to the outpatient clinic of a local hospital. Here, the evaluating psychiatrist ascertains that she suffers from a "personality disorder"—a long-standing psychological disturbance. He labels her with the specific diagnosis of asthenic personality, which is defined as a "behavior pattern characterized by easy fatigability, low energy level, lack of enthusiasm, marked incapacity for enjoyment, and oversensitivity to physical and emotional stress."[3] He prescribes treatment: a course of long-term individual therapy in the outpatient clinic, plus 150 mg of Elavil (an antidepressant drug) per day.

The medical approach to this woman's problems would have it that her "oversensitivity to physical and emotional stress" is a sign and product of her individual pathology, rather than a natural, individual reflection of a social environment that is unduly stressing. The host of complex economic, social, and psychological influences that have resulted in the formation of the symptoms are reduced to a pat formula: the psychiatric diagnosis. The assumption here is that this woman's problems can be diagnosed and treated in a way that is analogous to the diagnosis and treatment of, say, influenza. Furthermore, the assumption is that such treatment will effectively help her with the daily concerns that have brought her to therapy—that fixing this woman's head will fix her life.

Yet the "talking cure"—with or without the 150 mg of Elavil—is no cure for her and for millions like her. As R. D. Laing pointed out in *The Politics of Experience,* in no other branch of medicine is the patient's illness as hypothetical as it is in psychiatry. Presumably, in a truly medical situation, the patient's diagnosis, course of illness, symptoms, and cure are in no way affected by the doctor's predispositions, attitudes, feelings, and beliefs. (Although more recently, even in the medical sciences, many doctors have indeed come to recognize that disease may be caused not so much by invading organisms as by life patterns of physical, emotional, and environmental stress.) Thomas Szasz, Laing, and others have argued quite convincingly for the fact that there is no such thing as "mental illness"—that the diagnosis tells us more about the diagnoser than the diagnosed. Or, as Laing has put it, mental illness or health is judged by "the degree of conjunction or disjunction between two persons where one is deemed sane by common consent."[5] Without a systematic change in the life conditions of the woman with the "asthenic personality," her symptoms, and others like them are inevitable. (The social manufacture of female symptoms is the subject of chapters three and nine.)

The medical model has contributed to a social climate in which almost any human problem can be, and often is, seen as the consequence of individual pathology. Like myth 1, this has itself produced individual reactions which, in turn, are viewed as further symptoms of an illness: shame, guilt, low self-esteem, anxiety, and depression. The medical model has encouraged people to seek individual solutions to many problems that may not best be solved individually—or may not be amenable to individual amelioration at all. And it has discouraged people from finding more social or collective avenues of self-help. The woman in our example is more likely to think of going to a therapist than she is of organizing with others in her neighborhood or workplace for day-care facilities, though the latter may prove a better cure for her "oversensitivity" to stress than the former!

The medical model may be of some help to those who have the material options to make a private psychiatrist an affordable luxury. Taking an hour or so each week to explore one's inner life has been known to have beneficial results! (Though even here, a model with a health orientation rather than a disease orientation would be more helpful.) But for people of the lower classes, especially women—people whose emotional problems are most often rooted in the social arrangements and practices that have severely restricted their life options—the medical model can be destructive. For such people, the belief that they can solve by themselves problems over which they have no control as individuals has been known to have severely depressing results. The diagnosis of character pathology or mental illness itself constitutes a social stigma which often contributes to the worsening of their life conditions. Substantial discrimination on the part of employers, landlords, etc., still exists against persons with a psychiatric history.

Furthermore, the kind of treatment people of the lower classes get in the medical model system is likely to be very different from that offered to people of means. A long-term, individually guided journey to the mind's interior is only one of the possible treatments of the medical model. Others include crisis intervention, group or family therapy, mental hospitalization, electroshock therapy, and the prescription of "so-called" psychotropic drugs.

Poor people are less likely to be referred for private or public long-term individual psychotherapy and more likely to be treated with drugs, electroshock, or mental hospitalization. These treatments have little in common with individual psychotherapy—yet they are all logical extensions of the medical model system. The therapy patient who "fails" a course of individual therapy may at some point in her patient career come up against some (or all) of these practices.

The mental hospital or psychiatric ward is integral to the medical model, perhaps its center. It is the place where our typical working housewife outpatient might end up, should individual therapy and Elavil fail to cure her depression.

In *Mental Illness and the Economy,* M. Harvey Brenner has shown that admissions to mental hospitals go up proportionately as the economy declines, regardless of what other social variables are present and regardless of innovations in psychiatric care. He concludes that "mental illness" has more to do with economic decline than with individual personality structure or pathology.[4]

Thus the majority of patients in the state mental hospital system are people of the lower classes—those who are hardest hit by economic decline. In recent years it has been generally acknowledged—by experts and patients alike—that the back wards of state hospitals offer only shoddy custodial care and lead to an irreversible condition called "institutionalization." For the wealthy, or those with medical insurance, private psychiatric hospitals at least offer some therapy along with forcible chemical treatment. Private or public, the psychiatric ward is, for millions of women, the medical model's last resort. Yet a view from inside the inpatient ward shows us that too often the treatment itself becomes a disease of which the patient is never cured (see chapter two).

MYTH 3: THE EXPERT ■ The third myth follows from the first two: if the source of a person's emotional pain is a psychic disease or disorder, then only an expert in diagnosis and treatment is equipped to offer a cure.

As with physical disease, so with psychological disease— the doctor is the model of the Expert. The Expert is, above all, a *scientist:* a detached, neutral, benignly disinterested observer of the human misery that he diagnoses and treats.

Freudian psychoanalysis borrowed and adapted this model of the Expert from the natural sciences—hence, the well-known image of the psychoanalytic situation: the analyst with his note pad, seated behind the patient reclining on the couch. The patient's treatment was supposed to be furthered by this spatial arrangement in that the doctor became an even more "neutral" figure if he was literally not seen by the patient! (Freud himself often violated his own rule—getting into heated arguments with his patients and even having relationships with them outside of the analysis.) Though psychiatry has thrown out the couch, traditional or psychodynamic psychotherapy has retained the model of the Expert.

It is questionable, even in the natural sciences, whether objectivity is equivalent to disinterested observation. This notion is all the more dubious where the object of measurement is a person engaged in a relationship with another person, and the goal of that relationship is to alleviate the first person's emotional distress. The myth of the Expert leads to a denial of the effects on a person in pain of being "neutrally" observed as a patient with a pathology. (There is, in fact, nothing whatsoever neutral about this orientation!) The effects of this approach itself on the treatment are largely ignored. Typically, for example, neither the therapeutic relationship nor the outcome of therapy is studied or researched by psychiatrists.

Millions of men and women each day appear in their psychotherapist's offices. There, in one of the most intense and yet tenuous relationships, they learn from their therapists the meanings of their lives, past and present. They learn how to understand themselves in terms of the crucial aspects of their beings: love, work, and sexual identity. The myth of the Expert as the detached and neutral observer serves to cloud the fact that every therapist offers a world view to his patient—the terms by which the patient is to understand herself and her world. In this sense, every model of therapy is actually political in nature. The therapist's very choice of words, his choice of what to go after in therapy, what to analyze, what to stress and what to ignore: these are all political acts laden with meaning. There is nothing in the least neutral about this process. Of course this is more obvious in some cases than in others. If the therapist, for instance, regards his patient's homosexuality as sick or deviant and communicates this belief in the attempt to cure her, the coercion is readily visible—but only because we have a decade of an activist gay liberation movement behind us. The recent decision of the American Psychiatric Association to change the status of homosexuality from its original classification as a sexual deviation is a graphic example of just how political the so-called scientific judgments of the Expert actually are. (It is also an example of how social movements can have a crucial impact on the "scientific" realm.)

In reality, doctors, psychiatrists, and other Experts are hardly neutral toward their patients. Anyone who has ever heard the back room shoptalk among a group of psychiatrists would be struck by this fact. In contrast to the formal tone and language of the psychiatric case conference, psychiatrists often informally engage in a great deal of griping and whining about their difficult patients. All those hours of pretending to be neutral do, after all, take their toll, and therapists too need a place to ventilate their feelings!

Emotional self-disclosure is one of the cardinal taboos of traditional therapy. The therapist who reveals himself is by definition unprofessional—for professionalism hinges on the posture of distance. It is just this distance, the emotional withholding of the therapist, that is considered essential to his neutrality. Yet it is a male bias to think that this is so. In fact, there is nothing more inherently neutral or scientific or professional about emotional distance than there is about emotional connection or nurturance. Men in this society are trained to deny and cut themselves off from feelings in the interests of masculine discipline and strength. Women, by contrast, are trained to share their feelings and to nurture them in others. Emotional give-and-take is a distinctively female style in our culture. The traditional approach takes its model of expertise from the male style of personal intercourse. Yet it is precisely this style, typified by the (in)famous silence of the therapist, that is most damaging to people who are emotionally vulnerable—which means virtually every therapy patient. If you have been a patient in therapy and have had the experience of feeling that you are emotionally bleeding all over the rug while your therapist sits in stony-faced silence, then you know exactly how painful the "neutral" professional stance can be.

The traditional justification for the posture of distance is that if therapists reveal themselves to their patients they are somehow using them for their own ends. Traditional therapists seem unable to distinguish between sharing oneself as a person and exploiting the patient.

The value-free neutrality of the Expert is neither possible nor desirable. There is much evidence to suggest that the change-producing potential of psychotherapy is directly related to the empathic and supportive attitudes of the therapist—the very attitudes ruled out by the myth of the Expert.[6] The distance and disease orientation essential to the role of the Expert are destructive, rather than helpful, to patients of psychotherapy (see chapter two).

Just as myths 1 and 2 obscure the social roots of psychic distress, so the myth of the Expert obscures the social nature of the therapeutic relationship. The medical mystique surrounding the Expert conceals the basic fact that—whatever else therapy may be—it is fundamentally a relationship between people.

But just what kind of relationship is possible between the Expert and the Patient?

If you are a woman in traditional therapy, you probably know the answer to this question. As a patient, you've learned to expect the blank stare of the therapist as the norm for the therapeutic relationship. To expect or want any more than this, you learn early on in therapy, is a sign of your transference feelings—expressing early unmet needs and desires rather than any legitimate adult need for support, reassurance, or contact. To be a therapy patient is to accommodate yourself to the *lack* of such contact, to the absence of any sense of relationship to the person to whom you are baring your soul. To accept and adapt to this essentially lonely experience of deprivation of contact is your task as patient.

You learn to expect and adjust to the familiar silence of the therapist, punctuated by an occasional interpretation of your words. To the scrutiny of your words with no counterbalancing words of support. To the analysis of your current problems in the light of past events and feelings presumed to exist by your therapist—though often inaccessible to your own memory. To the knowledge that none of your questions about your therapist's life or feelings is considered appropriate—that all such questions will be left unanswered and instead analyzed for their unconscious content. To the profound sense that your own unconscious is visible to your therapist, that he can see through you, while you have only vague hints about the darkness within you. To the understanding that all of your disagreements with his superior knowledge are to be construed as resistance—a manifestation of your illness or neurosis. To the fact, fundamental and unshakable, that he knows you better than you know yourself.

In traditional therapy, Woman as Patient learns, with the help of Man as Expert, to adapt to a situation of Father Knows Best.

Not all traditional therapists fit this description. But those who do not are exceptional, unconventional, or eccentric. They are not playing by the rules. For this model of the male-style therapist is *explicitly* taught to all prospective practitioners of traditional therapy. The therapist in training learns just what kind of relationship is appropriate for the Expert and his patient. Among other things, he learns:

• To divest the patient's words of any current practical meaning; to regard everything she says as "material"—the conscious and unconscious manifestations of her illness; and to interpret her material.

• To interpret any strong feelings she may have toward him as transference, disregarding the possibility that these feelings may be related to him as a real person, or to his approach to therapy.

• To maintain a distanced and "abstinent" posture toward her; never to offer personal information; to throw all personal questions back at the patient and interpret why she asked. To make himself, as much as possible, a blank screen (especially in the mid-phase of therapy—where he is advised to be altogether silent).

• To watch closely for and interpret the patient's resistance to his interpretations—a sign of resistance to health. Her denial of her resistance is further proof of her resistance.

• To watch his own feelings toward the patient (countertransference), which are always considered to be a response to her transference feelings. None of the therapist's feelings toward the patient are thought to be autonomous—all are provoked by her pathology. Thus in watching his own feelings toward her, he receives clues about her illness.

• To define insight (the precondition for the patient's cure) as the patient's acceptance of the therapist's interpretations.

The prospective therapist may take his example from Freud, who tells this story in *Dora: An Analysis of a Case of Hysteria:* Dora's migraine headaches, depression, and nervous cough were diagnosed as symptoms of hysteria. In analysis, Dora's symptoms were interpreted by Freud as rooted in her Oedipal love for her father. After several months of this interpretation and no relief of symptoms, Dora left the analysis, insisting that Freud was wrong and he was not helping her. Freud's explanation was that Dora was taking "revenge" on him by trying to demonstrate his "incapacity as a physician."[7] This action was viewed as transference behavior and further proof of her neurosis.

Dora tried to defy the myth of the Expert: she told Father Freud that he didn't know best. For her effort, she was rewarded with the final weapon in the arsenal of the Expert— the Expert's last hex. She was told she would never be cured until she accepted her pathology as Freud saw it.

By definition, in the system of Father Knows Best, what the Expert says is true. By definition, the Expert knows it all and the patient is ignorant of the roots of her illness. This discrepancy in knowledge and power is thought to be the very basis upon which the patient's cure rests! By definition, the success of therapy depends on the patient's acceptance of the point of view of the Expert. Patient rebellions are construed as further manifestations of pathology. In essence, this amounts to a closed system of persuasion which constitutes a subtle form of brainwashing (a phenomenon most obvious in the inpatient setting).

By the terms of this system, the biases of the therapist are rendered invisible and consequently given even greater force. It is not simply the unique idiosyncrasies of the therapist that are in this way communicated as coercive influences upon the patient, but also the essential ideology of psychiatric therapy and practice itself.

I would suggest that where the traditional model of therapy has proven helpful or successful, this is largely a result of the therapist's *deviation* from, rather than adherence to, the cardinal rules of traditional therapy.

Should the therapist adhere to these rules, the myth of the Expert leads inevitably to a therapeutic relationship which is based on a fundamental inequality of power between doctor and patient. In therapy, as in other forms of Expert/Patient relations, the medium is the message: patients are taught to adapt to this type of relationship and, by implication, to accept similar forms of social relationships outside of therapy. The Expert/Patient relationship may prove helpful to a limited number of patients who identify with the power of the Expert's role—for example, male members of the upper classes. But adapting to a situation of powerlessness is bound to have negative effects on most patients, especially if social powerlessness has anything to do with why they are seeking help in the first place.

Once again, this means that the myth of the Expert is more harmful to women (and members of other socially powerless groups) than it is to men. For women who subscribe to myths 1 and 2, the lure of the Expert is bound to be very attractive. The image of the Expert as cool, detached, rational, omniscient, and powerful matches the cultural stereotype of masculinity. The image of the patient as ignorant, helpless, and emotional matches the cultural stereotype of femininity. Consequently, the myth of the Expert and his system of Father Knows Best is (to put it in psychiatric terms) "ego syntonic" for women and "ego alien" for men. What this means is that women are already socially prepared to accept as natural a relationship in which we see ourselves as inferior to and reliant upon an authoritative, powerful male figure. (This is, in fact, the model for the norm in male-female relations.) Women therefore find therapy easy to adjust to. Men, by contrast, find the therapeutic relationship more disarming and alien. (This explains what many therapists have observed: that women, by and large, make "better" therapy patients than men.)

In adapting to the Father Knows Best style of inequality in traditional therapy, women are positively reinforced to accept social domination in the rest of our lives. The experience of therapy itself makes it less likely that we will turn to more self-reliant or cooperative ways of solving problems. In effect, women are taught by the medium of therapy itself to collude in our own continued social subordination.

All three myths inherited from Freudian theory and practice work to reinforce each other. The person suffering from what she believes to be her own personal psychopathology appears to require the intervention of an Expert with medical training to provide the cure. The Expert cannot play his role as the one who cures without a passive, dependent Patient who knows that the cure can come only from someone more knowledgeable and powerful than herself. In effect, the Father Knows Best approach trains the Patient to let go of her sense of power as a person. However well intentioned, the three myths of the traditional system invariably result in a variety of practices that end up failing the patient, especially the female patient.

5. What's the Solution?

The problem is how women are seen and treated in the traditional mental health system. The failures of that system are multiplied in the case of women patients, for the overwhelming bias of the system is against women. The solution is a new approach to women and therapy. What's valuable in the old system can be preserved and transformed to meet women's needs. But the old myths must be overthrown. We must not be afraid to challenge the ancient bias against women head on: to develop new forms of theory and practice that are unabashedly pro-woman.

The rest of this book is devoted to this project. Hopefully, what will emerge is the starting point for a genuinely new therapy for women.

To understand how best to help women in therapy it is necessary, first of all, to understand who women are. And to understand who women are, one must understand the society in which women live. The task is to comprehend how what is "outside" a woman's head gets to be "inside" it; that is, how social structures come to be embodied in certain characteristic features of female psychology. Given the narrow definition of psychology that prevails in our society, such a task would not even be considered within the bounds of psychology proper. This, too, is part of the problem. For to understand the psychology of women, or of any oppressed or minority group, it is essential to change the definition of psychology itself.

Society as we know it has always been characterized by the domination of certain groups of people by other groups. The oldest form of domination is that of women by men. It has included the social conditioning of men and women along gender lines—the creation of specifically "masculine" and "feminine" persons. The woman's movement has shown that differences in sex roles are socialized, not innate, and that they can therefore be changed. But the term "sex role" may obscure the fact that male and female identities in patriarchal societies are profoundly different, and that these differences are socially produced in the interests of the dominating male group. Psychological differences between the sexes both reflect and perpetuate the structurally unequal distribution of power in the society. Men and women psychically structured along gender lines tend to see themselves in ways that do not threaten the social order but perpetuate it.

Traditional psychological theories of women have also reflected the interests of men. They have been theories made by men about women, made by the dominating group about the dominated. In this sense, psychology as we know it has also tended to reflect and perpetuate the subordination of women.

A genuinely new understanding of women must start with the perspective of the dominated group. A key question in this approach would be: What psychological characteristics do women have in common as a result of a shared condition of social domination?

Women develop a sense of self in a context of social victimization in a male-dominated society. In such a society, the normal feminine woman is the Victim. The Victim is the woman who has successfully adapted to a situation of social powerlessness. Such an adaptation is bound to be psychologically problematic. The Victim is the woman who sees herself through male eyes and thus learns to devalue, limit, and even hate herself. If the Victim often appears to be acting against her own best interests, this is because people who successfully adapt to their domination are bound to be self-destructive. They are bound to develop certain characteristic problems of identity, certain conflicts and "symptoms."

This is not to say that the Victim psychology of women is pathological. The problems inherent in developing a female sense of indentity in a situation of male domination are not the problems of a professionally defined group of psychological deviants. They are the problems of *all* women in a social context of female inequality.

A health-oriented and women-oriented perspective on the problems of woman as Victim must start with a new outlook on what have been traditionally seen as symptoms of psychopathology. From the perspective of women, rather than male practitioners, female symptoms might well be viewed as largely unconscious attempts both to adapt to and to rebel against the unhealthy psychosocial situation of being a woman in a man's world. Embodied in the symptom is the repressed rage of woman as Victim, a rage she has not been allowed to express openly. (Some of these typical female symptoms and conflicts are examined in chapters three, nine, and ten.)

A truly therapeutic approach to women's symptoms would look not to the pathology, but to the seeds of health and strength they contain. The most essential of these is the repressed anger that has found no socially acceptable outlet. With help, the symptoms of woman as Victim can be transformed.

The energy given over to such typical female afflictions as depression, anxiety, psychosomatic illness, sexual repression, fears of autonomy, and so on can be used *for* us rather than against us. To help women in this effort requires, however, a totally new approach to therapy.

A woman-oriented approach to therapy must dissolve the rigid line between Expert and Patient. It must start with the recognition of what a female patient and a female therapist have in common. And it must cultivate the shared experience of being female in a way that benefits the patient. *An emotional connection between the therapist and patient is a necessary precondition for any successful therapeutic work*, for therapy is essentially a relationship between people. The mystifications of the traditional Expert-Patient relationship must be abandoned in favor of a stress on the responsibility and accountability of both patient *and* therapist in a more equalized therapy relationship.

However useful certain techniques may be, the therapist's main tool in this relationship is herself. As we shall see, the therapist's use of her own feelings to further the patient's work in therapy is profoundly different from traditional therapy's exclusive emphasis on the patient's feelings alone.

A social model of therapy for women must comprehend both the limits and the potential of therapy. As long as basic structural inequities of power exist in society, large numbers of women will manifest symptoms of this inequality. Working to correct the social inequities is, in the long run, the only final cure for most forms of female emotional distress. Therapy may help people cope with certain intolerable social conditions, but it cannot improve those conditions unless it contributes to raising the consciousness of patients so that they will be less likely to tolerate them. On the one hand, this points to the necessity to demystify therapy so that people are no longer encouraged to believe that only individual psychological "treatment" can cure what ails them. On the other hand, this points to the by-and-large unexplored potential of therapy to be an instrument of social change.

The ultimate goal of a woman-oriented therapy is to help the female patient overcome the ways in which she colludes with her own oppression, and thereby to help her come to a fuller awareness of her power, both as an individual and as a member of a community of women. To reach this goal, therapy is fundamentally involved in surfacing the repressed rage embodied in so many female symptoms. How a therapist works with a woman's anger is a key element in whether therapy is essentially geared to her interests and needs. Any therapy that ignores the social roots of a woman's rage is bound to end up pacifying it. At best, such a therapy may be helpful in the short-run alleviation of symptoms. But in the long run, it reinforces the Victim psychology which keeps women producing more and more symptoms. Women need a therapy that will help us understand the personal and political origins of our anger and use that anger on our own behalf.

Therapy from a female perspective is not therapy from the "narrow" perspective of women. On the contrary, it is therapy from a wider perspective than before: one that *includes* what has been missing from the traditional male orientation. Compassion, empathy, intuition, nurturance: these are all culturally "feminine" skills which are actually essential to the practice of good therapy for women *and* men. Traditional therapy tends to ignore or devalue these skills while stressing the culturally "masculine" skills of intellectual mastery, discipline, control, and distance. In chapter ten, we take a close look at how a woman-oriented model of therapy works with certain typical female problems. This model of therapy is essential if therapy for women is going to be part of the solution, rather than part of the problem. But it is a model that can be equally beneficial to men.

Were this new model of therapy to be applied wherever therapy now occurs—in hospitals, clinics, and private psychiatric offices throughout the country—Woman as Patient and Man as Expert would die long overdue deaths. Given the enormous power of the mental health industry and its vested interest in maintaining this power, the institutionalization of such a new therapy is a rather distant prospect. The Father Knows Best system will not give up its stranglehold on people in psychological pain without a struggle.

But it is good to remember that there can be no therapy without patients. Woman as Patient has more power than she thinks. She may yet triumph.

CHAPTER

An Insider's View of Traditional Practice, or Everything You Always Wanted to Know About Your Shrink but Were Afraid to Ask

1. How to Be a Professional: My Psychology Training Begins

Not just anyone can be a psychotherapist. Most states require a lengthy and arduous training process which results in a variety of legal ranks: from counselor to psychiatric social worker to psychiatric nurse to psychologist to psychiatrist. The mental health industry, like other industries in this country, rests on a strict occupational hierarchy. As a rule, psychiatrists and psychologists are men; nurses and social workers are women. As in the larger society, so in the mental health field, men are on top and women are on the bottom.

Evidence from research in the field shows that traditional psychotherapy is generally no more effective than no treatment at all in curing people's emotional ills, and frequently makes people feel worse.[1] Despite this evidence, the myth is that the care of mental illness and disorders requires a special set of knowledge and skills known only to the Expert.

The Expert is white, male, and middle to upper class. He is not like you or me: he doesn't just help people, he treats them. In the mental health industry, the Expert is the psychiatrist. He is a Doctor. He makes diagnoses and prognoses, dispenses treatment, prescribes medications, and writes orders (which nurses carry out). While the social worker may see families at home, the psychiatrist sits behind a desk (or, in former days, a couch). From this superior vantage point, he administers the talking cure. His judgments are impeccable. His rare spoken words are highly expensive. He is as smoothly authoritative and aloof as a god.

The psychiatrist is the head of the mental health family—and Father Knows Best. In inpatient settings generally only the psychiatrist (or the psychiatric resident) presents a patient to a hospital audience made up of the various helping professions. In the end, he has the final power to formulate policy with respect to the patient's care. As the father of the family, he is the truth-maker and truth-sayer. What he believes filters down to the lower echelons of the mental health hierarchy as the final word.

The social worker is the psychiatric wife and mother. In inpatient settings, she is usually responsible for the general health and welfare of the patient's family. She may spend more time with the patient's family than the psychiatrist spends with the patient. Yet these hours are usually viewed as home visits or casework—not as psychotherapy.

The social worker works hard and is responsible, but has no authority. Such therapy as the social worker does is dubbed "supportive" or "reality-oriented"—as opposed to what the psychiatrist does, which is called "dynamic" or "insight-oriented." The social worker is rarely allowed to work with those patients who are considered capable of psychological insight. Her task is the support and maintenance of those who will never be "interesting" cases. "Interesting" cases require the superior intellectual equipment of the psychiatrist.

The mental health family is well-to-do enough to have a whole slew of servants: nurses who carry out the father's orders, dispensing medications and keeping constant watch on the patients. They do all the unglamorous work—from cleaning bedpans to keeping minute records of everything that happens.

The psychologist is the elder son. To make up for his lower status in the mental health hierarchy, the psychologist is a zealous overcompensator. He tries to outdo the psychiatrist by producing a mass of scientific research.

The experimental psychologist insists that he, not the psychiatrist, is the rightful Expert. He claims to have the highest possible knowledge of human psychology, gained through endless research hours in the lab chasing after white mice and brown monkeys. He thinks of the psychiatrist as a mere practitioner—a technician whose job is impossible without the important theories proposed by the experimental psychologist.

Similarly, the clinical psychologist prizes himself as the real Expert on emotional disorders. He comes fully equipped with the right tool for the job: an impressive battery of psychological tests which are mysteriously opaque to the psychiatrist. These tests empower the psychologist to render flawless judgments in the form of test reports so technical that even the psychiatrist can't understand them.

The rivalry between the psychiatrist and the psychologist has a decidedly Oedipal flavor. The son wishes to slay the father, or at least to share his spoils: power, money, prestige, and third-party payments. Father and son contend for the position of high command of the mental health family—which includes power over the family women (social workers and nurses) and children (patients). The Oedipal Battle of the Experts is fierce. But the father always wins.

It is unclear whether counselors are part of the mental health family at all. They are the illegitimate sons and daughters. They are found not in medical hospitals, but in storefronts, schools, community mental health centers, on the streets and, more recently, in women's health centers and shelters. They do the practical, necessary, but largely invisible labor that their more professional relatives shun: talking to drug addicts and delinquents, ex-prisoners and alcoholics, pregnant teenagers, battered wives and women seeking abortions. Counselors are definitely not Experts. They are not even in the running. They do not disclaim or report—they rap. Unlike all their mental health relatives, counselors have no professional association to represent them. They are not, when it comes right down to it, really pros. The mark of the pro is expertise combined with distance. To be the Expert on the <u>borderline</u> <u>personality</u>, it is not considered advantageous for the psychiatrist to *be* one. By contrast, it is often deemed helpful for the drug rehabilitation counselor to be an ex-junkie, or for the abortion counselor to have had an abortion. Counselors are disquietingly *like* their clients. They are more likely than their mental health relatives to be brown, black, working class, or female. They have less schooling and make less money. The line separating patient from professional tends to blur. For this reason, the pros of the mental health family find counselors vaguely embarrassing. Counselors sit at the outside of the family table, eating the scraps of peripheral respectability.

As an intern in clinical psychology and community mental health, I learned about this professional mental health hierarchy from the ground up. I was in a psychology training program, but my academic affiliation was to a counseling department—which, combined with my femaleness, put me way down on the hierarchy. The entire psychology department of the hospital in which I trained was a small and minor wing of the psychiatry department, a much larger unit run by men, with an almost exclusively male staff and residency program.

The scope and depth of my educational agenda as a psych intern were staggering. In two years' time, I was to learn how to evalute, diagnose, and treat patients. I was to become well versed in all of the various therapy "modalities": individual, couple, group, and family therapy. I was to work in every conceivable setting: the inpatient ward, outpatient department, the walk-in service for "acute" patients, and the community. I would be familiar with doing both child and adult therapy. Like a psychiatrist, I would know a great deal about medications— though I would not have the power to prescribe them. Unlike a psychiatrist, I would be able to administer a wide range of psychological tests. As an intern, I was encouraged to see myself as a student-practitioner and to begin to treat patients as soon as I felt ready.

When I began my internship program I was at a crossroads in my life. I had chosen this path deliberately and later than most, after years in the university, training as a literary scholar and teaching English. I was the mature student in my second career.

Still, I had the naïveté and sincerity of most aspiring therapists. I wanted to help people, to influence their lives, to be of use. I knew that the people I most wanted to help were *women*. I was set on developing the possibilities of an as yet unheard-of phenomenon—feminist therapy.

In my initial interview with the director of the program, I was heartened by the fact that the director did not seem put off by the fact that I had declared myself an out-and-out feminist. I thought this was a good omen.

I was wrong. I soon learned that, in the hospital, being a feminist was tolerable if it in no way entered into one's ideas about how to practice therapy. I learned that there were only two ways to practice therapy—a right way and a wrong way. The right way was called psychodynamic psychotherapy—a derivative of the master's original plan, Freudian psychoanalysis. The wrong way was any other way. I learned that a curious mind not wholly psychiatric in orientation was not only a disadvantage but a disgrace. I learned that being a feminist rendered me suspect in the eyes of my supervisors and jeopardized my standing as a legitimate student of psychology. I learned that I could trust no one with my feelings, for they would be used against me. I learned what it meant to be a mental patient and what it meant to be a mental health professional.

Above all, the program was dedicated to producing psychologists who would be unwaveringly professional. Interns were required to attend an overwhelming number of seminars, workshops, and supervision sessions designed to teach the basics of psychiatry, psychology, and professionalism. We were groomed to be pros down to our bones.

Our teachers never thought it necessary to define precisely what "professionalism" meant or why it was so overridingly important. It was taken for granted that everyone knew this already. But certain qualities of professionalism were clear from the outset. Professionalism had everything to do with appropriate behavior. In the psychologist's lexicon, "appropriate" and "inappropriate" were indispensable and all-encompassing words that, like "professionalism," did not need to be defined. It was considered obvious (and therefore not a fit subject for analysis) that appropriate behavior was behavior that was conventionally acceptable. Inappropriate behavior was behavior that was not conventionally acceptable. Conventions of behavior were not questioned by professionals—they were accepted and adhered to.

I soon learned that appropriate behavior for professionals meant conformity to the traditional psychiatric system.

To start with, professionals had to know how to greet the patient. This was no simple "how-d'you-do." It was a professional assessment. Meeting a person and conducting a diagnostic interview had little in common. In meeting someone, one learned about the person. In doing an interview, one learned about the person's illness. For instance, to start with, the therapist must ask the patient to describe her problem. What she says is *symptomatic* of her illness. Her problem is not what she thinks it is—her problem is that she is ill. What she says about herself—and also what she doesn't say—are symptoms of this illness. She doesn't, of course, know how telling her words really are. She thinks she's talking about her life, but she is really exhibiting her illness: its symptoms, etiology, course, and dynamics. All questions that the interviewer asks are designed to ferret out these features of her illness, past or present.

I was instructed that even without asking any questions, the skilled interviewer can learn all about the patient's illness by simply observing her: clues to patient diagnosis are everywhere. Start with appearance. Is she overly neat and meticulous? Probably obsessive-compulsive. Or a flashy and seductive dresser? A hysteric. Watch the way she enters the room: her gait, posture, and carriage. Is she stiff, rigid? Probably obsessive again. Or is she weighed down, with hunched shoulders and a concave chest? Then look for depression. Her facial expressions can communicate what you need to know about her mood and "affect" (the professional word for feelings). Is she flamboyantly expressive? Hysteric. Or is she bland, flat, or blunt (professional words for little-to-no expressiveness)? Then watch out for obsessive, depressive, or schizophrenic illness. Clues are everywhere, once you get the hang of it.

In this fashion, it is possible to come to an Expert opinion on the patient's past and present illness. Getting a detailed sexual, social, work, and family history helps delineate the dynamics of the illness more precisely. But finally it is imperative to do the mental status censorium. This tells the interviewer just how crazy the patient is at the time. Without divulging his intentions, the interviewer should ask the patient what she had for breakfast. What was her address five years ago? Count backwards from one hundred by sevens. Who is the President of the United States? What would you do if you found a stamped, addressed envelope on the street? What does this mean: "A stitch in time saves nine"?

A neutral observer of this interview situation who had not been informed beforehand that she was witnessing a psychiatric interview might well question the sanity of the interviewer. The interviewer reels off a series of unconnected, unintelligible questions. All of them are what we would call non sequiturs. They do not obey the consensual rules of communication that most sane people ordinarily follow: they are unrelated one to another, asked without any intelligible context, seemingly without purpose or meaning. They do not seem to have an explanation—and none is offered to the inquiring patient, except the peremptory reply that these questions are routine. Yet to the patient, they can only be seen as what psychologists and psychiatrists call "bizarre." Everything changes once the situation is known. The explanation is simple: it is not the interviewer who is crazy, it is the patient (potentially or actually). It is all for the patient's good.

This, then, was the cardinal lesson of professionalism: by definition, the patient is always sick, and by definition, the professional is always healthy. The professional's job is to search out, define, describe, and treat the patient's sickness.

It was not easy for me to sit through this lesson. I wanted to scream. I identified with the patient. This, I was soon to learn, was a symptom of my problem, as well as a cardinal sin against professionalism. I thought, if someone asked me all these questions, I would surely sense (apparently correctly) that my questioner thought I was sick. I would feel frightened, resentful, and on the defensive—which would cause my interviewer to see me as overly anxious or hostile. I would perceive the interview questions as an attack on my integrity. By the logic of the questions themselves, this would be considered evidence of my "paranoid ideation." It seemed unfair to treat people as crazy even before you knew anything about them— and then to view their reactions to this assumption as another aspect of their craziness! I wanted to say all this. But I sensed, without yet knowing why, that this would get me into trouble. I had to control myself. So I asked what I thought was a more low-key question: Would we be learning any other system of psychology besides this one, which (I added hastily) seemed to have such a pathology orientation?

Even with this considerably tamed-down question, I blew it. My supervisors gave each other a knowing look and then reassured me that, as we went along, the diagnostic interview would become easier for me to understand and to perform. With practice, I would soon feel more "comfortable with my role as a professional."

There was something insidious about this reply. My supervisors were right: I *was* uneasy about my role as a professional. Yet somehow their knowledge about my uneasiness served as a way to avoid answering my question altogether! It seemed that because of my anxiety about my role as a professional, the burden was on me and my feelings rather than on them and their ideas about professionalism, or their system of evaluating patients. In short, the problem was mine, not theirs. My question was interpreted, delegitimized, and forgotten. Having heard (correctly) the anger in my criticism of what I was learning, they were using that anger against me, as a sign of my pathology.

This way of treating me, I soon learned, was a vivid illustration of how a good therapist should treat a patient. My supervisors faulted me for "identifying with the patient." Yet in this instance, and for the rest of my internship, I was always treated like one. Like a patient, I was to follow certain rules. One rule was that I was not to be in control of the meanings of the words I chose to speak, particularly when those words were critical of what my supervisors wanted me to believe. Only those words that indicated obedience to the system of thought into which I was being initiated were taken at face value. All other words were interpreted to my detriment as indicators of my pathology and then dismissed. The first rule was: You are sick unless you obey.

The second rule was that my feelings were more or less opaque to me and understood accurately only by my supervisors, the Experts. Further, my feelings were irrational and had no relation to any actually existing current situation. They did not belong to a mutually understandable social world of communication, but to a chaotic inner world to which only my supervisors, as representatives of the psychiatric order, had the key. The second rule was: The Experts always know you better than you know yourself.

Following these rules was inordinately difficult for me, and more often than not I broke them. I had a habit of asking my supervisors irritating meta-questions about the philosophical premises and assumptions behind their teachings. These questions invariably got me into trouble, for they were almost always interpreted as signs of my hostility or anxiety. For my supervisors, my motivations were routinely suspect and therefore subject to constant scrutiny. Behind these questions, they thought, lurked some unconscious feelings that it was their job to interpret for my educational benefit.

It was not my supervisors' analyses of my feelings per se that annoyed me. It was how much these analyses were confounded with their arrogant use of power to repress all critical thinking. How much their use of psychological analysis reflected their own anxieties about being challenged. How much it was a weapon to delegitimize people—both patients and interns. The *feelings* of patients and interns were taken as basic, while their *thoughts* were often relegated to the category of "intellectualization" or "rationalization": defensive maneuvers of the ego that masked unwanted, anxiety-provoking feelings. (Supervisors' thinking about interns' thinking was not seen as intellectualization.)

This entire approach disturbed me not only because it reflected cheap psychologizing at its worst, but also because I began to see just how dangerous it was to persons called patients.

But if I looked closely at my own motivations, I had to admit it was not simply a passion for intellectual rigor that was behind my persistent questioning of my supervisors. They were right: I *was* hostile toward them. What they didn't see was that the professional rules with which I was expected to comply were hostile toward me!

At bottom, I wanted to get them. I wanted to resist. I wanted to say No. No to their patronizing arrogance. No to their power over me, a power that seemed unearned by wisdom. No to their illegitimate appropriation of total authority over matters of such importance as who people are and what causes their emotional pain. No to their ignorance of women's oppression and its psychic effects. No to their obedient, unquestioning acceptance of the status quo. No to their complacent exploitation of people's sufferings. No to their profound conventionality sanctified in the name of respectability and professionalism.

I knew that I was the person whom the professionals would treat, had I come to them in another context. My problem, as I was told repeatedly, was that I identified with the patients instead of the professionals. Yet I knew that one of the main things going for me as a future therapist was that I trusted my own insights and responses, and that to identify with professionalism in the way demanded of me was to destroy that trust in myself in favor of handing it over to them, the Experts. I was determined not to do that.

In the system of thought into which I was being initiated, such feelings on my part would be, and were, seen as totally irrational—symptomatic of the control issues of an obsessive-compulsive personality. Indeed, I did not want my mind controlled by the traditional system of psychiatric thought; and I was determined that this psychiatric labeling would not subdue me.

The last rule of professionalism was the clincher: Pretend that there are no rules and that everything you perceive is not really happening. The consequence of breaking this—the Emperor's-New-Clothes Rule—(or any other rule) was being labelled unprofessional. This label had the same force in the internship program as the word "pathological" had on the psychiatric inpatient ward. It had the ring of finality. It was unarguable. There was no appeal when this word was invoked. It meant total invalidation.

Like a patient, I was placed in an utterly untenable, no-win situation, the kind of situation that drives a person mad.

My internship had begun.

2. How to Diagnose Patients

The diagnosis of patients was crucial to the enterprise of being a mental health professional. Interns were required to master the art as quickly as possible.

To help us learn, supervisors practiced what I called the Diagnostic Detective Game. In this game, anything a patient said or did contained clues to his or her diagnosis. The clues were in the form of symptomatic behavior and speech. Virtually anything could be a clue. (I remember once being told that if we didn't like a patient, that was a diagnostic sign of something.) From all appearances, the goal of the game was to make an accurate diagnosis on the basis of the least possible evidence.

The Diagnostic Detective Game was not applied exclusively to patients. Interns were always fit subjects for supervisory diagnosis. In retaliation, interns secretly diagnosed their supervisors. Psychology supervisors diagnosed psychiatric residents and residents diagnosed psychology interns and supervisors. But there was one clear-cut rule: the mental health practitioner *never* diagnosed himself (at least not publicly). The point of the game was to distinguish the sick from the healthy. Hence the Diagnostic Detective Game was something the professional always played on someone else.

Nevertheless, it was virtually impossible for interns to resist the impulse to diagnose themselves. After the reading assignment on obsessive-compulsive neurosis every intern in the program was thoroughly convinced that he or she was an obsessive. Then, the following week's reading on hysteria invariably caused a diagnostic reassessment. Reading the literature on schizophrenia was a nerve-shattering experience for us all. While one intern suspected that he was perhaps much sicker than he had ever imagined, another confirmed that she was indeed as sick as she had always thought she was.

One of the major hurdles that interns had to overcome in learning how to diagnose patients was the impression that many patients were actually not very different from ourselves, and that what got labeled as symptomatic behavior, if not viewed in the hospital setting, might easily pass for normal.

Take, for example, the depressed patient. The symptoms of depression were easy to detect, for they were known to virtually everyone. Who did not, at one time or another, feel dejected, helpless, fatigued, hopeless, self-hating, and empty? Most people, if they were honest, had to admit that they even entertained thoughts of suicide at some point in their life. It was tempting to conclude either that most of us sometimes suffered from a mental disorder or that the depressed person was actually normal.

But precisely because the feelings and experiences of depression were so familiar, the diagnosis of depression demanded, all the more, that the distinction between the everyday garden variety depression and its "clinical" manifestations be rigorously maintained. Empathy was definitely *not* one's guide in diagnosis.

This distinction between a normal down and a clinical Affect Disorder often seemed to be somewhat arbitrary, to depend on who was doing the diagnosing. The depression expert who addressed me, the psychology student, told me that my depressions were "normal" and the patient's depressions were "clinical." But what if I were to show up as a patient in the outpatient department? At once, my depression would be transformed from a normal to a clinical one. The psychiatrist who diagnosed me might at the time himself be depressed. But because he was the doctor, not the patient, he was normally depressed while I wasn't. The key element in all this seemed to be who was asking for help and who was dispensing it.

Nevertheless, this primary distinction between the pathological and the normal was thought to depend on certain definite, objective criteria.

Take, for example, the criterion of duration of symptoms. It is considered normal to get depressed in response to an identifiable, external stress such as death. But an "excessive" reaction to such an event indicates that the depression is neurotic or psychotic.

My mother is the sole survivor of her entire family, which was exterminated by the Nazis. As I remember, she was depressed off and on for approximately the first ten years of my life. Was her depression normal or neurotic? Six months is the usual period mental health professionals allot for the normal mourning of a death in the family. In my mother's case, does one multiply six months by the number of family members she lost? And how much time does one add for the loss of her whole community and culture? By professional criteria, what is a normal, mentally healthy response to Nazi genocide?

Symptoms that last longer than the experts think they should are by definition excessive and therefore pathological. The criterion of duration of symptoms actually is a rather arbitrary judgment made by those who define the terms.

But the closer one looks at the terms, the more obvious it is how woefully contradictory, incoherent, or inadequate they are.

For another example, look at what experts consider to be a fundamental distinction in the causes of depression. An "exogenous" depression is a response to an identifiable external stress or event, while an endogenous depression is caused by an inter-internal chemical imbalance. According to these definitions, death is an external event, but conditions of life like poverty or sexism are not. Therefore it is considered normal to be depressed if your father dies, but pathological to be depressed if you have to cope with the exigencies and stresses of being a woman in a society that systematically subordinates women to men.

The diagnostician sets the terms. In so doing, he creates the reality he is defining. He tells us what is symptomatic and excessive, what is normal and pathological, what is internal and external, what is neurotic and psychotic, what is real and what is not.

Fundamental to this entire process is creating the distinction between ordinary experience and the symptoms of a mental disorder. But what is a "symptom"? The technical definition is "a specific manifestation of a patient's condition indicative of an abnormal physical or mental state."[2] This is simply a psychiatric tautology. In practice, a symptom is anything a psychiatrist or psychologist names as one.

The symptoms of depression I learned as an intern included increase or decrease in appetite, loss or gain of weight, constipation, sleeping more or less than usual, loss of sexual appetite, and fatigue. There are some who would say that these are all indications of a bad diet. But when they are dubbed "vegetative signs of depression," they take on an altogether different aura. It's all in the terminology. Because the terminology is defined by the experts, it is thought to be "objective"— that is, real. By this professional sleight of hand, virtually anything and everything one experiences can be turned into a symptom of something seriously sick.*

* Certain ironies are bound to ensue from this transformation of ordinary experience into diagnostic minutiae. For instance, as an intern I was taught that "paralysis of will" was a symptom of depression that could be relieved by the proper treatment: drugs. Give a depressed patient Elavil and her paralysis of will will often disappear. But there's a hitch. While suffering from paralysis of will, the patient is usually too stuporous to kill herself. But once the symptom is relieved, another symptom—suicidal impulses—is free to surface. The patient now has the energy to kill herself. Thus it is said that the treatment for depression often makes the patient well enough to commit suicide! Experts in diagnosis apparently do not find this way of thinking bizarre or illogical.

Once a symptom has been named, it exists as an entity that seems to require the intervention of an expert. The mental health professional effectively psychologizes reality and makes himself its sole legitimate interpreter. The entire system of diagnosis, with its intricate and often inconsistent technical terminology, legitimates the professional handling of those diagnosed. The experts generate the need for a special language. And the language generates a special need for the experts. And so the business of psychiatry goes on.

To learn the language of diagnosis, interns were instructed to read the vast literature on depression, schizophrenia, borderline personality, obsessive-compulsive neurosis, hysteria, and so on. We read assiduously. We took copious notes. But it was difficult to translate the terminological abstractions of the diagnostic system into empirical, observable behavior.

Early in my training, I learned that diagnosis could be learned more easily if I tried to *see through* the diagnostic system, rather than to use it directly. As an intern, I listened to the various categories of diagnosis not with an ear to what they said, but to how they were used. I paid attention to context, rather than content. I noticed which diagnoses were applied to which patients in "didactic interviews" (here the patient was interviewed before an audience of professionals expressly for the educational benefit of the latter).

In so doing, I made some simple observations. Educated, middle-class male patients were invariably diagnosed as obsessive-compulsive personalities. Women were most often hysterics (though more highly educated or male-identified women tended also to be diagnosed as obsessives). And working-class people, male or female, black or white, were almost always borderline personalities.

These elementary observations made, looking more closely at the diagnostic definitions illuminated the correlations. For example, the obsessive-compulsive personality is defined as:

> a behavior pattern . . . characterized by excessive concern with conformity and adherence to standards of conscience.

Consequently, individuals in this group may be rigid, over-inhibited, over-conscientious, over-dutiful, and unable to relax easily.[3]

What is most striking about this definition is how well it describes certain aspects of the ordinarily socialized middle-class male (including the mental health Expert himself!). Rigid cerebral machinations, lack of spontaneity, the inability to relax or let go, extraordinary tendencies toward domination (the psychiatric word was "control"), and an overactive sense of manly "duty": these are all products of the normal conditioning of middle-class men in our society. Yet they are all seen as the presenting symptoms of a personality disorder!

Hence, in professional case presentations, when a normal psychiatrist faced a neurotic obsessive-compulsive patient, it was sometimes difficult to tell who was who. This problem was overcome by labeling only the patient's behavior and not the doctor's. Thus, the patient's compulsive attention to detail was symptomatic, while the doctor's was not. The patient who tried to control the doctor had an issue with control, while the doctor who tried to control the patient was just doing his job.

The most obvious fact about hysterics was the one most ignored by my instructors: almost all hysterics are women. If one looks at the definition of hysterical personality, the reason becomes clear. These personalities are:

characterized by excitability, emotional instability, over-reactivity, and self-dramatization. This self-dramatization is always attention-seeking and often seductive, whether or not the patient is aware of its purpose. These personalities are also immature, self-centered, often vain, and usually dependent on others.[4]

Dependency, vanity, emotionality: according to Freud, these are the normal attributes of the normal woman! Thus the definition of hysterical personality seems to match the traditional male definition of normal femininity. (We examine the consequences of this double bind for women in chapter three.)

As for borderline personalities, this was the informal term

used by diagnosticians to describe patients who "bordered" on psychosis. Actually, the more technically correct term for borderline personality is <u>primitive</u> <u>oral</u> <u>hysteric</u>. The latter is a type of <u>hysterical</u> <u>personality</u>, only sicker.* Presumably, it takes some rather refined diagnostic skills to be able to distinguish between the two. But there was a rather easy way for me to distinguish a borderline from any other type of patient, for borderlines were invariably the least favorite patients of mental health professionals. When I first began to interview people who my supervisors told me were borderlines, I noticed that they were frequently people from the lower classes. They did not present the neat, clean, and orderly picture clinicians expected of those patients they called "good, healthy neurotics." They lacked bourgeois manners. They did not think or talk the way educated people do (hence their thinking was often labeled "concrete"). They were not psychologically sophisticated. They were sometimes hostile or passive-aggressive.

One of the main symptoms exhibited by borderlines was an overwhelming sense of urgency and anxiety, a kind of crisis orientation toward life. It seemed to me that, in most cases, this "symptom" was simply related to the actual life crises imposed by poverty. In a situation in which the basic amenities of life are not guaranteed, it is hardly surprising that people exhibit a sense of anxiety. This fact seemed to be largely overlooked by middle-class professionals who did not suffer from the same kinds of problems. Instead, the professional tended to see the borderline's needs as a symptom of his pathological fixation in the oral stage of psychosocial development.

Once I had established these basic correlations between diagnosis and sex and class, other diagnoses came even more easily. The diagnosis of <u>schizophrenia</u>, for instance, tended to boggle interns' minds, simply because there were more than ten different varieties of this illness. Schizophrenia was con-

---

* The choice between the diagnoses <u>hysterical</u> <u>personality</u> and <u>borderline</u> <u>personality</u> or <u>primitive</u> <u>oral</u> <u>hysteric</u> hinges on an intricate debate in professional circles having to do with whether the patient is fixated in the more primitive (hence sicker) oral stage or the more advanced genital stage of psychosocial development.

sidered a Thought Disorder. But contrary to popular stereotypes, one does not have to look, sound, or act "crazy" in order
to be a schizophrenic. One does not have to have active hallucinations or delusions. One simply has to have "psychotic
thinking." This kind of thinking was not always immediately
apparent to the observer. Many people might look and act just
like ordinary folks, but underneath they had a latent or underlying or incipient thought disorder. Symptoms of schizophrenia, we were told, included a heightened awareness of sounds
and colors, vivid dreams, and an increased interest in religion,
philosophy, art, and the meaning of life.

The diagnosis of schizophrenia was easy. It was the catch-
all category for mental illness: vague, impressionistic, and large
enough to embrace all forms of deviance, nonconformity, ec-
centricity, and creativity. It was the most popular diagnosis in
my training. The line between Us (professionals) and Them
(patients) was kept firm and strong largely through the use of
this diagnosis.

From here on, it was easy to embroider the fine points of
diagnosis by looking at the context of the diagnostic interviews
themselves, simply noticing which diagnosis was likely in a
given interaction between diagnostician and patient. For instance, if the patient was extremely wary of the interviewer,
she was a paranoid personality, and so on.

After about three months of using this system of diagnosis,
I was evaluated by my superiors. The most serious complaint
they had about me was that I did not wear a brassiere. This was
considered an acute lapse in professionalism. Professionals, I
was told, *never* make *personal statements*. Apparently, my not
wearing a bra was considered the making of a personal statement to my patients, whereas my supervisors' girdles, suits, and
ties did not speak personally.

Apart from this criticism, however, I was told that I was a
promising clinician. My strong suit, according to all my supervisors, was that I was already an expert diagnostician. Apparently, my elementary sex, class, and context correlations were
serving me well. I had a foolproof method of diagnosis. I was
on my way.

3. How to Do Psychological Testing

Psychologists learn that psychological testing represents one of the most advanced forms of scientific inquiry into the human psyche currently available. It is largely this conviction that distinguishes the psychologist from the psychiatrist. In the standing war between the two disciplines, the psychological test battery is the psychologist's major tool. No hospitalized patient treatment plan is considered complete unless it has been devised with the data input of cognitive and projective testing.

All psychology interns were required to complete one test battery the first year and two the second year. The testing with adults was performed primarily with hospitalized patients on the inpatient ward. Test results were written up and then given to the patient's team psychiatrist, who considered the results in developing his treatment plan for the patient. Test results could tell him whether the patient was a "suitable" candidate for therapy, what kind of treatment modality was most appropriate, what the patient's prognosis was.

In short, psychological testing was the psychology intern's entrée to real power over patients. We were expected to master the administration and interpretation of test results rather quickly. In this matter, the pedagogical technique by which we were trained might best be described as monkey see, monkey do. In case presentations, the intern would present the results of psychological testing on a particular patient, and both supervisors and interns would suggest their interpretations of the test results. The evidence for any particular symptom or disorder could be just about anything. Though testing was considered scientific and some tests involved an intricate scoring system, the actual task of test interpretation entailed a kind of free-wheeling, impressionistic spree on the part of the tester.

One time, we all discussed the test protocol of a seven-year-old child. On the Rorschach, this boy had seen a multitude of spiders in the inkblots. This was evidence of the child's hatred of his mother, said the supervisor, who was considered the expert in child psychology. The child hated his mother because he sensed that the mother hated him. Evidence for the mother's hatred of her son was the fact that she was a self-declared lesbian. According to the expert, this Rorschach seemed to prove how abused children of lesbians are.

We spent most of the supervisory hour embroidering on this mother-hatred theme. Approximately ten minutes before the hour was up, the intern who had administered this particular test battery realized that she had made an error. The test protocol we were looking at did not, in fact, belong to the seven-year-old son of the lesbian. It belonged to the twenty-year-old daughter of heterosexuals. The intern had just terminated individual therapy with this patient. Somehow, she had mixed up the test protocols.

This could have proved quite embarrassing for the child psychology expert. But he was not in the least nonplussed. Without any further ado, he reinterpreted the multitude of spiders on the Rorschach as evidence of this girl's "unresolved termination" with her therapist.

I soon became very astute in how to ascribe any response of any patient to any test question of any test as an indicator of some kind of pathology.

For instance, on the comprehension subtest of the Wechsler Adult Intelligence Scale, I asked patients, "What would you do if while in the movies you were the first person to see smoke and fire?" If the patient responded, "I'd scream," she had "poor impulse control." If I asked, "Why should we keep away from bad company?" and the patient asked me to define "bad company," she was hostile. On the Thematic Apperception Test (TAT), patients were instructed to tell a story based on certain pictures. Any patient who responded to the overwhelmingly depressing and bizarre pictures of the TAT with depressing and bizarre stories was considered psychotically depressed. On the Rorschach, patients were instructed to say what they saw in the inkblots. Conventional interpretations of the inkblots were only moderately neurotic but any response that manifested a more than conventional imagination (especially if the red, bloody-looking blotches were seen as red, bloody-looking blotches) was a sure sign that the patient was psychotic.

Psychotic disorders of thought and affect abounded in test results. *Never, in two years of administering and interpreting test results, to in- and out-patients, did I come across a test protocol that was considered to be normal.* This was true down to the last detail of the Cole Animal Test: "If you could be any animal at all, what animal would you most like to be and least like to be?" If the patient wanted to be a pussycat because pussycats had an easy life, she was overwhelmed by her dependency needs. If she didn't want to be a snake because they were poisonous and dangerous, she was terrified of her aggressive impulses. This, in combination with her poor impulse control (as ferreted out by her response to the question about the fire in the movie theater) was a deadly combination and made her likely to be either a suicidal or homicidal risk.

The fundamental and unquestioned rule of test interpretation was that everybody was sick. This was, of course, the same rule as in diagnosis and psychiatric philosophy in general. But it was brought to its most refined, sinister culmination in psychological testing. The major task of the psychological tester was to catch (via testing) the underlying psychotic pathology in what might mistakenly be seen as a person suffering from mere neurosis. If there were no hints in the diagnostic interview that the patient was crazy, this might simply mean that there was an underlying thought disorder or affect disorder that was masked by the patient's defenses but could be detected by administering inkblots and TATs, and asking questions like "How tall is the average American woman?" or "What's missing from this picture?"

As a psychological tester, my job was to reduce the complex human pain I witnessed to diagnostic simplicities. I would interview a woman who had intractable lower back pain which five successive operations had not cured, and I would have to write in my test report that she was a "hysterical personality with a distorted body image." Or I would talk to a working-class adolescent who felt that life was not worth living, and I would have to write "psychological testing reveals this patient to be a schizophrenic, schizo-affective type, depressed, with marked paranoid trends." Or I would talk to a black man raised in the ghetto by alcoholic parents, who suffered from the increasingly compelling idea that he was trapped in repetitive cycles of events from which there was no escape. And I would have to conclude that he showed "marked evidence of delusional thinking." I would hear about the daily pain of a working-class housewife who had been battered for years while her alcoholic husband drank away their income. And my report would say that she was "a borderline personality with acute conflicts in the area of dependency-autonomy." One time I interviewed a fifteen-year-old boy with two crevices in his cranium the size of tennis balls, the sinister marks of the pick-ax damage inflicted by his own father. Psychological testing, according to my supervisor, revealed the necessity for him to be in a long-term adolescent group where he could learn to sort out his "confusion about sexual identification."

There were occasional lighter moments—for example, testing a sixteen-year-old boy whose answers revealed an awareness of the absurdity of some of the questions he was being asked (Question: "What would you do if you saw a train approaching a broken track?" Answer: "I'd buy some popcorn, sit down on the sidelines, and watch the whole show blow up"). Sometimes it was even possible to establish a human connection across the vast gulf of professional insult between myself and my test victim. And there were some minor victories—like occasionally convincing a supervisor that the patient wasn't really a schizophrenic, she was just an adolescent.

But for the most part, I had to suffer and endure my role as the contemporary representative of the psychological inquisition. The more test batteries I administered, the more distraught I became. In professional lingo, I began to suffer from an increasing barrage of symptoms: anxiety, agitation, sleep disturbance, pathological rage, grandiose thinking, paranoid ideation, and the vegetative signs of depression. The weekly rituals of psychological torture I had to administer were driving me crazy.

Other interns too manifested mild to moderate to severe discomfort with psych testing. We were repeatedly reminded by our supervisors that the point of psych testing was to help establish the correct course of treatment so that the patient could be better helped. The most suitable treatment for endogenous depression was medication, while the best choice for exogenous depression was psychotherapy. Manic depressives needed lithium while psychotic depressives needed antidepressants or electro-convulsive therapy. Schizophrenics needed hospitalization; personality disorders needed individual therapy. There was a reason for testing, a method to all this diagnostic madness: treatment. But I soon learned that the treatment itself was often a form of madness.

4. How to Treat Patients

In the Middle Ages, madmen were thought to be carriers of the truth about the human condition in irrational form. They were the fools whose tales told all. But apparently the wise did not care to know the truth, for anyone thought mad could be herded into a boat with his kind and set out to sea.

By the early seventeenth century, the concept of madness had changed. No longer mad with the truth, madmen were now seen as morally depraved, possessed by the devil. Along with the poor. the unemployed, and criminals, they were incarcerated in houses of confinement. For the next two hundred years, they were caged like beasts. The treatment was thought appropriate to the condition.

It wasn't until the early nineteenth century that it occurred to anyone to distinguish between the criminal and the insane. The emphasis here was on the fact that convicts were being unjustly exposed to madmen. The stigma of the mad was greater than that of murderers and thieves. Thus began the era of the great asylums for the insane. The popular image of these madhouses as hideous snakepits is fairly accurate.

A half century later, the notion of "treatment" for the insane was first conceived. Before this, confinement and corporal punishment had been considered treatment enough. But now, new treatments emerged: inmates were immersed in scalding hot water and then wrapped in straitjackets and tied to their beds. Or they were given injections of insulin in doses large enough to induce insulin shock.

But today we live in an enlightened age of modern science. The insane are not viewed as morally depraved or touched with the truth but as victims of an illness. Social science has liberated the insane from the dark ages of the asylum into the white, clean-scrubbed halls of the modern mental hospital.

The old treatments are now looked upon in horror, as vestiges of ignorance and superstition. We no longer have ships of fools or madhouses or merciless floggings or insulin-induced shock. Instead, we have operations by which the frontal lobes of the cerebrum are cut off with a knife or laser beam, or burned off slowly with electrodes implanted by drilling holes in the skull.* Psychosurgery, in its first, crudest form—the lobotomy— was first performed in 1935. It enjoyed a brief heyday until it was largely eliminated by public outcry. In the last decade, however, it has reemerged as what a presidential commission calls a "beneficial form of therapy."

Insulin therapy has been replaced by ECT (electro-convulsive therapy, commonly known as "shock"). Now, instead of insulin, doctors administer shocks of 150 to 200 volts of alternating current to the brain. This technique has been so perfected that it no longer results in fractures and dislocations of the spine or jaw or in respiratory arrest, as it did in the late 1940s and 1950s.

---

* A government-appointed commission, the National Commission for the Protection of Human Subjects of Biomedical and Behavioral Research, issued a report in March 1977 that endorsed psychosurgery as a "potentially beneficial therapy" for people suffering from psychiatric and behavioral disorders, prisoners, involuntarily confined mental patients, and children. This report was later signed by the Secretary of the Department of Health, Education and Welfare. In effect, this gave the report the status of policy and thereby opened wide the gates for psychosurgeons whose scalpels had been waiting for the go-ahead. The most interesting aspect of this new policy is the targeting of children as an appropriate population for psychosurgery. Whereas in the past lobotomies were performed primarily on prison inmates and back wards chronic mental patients, the wave of the future is more and more psychosurgery for "depressed" or "violent" women and children.

MEDICATIONS: HOW TO PUSH DRUGS ■ Since the early 1950s, the decisive change in the modern treatment of the mad has occurred: physical straitjackets have been abandoned in favor of chemical ones. The era of psychotropic medication is here.

One does not have to be a therapy patient to get medications. One only has to have a mental disorder. "Meds" are a bona fide treatment in and of themselves, not simply an adjunct to therapy or hospitalization. The patient suffering from severe depression or anxiety may find medications a source of temporary relief. In such cases, the use of meds is warranted as long as the goal is to wean the patient from the drug as soon as possible. But as things stand, the psychiatric attitude towards meds invariably leads to drug abuse. In many cases, meds are prescribed automatically and patients are kept on a med diet interminably.

Everything is subordinated to the medication rule of thumb: *for every condition or symptom there is a medication.* And its corollary: for every side effect of a medication, there is another medication to counteract the side effect. Once this is accepted, the logic of the medication itself takes over: its effects and side effects are all that one need think about.

Hyperactive children are unruly. At school, they will not sit still. They twist in their seats. They have a low "frustration tolerance." Short attention spans, moving from one thing to another faster than the expert thinks is normal. Some hyperactive children are organically impaired. Others are simply too intellectually curious. Either way, they do not endear themselves to mothers at home or teachers in school. They have a mental disorder.

So I was taught by a local pediatric expert in a seminar on hyperactive children. She assured us that, contrary to appearances, the hyperactive child really *does* want to do what the teachers want him to do: "He wants to be acceptable seven days a week." To help him be acceptable, there is, fortunately, a simple and effective treatment: Dexedrine or Ritalin. The effect these drugs (which are called speed on the streets) have on children is opposite to their effect on adults. They slow hyperactive children down. Drowsiness is a side effect. But— no problem! The side effect can be cured with another "medi- cine": caffeine! Of course, caffeine tends to result in anorexia (pathological loss of appetite) and stunted growth. But—no problem! For this side effect there is another medicine: Periac- tin, which stimulates the child's appetite.

This is medication logic.

Under the sway of medication logic, no side effect is too damaging or uncomfortable or dangerous. No side effect is so bad that it can't be either tolerated because the benefits of the medication outweigh it, or alleviated through the use of another medication. The possible exception to this rule is death— which is listed as a side effect of several medications.

Take Thorazine, famous for its antipsychotic effects. Thor- azine is one of the phenothiazines, a group of major tranquiliz- ers. Though called tranquilizers, these drugs do not counteract anxiety. They counteract *thinking:* psychotic thinking, to be exact. They are routinely prescribed for patients diagnosed as schizophrenic.

Walk into the typical psychiatric ward and you may be greeted by the following sight: Some patients walk slowly, dragging their feet and staring vacantly ahead of them. Others are jittery and agitated, their eyes fixed upward, their mouths gagging or salivating, their facial muscles paralyzed into a masklike rigidity. Their speech is slow and their hands show a fine tremor. Some may be smacking their lips or sticking out their tongues. What you are witnessing are not, in fact, the manifestations of mental illness; they are manifestations of the *treatment* for mental illness! All of these bizarre movements and behaviors are the visible side effects of the phenothiazines.

One of these side effects is called tardive dyskinesia—in- voluntary movements of the face and mouth such as smacking of the lips or cleaving of the tongue to the roof of the mouth. With perfect dispassionate aplomb—the mark of the true Ex- pert—the typical psychiatrist administering such drugs will tell you that tardive dyskinesia represents permanent brain damage and that the side effects are therefore nonreversible.

In all of my training, I never once heard a psychiatrist even remotely suggest that he harbored any doubts about administering a drug that caused brain damage in his patients. Medicine is medicine. In return for having their thought processes chemically manipulated, patients must accept certain discomforts. In addition to the more noticeable ones listed, these discomforts include blurry vision, dry mouth, constipation, drowsiness, dizziness, interferences in menstruation or potency, urinary retention, allergies, skin rashes, and breast lactation.

To counteract the annoying side effects of these drugs, one need simply prescribe another drug: Cogentin. The side effects of Cogentin: blurry vision, constipation, dry mouth, and allergies. Sound familiar? The side effects of Cogentin are some of the very same as those Cogentin is designed to alleviate! (Apparently, since these side effects are less extreme than permanent brain damage, they are dismissed as insignificant.) Another side effect of Cogentin is psychosis. Thus the drug given to counteract the side effects of the drug given to counteract psychosis results in a side effect of psychosis. The solution to this medication paradox? Simple. First administer the phenothiazine plus Cogentin. Then increase the dosage of the phenothiazine to counteract the side effects of the Cogentin. And then, to counteract the side effects of the increased dosage of the phenothiazine, up the dosage of Cogentin.

By such trains of thought psychiatrists lose the thread of reason.

It is not that side effects do not trouble psychiatrists. Psychiatry's manner of overcoming them is rather ingenious, in its own way. The psychiatric rule of thumb about medications is not only to choose the "right" medication, but to choose the medication with the "right" side effects. For example, if a schizophrenic is paranoid, agitated, anxious, and generally difficult—give her Thorazine rather than Stelazine. A common side effect of Thorazine is sedation, whereas Stelazine doesn't usually have this effect. Thus Thorazine will not only get the patient to stop hallucinating, it will also guarantee that she not be troublesome to the ward staff. In this way, what could be a bothersome side effect is actually transformed into an aspect of the "treatment"! Such clever solutions to the problem of side effects are openly taught in training hospitals.

If all else fails, there is always the last in psychiatry's bag of medication tricks. If the side effects of a particular medication are troublesome—increase the dosage. Increasing the dosage actually decreases the side effects—temporarily, that is.

All of this might be amusing, if it weren't for the dire effects of medication logic on mental patients.

One such patient was Joe—an eighteen-year-old brought to the hospital by his father because the son was hearing voices. When Joe arrived at the hospital, he was a wiry, attractive young man, alert, agitated, and talkative. Three weeks later he had blown up like a blimp. His face and body were red and swollen beyond recognition. He had a skin rash all over his body and was suffering from hepatitis. He could barely speak. He was, in fact, close to death. But he was very compliant, and he no longer heard voices.

The doctors had a hard time figuring out what was wrong with Joe. His Thorazine had only calmed his voices down, not eliminated them. So they had given him Thorazine plus Stelazine to see if he wouldn't do better. Instead, he became very withdrawn and physically ill. So they dropped the Stelazine and Thorazine and replaced them with Haldol and Cogentin. But Joe only got more ill. At last, the doctors were forced to agree that Joe had drug-induced hepatitis and a systemic reaction to his medication. But to which? To the Thorazine? The Thorazine plus the Stelazine? The Haldol? The Haldol plus Cogentin? The Cogentin alone? It was virtually impossible to sort out this medication knot. Their only course of action was to take him off all psychotropic medications and substitute steroids to cure his medication-induced illness. One of the side effects of steroids is psychosis.

They discharged Joe on a diet of steroids only, with no psychotropic medication. He had been clean of phenothiazines for several weeks and was not psychotic. The doctors therefore thought of Joe as a success story.

Joe's is the typical story of a routine psychiatric overdose. When I asked the young resident who treated Joe whether Joe's close brush with death had led the resident to question the virtue of large doses of phenothiazines piled on top of one another, he looked quite genuinely surprised. His young face was innocent of all guile. His answer was simple. "Even penicillin has side effects. Do we let a patient's infection go, just because penicillin has side effects?" I knew that this resident would one day make a good psychiatrist, for medication logic was in his bones.

Lithium is a chemical that replaces all sodium in the body. Lithium treatment was developed in 1949 by an Australian doctor who noticed that it made guinea pigs lethargic. From this he extrapolated the ingenious idea that lithium would be an excellent cure for manic depressive illness, manic type. Lethargy would counteract the mania.

Since the development of lithium treatment, psychiatry has jumped on the lithium bandwagon. Like electroshock therapy, its actual workings are unknown. Among other things, lithium causes diarrhea, nausea, abdominal pain, vomiting, and pathological thirst. In too high a dose it produces tremors, slurred speech, convulsions, coma, and death. Given these side effects, it is not surprising that lithium works best in counteracting mania and not as well in conteracting depression. Nevertheless, it is routinely prescribed for manic depressives, many of whom have never experienced a manic episode but who are simply severely depressed.

The obsolete name for schizophrenia is dementia praecox. Before the advent of psychotropic medication, it was a rare mental disorder. Psychiatrists did not even presume to understand it. But after the development of the phenothiazines, "schizophrenia" (the more up-to-date word for dementia praecox) became a widespread disease. Suddenly, in psychiatric wards and hospitals throughout the country, schizophrenics appeared in epidemic proportions. The diagnosis become more and more widely used as the "treatment" for the illness became more and more available through the pharmaceutical companies.

Similarly, now that psychiatry has discovered lithium, there are more manic depressives than ever. It is without a doubt the fastest rising diagnosis in psychiatric circles.

Unlike other psychotropic meds, lithium is prescribed for one's entire life span. But a patient cannot simply pop lithium on her own. She must go to her psychiatrist's office weekly and have her blood carefully monitored. Only a certified M.D. can administer lithium, for too high a dosage can lead to death. Hence the great advantage of lithium to psychiatry: it makes the patient not only drug-dependent for life, but doctor-dependent for life.

Just as the key element in who gets labeled neurotic is who is doing the diagnosing, so the key element in what gets called a medication is who is doing the prescribing. Seconal is a severely addictive barbiturate. The withdrawal symptoms can be lethal. A pronounced barbiturate addiction, say the experts in drug dependence, often leads to psychosis. Seconal, called "blues" and sold on the street or under the counter, is viewed in professional circles as a bad drug which indicates the user is a drug-dependent personality, probably psychopathic in type. But according to these same experts, when Seconal is prescribed by a certified psychiatrist, it is medicine for sleep disturbance and indicates that the prescriber is a respectable professional.

Medication logic is compelling. People who are addicted to the drugs they like and have decided to take are sick. People who are addicted to drugs they don't like which have been prescribed for them by others are getting better. People who prescribe the pills that make people sick are making people better. And finally, people who think that the pills that are making them sick are making them sick, are sick.

The Experts who abide by such logic do not consider such

thinking evidence of "impaired reality testing" or a "psychotic thought disorder." Nor do they tolerate any challenge to their reasoning. By medication logic, any such challenge is viewed as itself evidence of a psychotic thought disorder.

Peter was a young man on the inpatient unit who offered such a challenge. He refused to take his meds. Unlike some patients, who "tongued" their meds (slid the pills under their tongue, pretended to swallow them, and later spat them out), Peter's refusal was direct and outright. He told the staff that he believed in eating well (a diet of whole, organic foods) and in not polluting the body with useless, harmful drugs. All the staff's concerted efforts to persuade Peter that he was ill and that his medication was good for him were to no avail. When pushed to take meds, Peter railed at the staff that meds were an "ignominious destroyer, born of ignorance," and that his doctors knew nothing about the human body. In his record, the doctor noted: "Because of Peter's intricate delusional system, he refuses to take meds."

In the treatment of patients, medication logic always prevails.

THE INPATIENT WARD: EYE OF THE STORM ■ As a psych intern I was required to do a rotation on the inpatient ward in the hospital. It was considered an open ward. There were no bars on the windows or locked doors, and no involuntary admissions, as there are in wards for hard-core "psychotics" considered dangerous to themselves or others. Incoming patients had to promise at the door that they would not kill themselves or do violence to others or to the property. In return, they got to live in an environment considered optimally therapeutic for moderately disturbed patients who had voluntarily submitted themselves for treatment.

When I started out in my rotation on the ward, I was nervous. I had never worked with psychotics and I wasn't sure what to expect. I was reassured by my supervisors, who told me that many of the residents who headed the treatment teams on the ward had never even had a psychiatric rotation in medical school. They were going in cold, whereas I was going in armed with my knowledge of diagnosis. Somehow, this did not reassure me.

All my doubts were confirmed by what I saw on the ward. Most of the patients were lonely, scared, depressed or angry. Some were certainly very disturbed or disoriented. Their "psychotic" labeling made them eligible for high doses of drugs which only worsened their problems.

My first morning on the ward, I was unprepared for what greeted me. There were no cries of anguish, terror, or rage, just a deadly, eerie silence.

The first sight I saw was an elderly woman of approximately seventy years with white hair and a body so thin she looked like a stick figure. She was strapped to her chair by two leather bands, one on each wrist. A nurse was feeding her as she cried continuously.

Slowly, patients began to enter the day room where Morning Meeting was to begin. Some looked swollen and placid. Others seemed to have nervous tics in every part of their body. Many dragged their feet in a strange, disturbing way (I learned later that this was the famous "Thorazine shuffle"). The overwhelming impression in the faces of the patients was a look of terrifying vacancy.

Later, after I'd seen some patients come in on Intake, I began to realize that patients did not come into the hospital looking this way. They came in looking scared but alive. The first treatment dispensed to these newcomers, one and all, was meds. And it was this drug-induced death-in-life that I saw in the faces of the patients on that first morning.

After all the patients were assembled, Morning Meeting began. The Charge Nurse began to read her report on how the patients had fared the evening and night before. Throughout this reporting, Mrs. D., the white-haired lady strapped to her chair, was making writhing movements with her body. Her eyes were raised heavenwards in a gesture of helpless appeal. Her mouth made small, muted, moaning sounds. It was hard to listen to the Charge Nurse's Report. The surrounding patients seemed acutely uncomfortable, most of them staring down at their laps and rather pointedly *not* staring at Mrs. D.

Mrs. D. was considered organically psychotic. She was incapable of speaking. When the charge nurse came to the part of the report which referred to her, Mrs. D.'s eyes rolled around in her head and she struggled against her leather restraints. Without words, her message was painfully clear: "Please get me out of this chair. Set me free." The nurse next to her cooed soothingly.

At this point, Mr. M., an elderly gentleman with a dignified air, shouted, "How long must we sit here and watch the deterioration of this human being tied to her chair?"

The Charge Nurse interrupted her reading to reply. "We all share your feelings of frustration at Mrs. D.'s severe illness."

Mr. M. grimaced but kept silent. It seemed to me that this was not what he meant at all. He was not frustrated with Mrs. D.'s severe illness; he was frustrated with Mrs. D.'s treatment, with watching her so helplessly trapped.

The Charge Nurse finished her report. Dr. T., the Chief Resident, now stood up and whispered to a middle-aged woman beside him. She then stood up too. The vacancy which I had seen in so many patient faces haunted hers. But on top of it was a thin patina of cheerfulness which seemed bizarre in the context of the environment to which she was now being introduced. "This is Mrs. N.," said Dr. T. "She is a fifty-eight-year-old white female who was admitted last night following a suicidal gesture in her home."

The fabricated smile on Mrs. N.'s face widened apprehensively. Her smile would no doubt be labeled inappropriate by ward staff. But I recognized it as the mark of a woman who was, above all, trained to act appropriately female in social situations ("Smile and be nice") and whose training had finally caught up with her.

Dr. T. continued. "Mrs. N.'s husband passed away three weeks ago and she has been acutely depressed ever since. Her three children are all grown and in school, and her social contacts somewhat limited at this time. She is oriented to person, time, and place, her memory is intact, and she shows no active signs of hallucinations or delusions at this time. But she is severely depressed and suicidal and will be on one-to-one supervision until she feels better. We hope that you will all try to make Mrs. N. feel at home here and help her to talk about her loss."

Mercifully, Mrs. N. was now allowed to sit down. Throughout this public airing of her private grief and her mental status, she had bravely faced the throng of strangers without flinching.

In the weeks to come, I was to learn that this public presentation of the patient's psychic state was a routine part of ward life. It extended beyond this initial introduction into all aspects of what a patient said or did. Even a patient's private statements to her one-to-one individual therapist were considered open to the staff/patient "community." The much vaunted confidentiality which was so highly respected a feature of outpatient therapy no longer held for hospitalized mental patients. On the contrary, the stripping away of a person's privacy, in both its physical and emotional aspects, was considered an important part of a "milieu" approach to the treatment of hospitalized mental patients. Just as in the bathrooms there were no locks on the stalls (and in some cases no doors), so in general there was no emotional or physical space which was sacrosanct for the inpatient.

After Mrs. N.'s introduction, there was a deadly silence in the day room for several minutes. The silence was broken by the Charge Nurse, who asked, "Doesn't anyone have anything to say this morning? Any response to Mrs. N.? Or other patient issues to be discussed? Surely there's been enough going on on the ward lately?" Her question was a command: patients must now speak their minds. They all shifted in their seats.

Finally, Mr. M., the elderly dignified gentleman who had objected to the treatment of Mrs. D., broke the silence. "I don't understand why we have to subject ourselves to this every morning. Everyone knows that Morning Meetings are boring, useless, unnecessary, and fruitless. No one gets anything out of them. I really don't see why we have to sit here."

It seemed for the next moment everyone held their breath. Then, slowly and hesitantly, another patient spoke up. He was a thin, wiry young man with heavy dark-rimmed glasses, wearing a white shirt and black slacks that seemed two sizes too big for him.

"Yes, why do we?" he asked. His voice conveyed a curious mixture of deference and defiance.

Again, silence.

It was a staff nurse who broke it this time. She looked pointedly at Mr. M. and the young wiry man and then around the room to see if anyone else was going to say anything. Then she cleared her throat.

"This complaint has been raised before. And we've explained that the function of morning meetings is to introduce new patients, to keep the community abreast of how different patients are doing, to help one another to acclimate ourselves to the ward, and to bring up important patient issues that need to be addressed. You all know that. So what's *really* going on here today?"

Mr. M.'s question was put in its proper place: diagnosed as an avoidance of the "real" issue. Some patients looked vaguely disgruntled. But for the most part, everyone simply maintained the look of complete blankness to which I was now getting accustomed.

The air seemed charged with some unnamed tension. Then, when it seemed that the tension was no longer tolerable, a young woman in her twenties with matted blond hair and a look of practiced meekness, spoke up.

"Perhaps it's difficult for us to talk this morning because Mrs. D. is still so sick and that raises everyone's anxiety. And then, on top of that, the new patient, Mrs. N., is severely depressed. Maybe we're all having a hard time responding to her. So many of us are depressed that it's kind of hard to take another depression."

The staff nurse smiled and nodded approvingly at this patient. Her unmistakable cue ("Yes, very good, this is the proper way to express yourself") was taken up by several other patients. Some talked about their own feelings—but in a distanced, abstract way that was unnervingly reminiscent of the way staff talked about patients. Others tried to bring out the feelings of fellow patients by mimicking the intrusive style of psychiatric staff. The major technique here was divulging statements which had obviously been made by fellow patients in private—that is, telling secrets.

This was the Show and Tell Feelings Game. In this atmosphere of coerced intimacy, the "good patients" were those who sounded most like the psychiatric staff. And the "bad patients" were those who sat in silence or, worse still, criticized the game.

Lucy A. was one such patient. "Why, I'd like to know," she now asked, with no attempt to hide her contempt, "are we all required to fink on each other at Morning Meetings?"

At this, several patients looked visibly agitated. Others were clearly pleased but tried to hide it. Mr. M. nodded. The staff maintained its look of studied nonexpressiveness.

One of the residents rallied. "Why are you so distrustful of patients and staff, Miss A.?"

Then a female patient—one of the good ones—piped up with her answer to the resident's question.

"I think Lucy is really paranoid. She's always thinking people are out to get her."

"People *are* out to get me," Lucy shouted. "Why do you think I'm in here?" Miss A. was referring to the circumstances of her hospitalization. She had been brought to the hospital by police after assaulting a man who had tried to rape her.

"Well, nobody ever tried to rape me. What do you think you're doing to provoke it?" countered the same good patient.

Lucy glared at her and then launched into a heated diatribe against men. Men were rapists at heart, if not in action. Rape was on the rise, especially now after the women's movement. The world in general was dangerous for women, especially poor women.

When she had finished, the Chief Resident, with a look of enduring patience, said, "There's no money in establishing all of this as sociological fact, Miss A."

I had to suppress a smile at the doctor's unconscious pun. Indeed, there was no "money" for the doctor in Lucy's attitude about psychiatry. She simply refused to see herself as a Patient. She did not consider herself sick. She was overtly angry, aggressive, and belligerent. She would not play by the rules of the game. She conveyed an Us-vs.-Them attitude about the inpatient ward: exhibiting great loyalty to patients and openly criticizing the staff. Staff response to her behavior was usually the same as on this first occasion: they would ask pointed questions about her childhood and about her feelings toward members of her family.

"What are your feelings toward your father?" was the question asked of her this morning.

Lucy replied without the slightest hesitation. "I hate my father. He was always drunk. He stank. He was really into guns and tried to kill me once with a shotgun. What do you think I feel about him?"

There was no bulldozing Lucy with psychiatric interrogations. She was an openly man-hating angry woman who refused to bow her head. Nevertheless, her initial question about patients being required to fink on each other had been effectively evaded. She could not raise a patient rebellion by herself, and the other patients seemed too well trained to take up arms with her. Yet she had clearly disturbed the smooth functioning of Morning Meeting. Both staff and patients alike seemed relieved when the hour for Morning Meeting was up.

That same afternoon at the Staff Meeting, when Lucy's name came up, the Director of the ward summed up her case: "Anyone who doesn't believe in the childhood causes of mental illness after Miss A.'s case," he said, "surely has something wrong with them." So much for Miss A.'s criticism of ward and staff. Dispelled at once, with a quick wave of the pathology wand.

In the following weeks Lucy gained a reputation among

staff as a difficult patient. Patients as overtly defiant as she was were often fated to be pink-papered (involuntarily committed to a state hospital) as homicidal risks. But Lucy was diagnosed as borderline and therefore not seriously enough ill to be pink-papered. There was no way to dump her from the ward except for the staff to acknowledge that psychiatric hospitalization was not working in her case. Three weeks later, Lucy was discharged from the hospital—a treatment failure. She was psychiatrically incorrigible.

Other patients did not fare as well. At the afternoon Staff Meeting, the case of Frieda C. came up. Frieda was one of the silent ones on the ward. Because she was loath to talk at meetings, she was considered manipulative. Because she was considered manipulative, her meds were upped. She clearly could talk freely when she wanted to, because staff had seen her communicating intensely with her boyfriend during visiting hours. Consequently, she was regarded as paranoid because she did not trust the staff. The consensus at this staff meeting was to take away Frieda's visitor privileges. She was no longer allowed to see or talk to her boyfriend on the ward.

Over the next few weeks, Frieda "decompensated" (the technical word for going crazy) rapidly—that is, she became, according to psychiatric assessment, more and more flagrantly psychotic. She talked wildly of being in prison and accused the hospital staff of persecuting her.

It became clear to me that first day on the ward that what I had thought to be the somewhat exaggerated fiction of *One Flew Over the Cuckoo's Nest* was, in fact, a fairly accurate representation of business as usual on the inpatient ward.

From that moment on, I saw clearly what my role on the ward would entail. In order for me to help patients, I would have to help them play by the rules. First of all this meant that they were to act as though they believed in their diagnosis as the sacred truth of their personality. They were to talk up at meetings about their feelings, whether they trusted the staff or not. And they were to acknowledge that the staff was helping them. In this way, by making the staff feel better, they could get to leave the ward as soon as possible. The hard part was to convince them that acting crazier and crazier, though it was positively reinforced on the ward (since it was the "craziest" patients who got the most staff attention), was actually a self-defeating game. For the kind of attention patients received for acting crazy only furthered their problems.

But this was in the future. My first day on the ward, I had not yet adjusted to what I was witnessing. That whole day I was overcome by the early morning image of Mrs. D., strapped to her chair and drooling while desperately trying to get the staff to free her. There was little hope of her recovery. Legally, restraints were allowed to be used only in cases of danger of the patient's harm to self or others. Because Mrs. D. could not speak, she was considered dangerous to herself. Her body language was clearly not seen to be a manner of communicating. I wondered what would become of her.

That same afternoon, I saw her in the day room, still trapped in her chair. This time, a nurse was combing out her aged white hair and rolling it into curlers. With each yank of hair into the roller, Mrs. D. grimaced and cried. A male nurse sauntered over and, seeing Mrs. D. so visibly upset, he chided her:

"Now, now, don't you see that the nurse is trying to make you pretty? Don't you care? Answer me! Don't you care?"

Mrs. D.'s answer was clear. She cried and winced. The nurse continued to roll her hair and tried to soothe her.

"Now, now, honey. Appearance is important."

My experience on the inpatient ward taught me that treatment offered virtually no hope for Mrs. D. But the rituals of feminine self-improvement were mandatory.

HOW TO PRACTICE PSYCHOTHERAPY ■ The core of my training in how to treat patients was how to practice psychotherapy. As an intern, I worked with couples, groups, and families. But for the most part, I worked with individuals. Individual therapy, in traditional circles, is still generally regarded as the most respectable and inherently beneficial form of therapy. Despite the inroads into this view wrought by advocates of couple, family, and group therapy in the last decade, individual therapy remains the bulwark of therapy practice.

I learned that there was far more to the practice of therapy than meets the eye. As a therapist, one did not simply sit and listen and respond. One had to know what to listen for and how to understand what one heard, and when and how to respond in an effective manner. The therapist was a skilled professional, not a lay listener or friendly ear.

Indeed, truly listening to someone's pain with one's full concentration is a difficult art, as anyone who has tried to do this for even a short period of time well knows. Though some people seem to have an innate talent for this art, it is nevertheless something that can be learned. (Women in our society, for instance, are generally much more skilled listeners than men because throughout the socialization process in appropriate sex-role behavior, females receive specialized training in how to be "receptive.")

In two years of training as a therapist, however, there was not a single seminar, workshop, or supervision session devoted to the practice of listening skills. Being receptive as a therapist was not the point. The point was first mastering a certain body of knowledge and then learning to analyze everything a patient said and did in light of that knowledge. The Freudian-style therapist did not listen *to* a patient's *experience*. He listened *for* a patient's *pathology*. Thus in training, one spoke of analytic skills, not listening skills. The model of the therapist was a keen intellectual mind who could process everything he heard into the proper Freudian categories with great ease. The model was not someone who could intuit well what a person felt or who could respond with compassion, validation, or understanding. The model, in short, was male, not female.

The professional therapist had to absorb an enormously technical literature and learn how to apply it in practice. One had to know how to interpret material and transference, as well as how to interpret resistance to both material and transference. One had to know how to use suggestion and clarification and how to encourage catharsis. One had to know how to recognize the various kinds of transference resistances: about the patient's search for transference gratification, about generalized transference and defensive transference and acting out. One had to know how to recognize when one was in the initial, mid, and late phase of therapy so as to know exactly what to expect from the patient and how to behave as a therapist in each phase.

In practice, the professional's responses to the patient in therapy had to be extraordinarily subtle in wording and timing. Therapy was no hit-or-miss affair. The results of therapeutic mismaneuvers could be potentially lethal.

For instance, I learned that in doing therapy with a borderline patient, the therapist must always keep in mind that borderlines tended to think concretely and act accordingly. Never say something like "Have a nice vacation" to a borderline. One therapist made the mistake of doing so. His patient was so concrete in her thinking that she took his friendliness as an order. She could not bear to tell him that she had not lived up to his mandate. So rather than tell him she had a lousy vacation, she killed herself.

How, I wondered, did this therapist know that it was his "Have a nice vacation" that had spurred his patient to suicide? Surely, there were some other variables involved—some other factors in the therapeutic relationship (not to mention the patient's life), outside of his passing remarks, that had motivated her. There's no asking a dead woman. But Experts simply *know* these things.

We had been duly warned: watch your words. ("The patient," said one of my supervisors, "may kill himself to spite you.") It did not occur to most interns to question the Experts' wild sense of their own power which, if exhibited by a patient, would undoubtedly be diagnosed as "grandiose thinking." The lesson was deeply embedded: therapy was not a matter of trusting your gut responses. Throw intuition to the winds. Patients were too ill to be treated like regular persons. Do so at your patients' peril—and your own.

This lesson in the importance of not being earnest had the

effect of rendering most interns largely impotent when it came to meeting their first patients. Nevertheless, it was of singular importance in confirming the trainee's devout loyalty to professionalism. Trainees learned that following their hunches, or relying on common sense, empathy, or compassion, could have disastrous consequences. Instead, the bona fide therapist came to the practice of therapy armed with the only reliable tools that the professional could trust: diagnosis and a trained ear for the predetermined process of therapy known only to the Experts. In this way, the intern was convinced that helping people was something only a trained professional could do. Furthermore, by this same route, professionals convinced themselves of the rationale for charging fees like seventy dollars an hour. Professional help was worth every penny.

Once it was established that the practice of psychotherapy was essentially esoteric, everything else followed. Like medication logic, psychotherapy logic was impeccable.

The most important aspect of the practice of therapy was a deep understanding of the workings of the transference relationship between patient and therapist, and of how to manipulate it. Transference, as we may recall, was the process by which the patient transferred to the therapist feelings and attitudes that were not appropriate to the therapist but belonged instead to significant figures in her early life. Much of the insight to be gained from long term, insight-oriented therapy was thought to reside in the patient's increasingly conscious knowledge of this transference. The patient who came to see that her feelings toward her therapist were in no way related to him but had everything to do with unresolved conflicts engendered in early childhood was making progress.

To further the therapy, therefore, it was considered essential for the therapist to maximize or enhance the transference. To do so, interns were instructed to take an "abstinent" posture toward the patient. This meant that the therapist must suppress himself as a person; withhold any opinions, feelings, and responses toward the patient; and abstain from offering the patient anything that might gratify her transference needs and feelings. She might, for instance, want to be comforted or praised, and ask for this either directly or indirectly. Whatever you do as a therapist, we were warned, *don't give her what she wants!* If you do, you will only cause her unconscious feelings to submerge, and you will therefore never get to the *real* issues and conflicts involved. Instead, the therapist must invite the transference by *intentionally frustrating the patient.* This will cause the patient to *regress* and, in this manner, the therapist will get at the real issues which are interfering with the patient's present behavior.* (Asking for praise or comfort was apparently regarded as an "issue"—something that interfered with the adult functioning of the patient. Adults were not supposed to ask for help, or to need. Only people with fixations in early stages of development ask or need.)

To be sure, we were taught that it was important for the therapist to forge a therapeutic "alliance" with the patient. The emphasis here was on getting the patient to trust the therapist so that she would accept his interpretations with a minimum of resistance. Through this alliance, the therapist trained the patient to examine herself in the light of his theory of her. The work of therapy consisted of the patient emoting in the presence of the therapist, who remained "blank" or "neutral." He was the clear screen or mirror upon which she projected all of her unconscious wishes and feelings from her past.

This was the "Nobody Home" approach to how to be a therapist. The personhood of the therapist was seen as an unwanted intrusion in the therapeutic process. Not the therapist's

---

* One might consider the possibility of a new diagnosis to be added to the Diagnostic and Statistical Manual—that of *professional personality.* Found among therapists as a group, this character disorder is characterized by the therapist's alienation from his own inner life and his fear of his own emotions. Such people obtain emotional satisfaction through the vicarious experience of others' emotions—particularly in a situation in which the rules are that the other person is obliged to unearth and communicate her feelings, while they are not obliged to reciprocate. The therapist with this disorder is emotionally distant, withholding and taciturn. While he may claim that his withholding is necessary to his patients' well-being, in reality it is a symptom of the repressed anger which he harbors at his patients for their dependency on his help.

compassion, but his professional distance and neutrality were thought to be the absolute requirement for therapeutic work.* (Some Interns found this manner of practicing therapy difficult. They tended to bungle things by forgetting themselves and responding more naturally or warmly to patient requests. They were cautioned in supervision to watch this tendency, known as "overidentification with the patient.") Fortunately, most therapists cannot possibly carry off this approach to a relationship, though they do give it a good try. It is precisely when therapists fail at this role—because it is almost impossible to eradicate themselves entirely as persons—that therapy in the traditional vein is at all effective.

I learned that some patients (borderlines and more serious personality disorders) could not tolerate this heightening of the transference relationship. Unlike "good, healthy neurotics," these more disturbed patients were too regressed to begin with. To regress them even further could cause them to decompensate. In such cases, "dynamic" or "insight-oriented" psychotherapy was abandoned in favor of "supportive" or "reality-oriented" therapy. In the latter, it was advisable to minimize the transference: deemphasize dreams and unconscious material and concentrate on more concrete, day-to-day, conscious issues. The therapist was more real, less of a transference object.

Patients who exhibited overt anxiety or hostility toward the professional stance of abstinence were seen as inherently sicker than those who complied and adapted. By this curious twist of logic, such patients were entitled to talk about their daily problems without necessarily having these interpreted as manifestations of early unconscious conflict. But this was only because they were too sick to tolerate "insight"! Apparently, if

---

* I am reminded of a line from R. D. Laing's *The Politics of Experience:* Any theory [of therapy] not founded on the nature of being human is a lie and a betrayal of man [sic]. An inhuman theory will inevitably lead to inhuman consequences—if the therapist is consistent. Fortunately, many therapists have the gift of inconsistency. This, however endearing, cannot be regarded as ideal.[5]

such patients knew the truth about themselves, they would flip out or commit suicide. They were too crazy to be granted the gift of self-knowledge, which the more highly valued insight therapy had to offer.

But supportive therapy was in many respects somewhat of a misnomer. Giving a patient support hardly meant that the therapist should be more responsive. In all cases, the therapist was to remain *professional*. The borderline who wished to explore her dreams was just as misguided as the good healthy neurotic who wanted to talk about day-to-day reality problems. In both cases, the therapist must disregard what the patient expressly wanted and steer her into what she really needed. In short, the therapist was never to abandon one of the cardinal rules of professionalism I had learned early on: The Expert always knows the patient better than she knows herself.

This rule applied as well to the question of how often to do therapy. Increasing the frequency of therapy, we were taught, increased the patient's anxiety. Only the patient with good "ego strengths" could benefit from this, whereas the weaker, more dependent patient might easily decompensate. Apparently, only the strong could take the assault on one's ego that therapy offered. Unfortunately, the weaker, more dependent patient, who was least capable of tolerating the anxiety of more frequent therapy, was precisely the patient who was more likely to ask for it. Thus we were cautioned not to let ourselves be "manipulated" by the neediness of dependent patients. Here again, the professional worked counterintuitively. The rule about frequency of therapy was: Give to those who have; withhold from those who need.

In practice, "good healthy neurotics" who could benefit most from therapy three, four, or five times a week generally turned out to be middle- and upper-class patients who could afford it, whereas the more dependent (orally fixated) borderlines, as we have seen, were more likely to be lower class. Hence this rule worked out quite lucratively for the aspiring therapist.

As transference was central to the process of therapy, so

too, was countertransference—the therapist's feelings provoked by the patient's transference. As a training example, we were told the following therapy anecdote: While a patient was telling a story, her doctor fell asleep. Falling asleep was the doctor's countertransference. In the next session, the doctor made good use of it. He said to his patient: "There must have been something in what you were saying or doing that made me fall asleep. What do you think it might have been?" In the explorations that followed, it was discovered that the patient was transferring onto the therapist early sexual feelings that she had had toward her father. As a teenager, this patient would stimulate herself sexually in her father's presence by putting her legs together and moving her feet. It was this movement in therapy that had "hypnotized" the therapist and caused him to fall asleep! (The patient's movement of her feet was considered an "acting out" of unconscious feelings in therapy).

In another training anecdote, we were told about a New York analyst whose patient stopped talking. For six months, patient and analyst sat in silence for the duration of every session. Finally, the analyst had had enough and told his patient he was angry at her. It was only after this expression of the therapist's countertransference feelings that the patient felt "safe" enough to continue talking, for she saw that her own anger would not kill the therapist.

Both of these anecdotes were given to elucidate how the aspiring therapist must both recognize and use his countertransference feelings in the service of the patient.

When the patient has worked through all of her unconscious conflicts, the termination of therapy is at hand. However, the therapist must be cautious about the patient's desire to terminate. Often a patient will suggest termination as a way of avoiding some issue that is too threatening for her to handle. Or a patient will want to terminate as a way of acting out her transference. The patient who, for instance, insists that the therapist is no longer helping her and feels that she is wasting her time is acting out her transference anger. It is wise to warn such patients that a premature termination can be injurious to all the therapy they have done so far.

The true point of termination arrives only when the patient has completely and successfully worked through her transference relationship. At this point, the patient relates to the therapist less as a "transference object" and more as a "real" person.

The contradictions in these lessons in psychotherapy boggled my mind. First, transference was defined as the patient's feelings that were inappropriate to the therapist as a "real" person. Yet simultaneously, therapists were instructed never to behave like real persons in therapy! Therapy was defined as the process by which the patient gradually came to shed her transference neurosis and to see the therapist for who he was. But who *was* he? Someone who sat in a chair taking notes while she spoke her innermost feelings. Someone who rarely if ever responded directly to anything she said. Someone who sat in silence while she searched inside herself for the most painful emotions she could dredge up. Indeed this was not the behavior of a "real" person. What was the appropriate response to someone who acted this way? Walk out and never come back.

How could the therapy patient come to see her therapist as more and more of a real person if he never acted like one? By these rules, the patient was doomed to be a patient eternally. (Indeed, none of my supervisors seemed concerned about stories of interminable therapy cases which continued for ten, even twenty and twenty-five years.)

Toward the end of my training program, interns were treated to something new. By contrast to the more conservative psychoanalytic approach to therapy we had been learning, we were exposed to different approaches to therapy practice. Toward this end, we were invited to attend seminars given by experts in the growing field of couple and family therapy. Family therapy was considered a fairly radical approach to pathology: instead of focusing entirely on the individual patient, it looked at the entire "system" in which the patient functioned —the family.

The guest speaker was a leading light in the family therapy field. He spoke about the family "system" and how usually one person in the system came to be the "identified patient." But to understand and treat the problem, one had to understand and treat the whole system. When a couple or family came to therapy, they were calling in a third person for help. This third person then became part of the system.

What was the therapist's role in this system? "When the therapist joins the field emotionally," he said, "he changes the field." Therefore, the therapist must guard against contaminating the system. He was there to observe and analyze, not to join.

"In an effort to stay out of it," he said, "I tell my patients to talk and pretend I'm not there. I observe, take notes, I don't look at them, I look somewhere else. What I'm trying to do is calm down the emotional reactivity by keeping cool, calm, and intellectual. That way I won't get involved in the field."

By ignoring the patients, this therapist convinced himself that he was not affecting them. Was this the therapist's intricate delusional system? No. This was the cutting edge of recent theory and practice in the field of psychotherapy.

To illustrate his practice, we saw a videotape of a couple's therapy session. The therapist was true to his word. For the most part, he completely ignored the couple and let them go at each other for most of the hour. When he did raise his head to speak, his words were invariably addressed to the male partner in the couple. He talked with the husband about what he thought was wrong with his wife, who was diagnosed as schizophrenic. And then he talked to the wife about what was wrong with her. Later on, after the videotape, this therapist commented that the problem with this couple's system was that the woman was smarter than the man. She was always asking her husband to substantiate what he said. This, naturally, drove the husband wild. Were it the other way around—the husband asking the wife to substantiate what she said—then everything would be "normal." Hence the problem with this system. It was not normal.

If this was the "system" approach to psychotherapy, it was clearly the same old system: Father still Knows Best.

3

Traditional Therapy and Women

In her ground-breaking book, *Women and Madness*, Phyllis Chesler compared psychotherapy and marriage, suggesting that women turn to male therapists as they do to husbands, in search of personal salvation through the presence of a benevolent male authority. The middle-class woman finds in therapy a comfortable, socially approved alternative or adjunct to marriage, a relationship that reinforces the cultural meaning of what it is to be a woman. Both marriage and psychotherapy, said Chesler, can be viewed as "re-enactments of a little girl's relation to her father in patriarchal society."[1]

Written ten years ago, Chesler's analysis was an eye opener. It showed how both traditional marriage and traditional therapy enforced feminine helplessness and passivity. Chesler's main point was that traditional psychotherapy and psychiatry in general were institutions of social control through which women learned or relearned how to be "feminine"; and that women who did not learn this lesson properly or who rebelled against it were considered sick or mad.

As we have seen, the traditional therapy relationship is one in which a powerful, impersonal (culturally masculine) Expert acts upon a vulnerable, emotional (culturally feminine) supplicant. The therapist is the authoritative father. The patient is the ignorant, helpless child. The therapy process is thought to reach its completion when the patient has fully absorbed the insight proffered by the therapist. In short, therapy terminates when the "feminine principle" is mastered by the "masculine."

The social archetype for this Father Knows Best model of therapy is the relationship between the father and his children in the classic patriarchal family of the Victorian era. The rule of the father in this family, even at its most benign, undermined the autonomy of both male and female children. But there was a crucial difference in the effect of this rule on males and females. Little boys could grow up to be fathers themselves, to wear the robes of power. Little girls could only marry power. Symbolically speaking, the son could kill the father or succeed him. The daughter had to bow her head to the father's successor.

The psychiatrist in traditional therapy is the last in the line of these (at best) benevolent patriarchs.

The patriarchal power of the therapist is thus more intense and destructive for the female patient. The passive, unknowing, and helpless female who turns to the male for what she is taught to believe does not exist within herself (skill, knowledge, power) has been the accepted norm for the relation between the sexes in our society. Traditional therapy, in this context, has often been the attempt to finish off the socialization of femininity which begins in the family. Its unwitting goal has been to continue the work of the family in keeping women powerless.

Thus the doctor-patient relationship of traditional therapy is less alien to most women than it is to most men. The traditional situation of Woman as Patient—in which she is encouraged to see herself as someone who is acted upon, rather than someone who acts—corresponds to and reinforces the Victim psychology of women (see chapter nine). Woman as Victim easily becomes Woman as Patient. Once a woman comes to therapy with the identity of a patient, she has already (at least partially) surrendered the part of herself she will most need in order to help herself: her power as a person.

One result is that Woman as Patient often becomes proficient at playing the traditional therapy game: she learns to talk endlessly about herself while longing to be someone else. In this game, the patient's self-preoccupation becomes self-escape. The therapist is credited with the power to remake the self that the patient wishes to escape. In awaiting the magical day that the therapist will rescue her from the ordeal of her own identity, Woman as Patient loses the freedom of exerting her own will to change.

The traditional therapist may advise Woman as Patient that he can only help those who help themselves. Or he may tell her that the fantasy that someone else will "save" her is just magical thinking, or just the operation of her transference. But the very form of the traditional therapy relationship works against the therapist's assertions.

To keep women feminine, therapy has relied not only on the structure of the therapeutic relationship, but on the Freudian psychology of women. Until recently, this theory has been the undisputed view of women in both professional psychology and popular culture. Since the advent of the women's movement, both the theory and the feminist critique of it have become fairly well-known.[2] But it bears repeating that psychic and social powerlessness was the hallmark of Freud's definition of the normal woman.

Freud essentially pictured three kinds of women. The first woman was hopelessly devastated by the fact that she didn't have a penis. She renounced her sexuality. She was "neurotic." The second woman continued to behave as though she had a penis. She imitated male behavior and avoided the "wave of passivity" that normal women should undergo. She refused, in short, to become a woman. She had a "masculinity complex." And the third woman did the best she could without a penis. She developed an exclusive dependence on men and (especially male) children. She was "normal." The signature of a woman's normality was her adaptation to a male-defined and male-centered form of female sexuality in which her highest achievement was the production of male babies. The normal woman adjusted well to her inferiority, diverting her envy of men into the pursuits of home and family. By nature, said Freud, she was vain, passive, masochistic, narcissistic, and suffered from excessive shame and an undeveloped moral sense.

Freud succeeded in "scientifically" enshrining the subordination of women to men as psychological law. In viewing femininity as female nature, the Freudian psychology of women effectively discouraged any rebellions against it. To be considered normal, women had to be feminine in the Freudian sense. Women strong enough to resist the magnetic pull of female socialization and fight for themselves as persons were viewed as abnormal. Femininity was the model of female mental health. In the prevailing model of therapy derived from Freudian theory, the therapist was there to cure woman's ailing femininity.

In the decade since *Women and Madness,* ideas about women, marriage, and psychotherapy have changed. The Freudian norm of femininity has been seriously challenged. The classical patriarchal family (which has been consistently undermined since the Victorian era) has come to coexist with other forms of family life. And the classic doctor-patient relationship of psychoanalytic psychotherapy is no longer the *only* form of therapy; it has been reduced to one among many kinds of therapies currently available.

These changes have come about partly because women have rebelled. We have insisted on defining femininity and female psychology for ourselves. We have demanded changes in the organization of sex roles within marriage and the family. And we have increasingly insisted on therapy that doesn't simply add to the forces already ranged against us. When I was an intern in psychology ten years ago, male psychiatrists were still teaching that women were not well adjusted unless we married and had children. To the extent that some traditional therapists have changed these attitudes about women, and are now tailoring their views to the age of the "liberated woman," they have done so only because women have been defying Freudian views of femininity as well as the traditional system of therapy. We should not underestimate the influence of economic factors in encouraging therapists to change their theories. As increasing numbers of women challenge and refuse to hire therapists who ascribe to a double standard of mental health for men and women, therapists will find it good business to change their standards.

But the problems of Woman as Patient in traditional therapy are not a thing of the past. While humanist or growth therapies now offer an alternative to the traditional model (see chapter six), traditional therapy remains the prevailing model of therapy in this country. It still commands the majority of therapy patients—and those patients are still mostly women. And it remains an unequal relationship dominated by masculine authority. There has been no reduction in the power wielded by the doctor in all fields of medicine, including psychiatry. The doctor is still thought to possess the male power and knowledge the patient lacks. The model of this therapy relationship is still taught in graduate schools, internship programs, hospitals, and institutes throughout the country.

It is likewise mistakenly optimistic to think that the dangers of the Freudian myth of femininity for women in therapy have altogether disappeared. We must bear in mind that only the newest crop of therapists who have attended graduate schools in the last few years have had the opportunity to study female psychology from a feminist perspective. In the meantime, the Freudian and psychoanalytic theories of women continue to be taught in orthodox graduate departments and postgraduate institutes. Most psychiatrists practicing today have been schooled in these theories.

It is also questionable how many therapists have changed their traditional views of women outside of the major cities in which the women's movement flourishes. As recently as 1978, I participated in a panel discussion at a women's conference in Missoula, Montana, in which a local psychiatrist told an audience of feminist women that women needed therapy because they were basically vain, narcissistic, childish, and dependent.*

One of the main ways that Freud's theory of women continues to shape traditional psychiatric attitudes and practices toward female patients is through the use of the diagnosis hysterical personality. Freud defined the normal woman as vain, narcissistic, passive, masochistic, overly emotional, and childishly dependent. This definition corresponds almost exactly with the current psychiatric definition of hysterical personality as a disorder characterized by immaturity, vanity, narcissism, seductiveness, and dependency. Not surprisingly, as we may recall from chapter one, hysterical personalities are almost always women. Should a woman who would be considered normal by Freudian standards enter a psychiatrist's office, she is likely to be diagnosed as hysterical!

Freud himself had a hard time distinguishing the "normal" from the "neurotic" woman: they ended up looking very much alike. He admitted that the attainment of mature, normal femininity seemed to be a difficult and treacherous journey which few women completed successfully. Most women became neurotic.

Freud treated large numbers of these neurotic women, all diagnosed as having hysterical neurosis: a condition in which

* Anyone who doubts that the Freudian legacy for women is still very much alive might take a look at *Obstetrics and Gynecology,* a textbook widely used in medical schools throughout the country. It tells us that "the traits that compose the core of female personality are feminine narcissism, masochism, and passivity." These are none other than the three psychological traits that Freud designated as fundamentally feminine.

In this same textbook, the future doctors of America are advised to treat their female patients as docile children, helpless creatures of their biology who are totally dependent upon the benign paternalism of their doctors in order to survive the major events of their lives: labor, childbirth, and menopause. Women are presented throughout as "hysterical personalities" whose physical symptoms are to be viewed as evidences of emotional disorders.

Furthermore, the text tells us that, as masochists, women require pain and suffering, that female sexuality normally involves a "masochistic surrender to the man"; that "there is always an element of rape" in the sex life of the normal woman. Finally, "the [normal] woman gives up her outwardly oriented active and aggressive strivings for the rewards involved in identification with her family and . . . sacrifices her own personality to build up that of her husband."[3]

the woman exhibited gross symptoms of the voluntary nervous system that were thought to be psychological in origin (for example, blindness, deafness, paralysis). In the nineteenth and early twentieth centuries, such conversion symptoms, as they were called, were quite common among women. (There were virtually no male hysterics.) But in contemporary times, these somatic signs of underlying conflicts have become more and more rare—largely because the repression of women's emotional and sexual lives has eased up. Thus nowadays, psychiatrists are less likely to diagnose a hysterical neurosis than in Freud's day.

But this doesn't mean there are fewer *hysterics* around. While the diagnosis of hysterical *neurosis* has decreased, it has been supplanted by the diagnosis of hysterical *personality*. Thus, in Freud's time, to be diagnosed as a hysteric, a woman had to be showing symptoms that often severely impaired her ability to function. But nowadays a hysteric just has to look and act like an ordinary "feminine" woman, perhaps somewhat exaggerated in her femininity.

The culmination of the Freudian legacy for women is the psychiatric double bind: in order to be normal, women must embody a set of characteristics that are then diagnosable as pathological by psychiatric experts.

The clincher in this double bind, as we have seen, is that any woman who defies (consciously or unconsciously) the conventions of normal femininity is also seen as pathological. The case of Lucy on the inpatient ward is a good example. Because Lucy was overtly angry, aggressive, and verbally challenging— that is, because she exhibited "masculine" rather than "feminine" behavior—she was considered to have a serious borderline character disorder. Her rebelliousness against normal femininity was taken as a sign that she was even more pathological than the ordinary feminine hysteric.

Clearly psychiatry has had, and continues to have, a double standard of mental health for men and women—a standard which ends up devaluing women. In this it has both reflected and contributed to women's inferior position in society.

Up until the last few years, the only way that a woman could be considered normal in our society was to become psychologically subservient to men. To win the approval of those who had power over her, she had to give up all hopes of having power herself. To be recognized as feminine, she had to obliterate herself as a person. To be loved by men, she had to learn to serve them. To get her needs met, she had to exhibit only those needs that were appropriate for "feminine" women; and even here she had to be careful not to need too much, lest she be seen as hysterically dependent on others. To be seen as a woman she had to make herself invisible as a person.

The normal woman was the happy housewife whose family discovered that she was a hidden alcoholic. She was the woman who had everything—home, husband, children, material comfort—and felt that she was slowly dying inside. She was the romantic woman who gave up everything to keep her man, and fell apart when he left her. Or she was the career woman who preferred the company of men and felt superior to other women. She was the heterosexual woman who was homophobic, or the closet lesbian who never felt quite right as a woman. Isolated and divided from other women, she felt complete only when she was dominated by a man. She was the woman who consciously and unconsciously refused to admit how angry she was and why.

These "normal" women have been the inevitable result of a society in which men dominate women. Women have learned to accept this domination by being systematically deceived into believing, both consciously and unconsciously, that the social condition of female powerlessness is "feminine"—that powerlessness is normal.

The raw data upon which Freud drew his conclusions about female psychology were the conflicts that women had about being normal women. Indeed, many of his female patients were engaged in both overt and covert rebellions against normal womanhood. These rebellions were inevitable in a society in which the development of woman as a feminine being was largely incompatible with the development of woman as a person in her own right. The Freudian norm of femininity, in which woman is seen as an incomplete and mutilated man, is a simple reflection of woman's traditional dilemma: to be a woman, she must behave as a mutilated person; to be a person she must see herself, and be seen by others, as a woman who mistakes herself for a man.

Specific norms of femininity have varied, to some extent, historically and culturally. They have also varied, to some extent, with a woman's race and class. But whatever the variations, they have always been male norms. And they have always been norms that devalue women in comparison to men. In this sense, woman has always been socialized to be Woman as Victim.

Consequently, without a strong feminist movement, it has been difficult for women to see ourselves in our own terms. Each stage of a woman's existence, including the most intimate aspects of her bodily and self awareness in menstruation, sexuality, childbirth, and menopause, has been partly shaped by the masculine cultural artifact called femininity. In the absence of a social movement by which women can begin to discover ourselves and each other, to know who we are apart from the male image of what a woman is or should be, it has been more or less inevitable that women see ourselves as men see us.

This male identification, or identification with woman-as-seen-by-man, has been the gauge of the culturally feminine woman. The feminine woman has been the woman who accepts that her aspirations can know no greater fulfillment than the entrapment of a suitable man to fill her up. She has been the woman who thoroughly relinquishes her right to any ambition of her own. She has been the pregnant woman who dreads having a female child and prays for a boy. She has been the woman who knows that her job is to clean house for her husband and who doesn't question the assumption that housework is a function of her nature, rather than socially useful but unpaid labor that benefits men as a group. She has been the woman who experiences her greatest moments of sexual pleasure at the point at which she feels most sexually dominated—or the woman who feels little pleasure at all, but fakes it. She has been the woman who has lunch with the boys and laughs, when they do, at the "dumb" office secretaries. She has been the woman who accepts the myth that competence in the public world is incompatible with being a woman—and who therefore gives up the public world to remain female or enters the public world by imitating men. She has been the woman who feels flattered when she is treated like a body without a mind. She has been the woman who desperately tries to mold her body to men's liking—following all the styles and being on a constant, self-enforced starvation diet—but who hates her body. She has been the woman who confuses male paternalism with respect. The feminine woman has been the *man-made woman,* the woman who sees herself through male eyes.

Some of these specific manifestations of femininity are in the process of cultural decline. Others continue more or less unchanged. But unless women engage in the self-conscious process of collectively defining ourselves from our own point of view, femininity will remain what it has always been: a state of consciousness in which female identity is partly determined by what men need and want from women.

In learning to see ourselves as men see us, we have learned how to devalue, limit, and hate ourselves. The dilemma of being a man-made woman has been experienced in isolation, as a personal problem. The internalization of the cultural tension between the attainment of femininity and personhood in the modern age of psychology has been manifested in what appear to be irrational, personal conflicts or "symptoms."

Women in therapy and out are often beset with these symptoms. We have recurring headaches or stomachaches or backaches or menstrual pain. We alternate between eating too much and starving ourselves. We don't want sex but pretend we do, or we want sex but find it unsatisfying. We bite our nails or slash our wrists. We are terrified of being alone. We beat our children, whom we love. We feel guilty, not about something specific, but as a permanent condition. We cry hysterically for apparently no reason. We feel incapable of integrating work and family. We feel empty and lost and panicked and worthless. We hate our bodies. We are depressed. We feel powerless.

These are the symptoms of femininity. Most women have experienced one or several of them, or know women who have. The symptoms are systematically socially produced. Yet they are experienced as, appear to be, and are diagnosed as wholly individual and personal. Thus the "cure" that traditional therapy peddles for the relief of these symptoms is part of the problem. Traditional therapy confirms the man-made woman in her most deeply internalized conviction of personal failure.

From the dominant (male) point of view, female symptoms are indications of pathology. But from the submerged (female) point of view, they are often manifestations of the victim psychology of women. They reflect women's ambivalent adaptation to and rejection of normal femininity. Just as the women whom Freud examined rebelled against their feminine lot, so do women today. And often, we still do so through the creation of symptoms that manifest our rebellions without openly declaring them.

Despite the rise of feminist ideas, the symptoms of femininity persist. Old patterns of socialization do not simply disappear with new ideas. In fact, an accurate measure of how the traditional norm for femininity continues to create problems for women is the persistence of traditional female symptoms such as depression, psychosomatic pain, and so-called frigidity.

The hidden component in female symptoms is a powerhouse of suppressed rage. Women have learned to convert anger into symptoms that allow us to be feminine and to rebel against femininity at one and the same time. Normal femininity, in this sense, is a treasure chest for traditional therapists, guaranteeing that Woman as Patient will endure and keep on paying for therapy.

This is not to say that women have not changed or are not changing. On the contrary, in the past decade we have been collectively defining ourselves from our own point of view on a grander scale than ever before in history. The traditional definition of normal womanhood epitomized by the Freudian norm is being actively challenged. Male and female psyches are in a state of upheaval. More people than ever before are questioning what it means to be masculine and feminine.

As a result, the Liberated Woman has arrived on the cultural scene, embodying a new norm of femininity. This new norm reflects the ambiguities of the position of women in our society today. On the one hand, the image of the Liberated Woman is freeing: she is the woman who has been emancipated from the tyrannical force of sex roles. But on the other hand, the image of the Liberated Woman reflects how male society has assimilated and pacified the potentially revolutionary message of the movement for women's liberation. The Liberated Woman, in this sense, is compatible with a society which has made only minimal concessions to the demands of women for full, structural equality with men.

According to this new male cultural standard, the Liberated Woman has all the traditional masculine virtues: intelligence, competence, rationality, discipline, a keen business sense, the capacity for hard work and team loyalty, even an athletic body. At the same time, through some act of cultural grace, she retains the old feminine virtues without which a woman in our society is still not seen as a woman: nurturance, beauty, and sexuality. Though she is every bit as capable as a man, she is still sexy after all these years. Her masculine virtues, when embodied in the female form, attain a distinctly feminine sexiness they didn't have before. She is a far cry from Freud's normal Victorian hausfrau. She is no longer required to have male babies. But she is still required to keep her body beautiful for men. She is still essentially identified with her body. Now, as always, she continues to pay the price of this identification, including rape and battering. The feminine woman is still Woman as Body (see chapter nine).

What this society has not yet accepted is the terrifying possibility of an actual equality of the sexes which would make the words "masculinity" and "femininity" obsolete. The norm of the Liberated Woman reflects a significant broadening of the old psychic restrictions. But there is still a cultural necessity for women to remain feminine (and for men to remain masculine).

Furthermore, the Liberated Woman is still, in some ways, a standard for femininity that ends up subordinating women to men. In reality, as opposed to media image, she is still oppressed. At work, she is more likely to be a secretary than an executive. Her fulfilling career is often a low-paid, insecure position in the pink-collar ghetto. She is much more likely to take orders than to give them. If she does give them, she almost always gives them to other women. She still gets less pay and has less chance of upward mobility than a man. And the Liberated Woman at home still does most of the housework and retains primary responsibility for the children.

Yet despite all this, the Liberated Woman is not pictured as harried, bedraggled, or angry. She is pictured as fulfilled and complete. Like other norms of femininity, the Liberated Woman image reflects, in part, the societal demand that women accept the status quo. The feminine woman, whichever way she is defined, does not rock the boat.

This is not to say that the Liberated Woman doesn't have some things to be happy about. In the heyday of the "feminine mystique," the career woman was pictured as a dried-up old spinster with no sexuality or family life. She sacrificed the joys and requirements of femininity in order to be like a man. But since femininity and masculine-style work are no longer seen as necessarily incompatible, the Liberated Woman is not required to make this kind of sacrifice. She is not only allowed but encouraged to "bring home the bacon, fry it up in a pan, and still make you feel like a man" (in the words of a TV advertisement). In short, the Liberated Woman is supposed to be and have and do it all—the Liberated Woman is Superwoman.

The old norm of femininity coexists with this new mythic ideal of Superwoman. But the personal fulfillment of Superwoman can easily coexist with the continued oppression of women as a group. For by definition, only a few women will ever make this mark. Despite the ideological advances of feminism, the Liberated-Superwoman takes her place in a society that has not yet made the basic socioeconomic changes it would take to liberate women as a group. Though, in theory, Superwoman is confronted with more life choices than ever before, the achievement of these choices remains almost as difficult as ever. This is because, for the most part, the personal and cultural changes in attitudes about femininity in our society have not been met with significant political and economic changes in the structure of social institutions. In the family, new attitudes about sex roles are reflected in a piecemeal way. Women who wish to establish an equal partnership in marriage and family life are still dependent on finding the "right man" to support them in their endeavors. (The feminist version of the right man is the man who is devoted to women's freedom. I would venture to say that this makes a good man as hard to find as ever.) Those women who choose lesbianism continue to suffer the social and economic consequences. Without a social transformation of family life (for instance, in the form of wages for housework), these individual attempts at social change can go only so far.

Changes in sex role attitudes in the workplace are even more limited. Though more and more women are entering the labor force, jobs continue to be sexually segregated, with women in the lowest paid, most insecure, and nonunionized positions. The assimilation of women into the labor force has not resulted in the clear-cut victory of more economic independence for women as a group. Of the increasing number of female heads of households, for instance, more and more are becoming impoverished. Economically, women as a group are more wretchedly poor than they were before the advent of the women's movement. (See chapter nine, "Women and the Labor of Relatedness," for an analysis of how women's socioeconomic position affects the formation of female identity and results in specific emotional problems for women.)

The tokenism by which a small minority of women are

allowed greater access to formerly all-male positions of power in business and government serves to mystify the fact that satisfying labor outside the home is still as distant a prospect for most women in our society as it is for most men.

Thus despite the ways in which it has led to greater freedom of choice for men and women, the ideology of feminism continues to be in conflict with the traditional values and economic structure of our society. It is too early to tell how that conflict will be resolved, for the battle is still in progress. The New Right, the "Moral Majority," and the Reagan administration actively threaten recent gains in women's rights. History shows us that radical ideological departures such as feminism often occur in waves which surface with enormous energy and then gradually resubmerge under the force of social reaction. Judging from the dismal fate of the ERA, this society may not yet be committed to accepting even the basic principle of equal rights for women, much less to achieving those rights in practice.

In short, women as a group are not yet equal to men as a group in our society. In this sense, the *real* liberated woman has not yet come into existence. Without the socioeconomic changes necessary to accommodate her needs, she will not do so. Feminism will be yet another value system, rather than an instrument of overall social transformation. In a society not yet committed to reorganizing the structures of social institutions to meet women's needs, the Liberated Superwoman's task (to succeed in the way that men have, while continuing to succeed in traditional feminine ways as well) is barely possible.

There have always been women who have managed to defy both the conventions and the organization of a society based on the subordination of women. Certainly, we can foresee more and more women carrying off this new ideal and feeling more whole than ever before. At the same time, as the mythic idea of Superwoman more and more establishes itself as the new norm for femininity in our society, I foresee a whole new host of problems for women as a group. The Superwoman ideal has already led to a new set of conflicts for women who wish to be liberated and blame themselves for not making it * (for an example, see chapter ten's section, "Dependence/Independence: Dilemmas of the 'New Woman' ").

Women in the 1950s who failed to meet the Freudian norm of femininity were diagnosed as neurotic. My prediction is that, as the Liberated-Superwoman more and more becomes the established norm for femininity, the psychiatric establishment will once again declare women who do not meet the norm mentally unhealthy. What will remain essentially unchanged in all of this is the fact that the norm for mental health for men and women will still be equated with masculinity and femininity, respectively. There will still be a double standard for mental health. (Men will not have to be Supermen: they will just have to be men.) And women who live in a situation of sexual inequality will continue to pay the psychic costs.

* In a *Boston Globe* article headed "Superwoman, Class of '82: Her Choices," a Wellesley college senior was quoted as saying: "They tell us at Wellesley that we don't have to be Superwoman but 'you may as well try.' If that's what I have to be when I grow up, I don't want to grow up." (See *Boston Globe*, May 23, 1982).

4
CHAPTER

Polly Patient:
An Introduction

This book is divided into three major parts. The final chapter of each part traces a "day in the life" of Polly Patient in a typical therapy session in the traditional, humanist, and feminist modes, respectively.

Polly is not a real person, but a composite of many real women whom I have seen over the past ten years of doing therapy. She is the woman whom traditional psychiatry would diagnose as "hysterical personality." As a patient, she would no doubt be familiar to many therapists. As a woman, she is likely to be familiar to many women and men—both in and out of therapy. Polly is Woman as Victim. She is familiar with feelings, and she is practiced in using them against herself. Whatever Polly feels, she feels that she shouldn't be feeling it. Mostly, her feelings cluster painfully in the range of sadness–hurt–fear–shame–self-loathing–helplessness–despair. Anger is not generally a part of this spectrum and intrudes itself into her consciousness only rarely, often against considerable resistance. Even when she does let herself feel it, it is almost always the anger of the Victim: the frustrated rage of the child in the face of unconquerable parental forces. The anger of impotence. Brittle and fragile as an icicle, it is anger that soon loses its contours and melts into the habitual lake of self-contempt and despair. Or, as Polly herself is more apt to call it, depression.

The major ingredients of depression—an abiding sense of powerlessness and self-hatred—are so routine for Polly that she may not recognize them as separate, discrete feelings. She is used to sleeping poorly—waking early or not being able to fall asleep at night. She is accustomed to an assortment of pills for sleeping and calming herself (ranging from over-the-counter buys to the tried and trusted Valium).

Polly explains her depressions the same way she explains almost everything about her life: she is sure that she is in pain because she isn't good enough. Whether it's that she is earning too little money as a low-paid secretary in a generally under-paid occupation, or that an acquaintance has just committed suicide, or that the man she is with turns out to be a liar—whatever the problem, Polly sees herself as the root of it. She assumes that if she could only pull herself together and be perfect, then she would deserve to get what she wants. But she is never sure what she wants. Superficially, Polly may some-times look like someone who likes to blame others for her prob-lems (especially her mother). But, at bottom, Polly believes that everything is her own fault and her own doing. She doesn't know the limits of her power.

At the same time, Polly scrupulously avoids exerting what little power she has and might use to prevent herself from get-ting repeatedly victimized in her relationships. Because she feels powerless and is terrified of her anger, she is the perfect victim. Polly is compulsively "nice": the kind of person who is an easy target. She is always feeling sorry for people. Her com-passion extends to everyone but herself. She is tempted to take in any stray cat that crosses her path—the sorrier the specimen, the stronger the temptation. Her compassion for men often fol-lows the same rule: a man in need of her has found the goose that lays the golden egg. She is often so busy nurturing that she fails to see, or act on, the ways that men (and women) are taking advantage of her. Standing up for herself seems less important than being needed. Moreover, she tends not to trust her own perceptions about her relationships.

As for her own needs, Polly is likely to describe herself as "needy"—a way of expressing her conviction that her needs are unjustified or out of scale. Polly is always hungry—and always on a diet (or just off a diet, or just about to be on one.) It is the same with emotional food. She wants but doesn't take in. She needs but doesn't believe she deserves when she gets. Getting makes her feel guilty.

Polly is obsessed with "relationships"—by which she means relationships with men. She often has close women friends, but they are not what counts. She tends to take these friendships for granted and doesn't work on them in the same way she does at "relationships." When she thinks of intimacy she thinks of men, though there are things she will tell her women friends that she wouldn't dare tell her male lover.

Polly has ambivalent feelings about sex. She always looks forward to it eagerly but is often disappointed. The anticipation of sex with a man is itself a turn-on. But oddly, once her genitals are involved, she tends to withdraw and become detached. She often has the feeling of looking down on herself, watching herself make love: judging how "good" she is, trying to do all she can to please her partner while ignoring what she wants for herself. This sense of detachment bothers Polly, but she tries not to think about it. She is rarely orgasmic, but is not above faking it with a lover. In fact, she takes some pride in the fact that most men she's slept with have had no idea of how distant she really was. (The other side of this is a strong feeling of contempt that she harbors against these men, but she tries not to think about this either.) The part of sex that Polly likes most is the kissing, cuddling, and hugging—the feeling of being close to someone. Foreplay is often more emotionally and sexually satisfying than actual intercourse. But again, Polly does not actively admit this to herself. Underneath, there is a gnawing fear that despite her superficially sexual appearance, she is actually "frigid."

Polly is a woman who worries about her looks—whether she is "plain" or "pretty" by conventional cultural standards. She follows the fashions, whether she can afford the expensive department store items or only their cheaper, bargain-store imitations. Her nightmare is there in the noticeable wrinkle, the sagging breast, the bulging thigh.

Many of Polly's characteristics appear in woman of any age. But in order to give Polly some real shape, I have had to make some of her features more determinate. I have made her, like many of the women I see in therapy, in her mid-twenties to mid-thirties and single. And like most of the women in private, individual therapy (because they are the only ones who can afford it), she is middle class and educated. She is intelligent, but she thinks of herself as stupid. She has chosen not to marry, though she doesn't think of this as a choice so much as an unwanted and dismal fate. She has always maintained her economic independence—earning her own living rather than relying on a man, but thinks of herself as dependent. Like millions of working women, she is a secretary.

Finally, Polly is an experienced therapy patient. She has suffered from sometimes devastating and paralyzing bouts of depression. She has been in therapy, on and off, for years. Sometimes she comes to me with her diagnosis in hand ("I am a borderline personality"), having read the psychiatric textbooks and internalized the contents. Even if she hasn't actually gone this far, she is most certainly psychologically acute and aware. She is always ruminating about and analyzing herself. She has read numerous self-help psychology books, and "psyching people out" is what she does over coffee with her female friends and in her spare time.

Now for a note about the therapy sessions themselves. I have tried to describe typical sessions. By "typical" I mean that they represent the major therapy strategies practiced by the therapist and the likely responses of the patient to these strategies. For the purpose of elucidation, all three therapy sessions are "telescoped"—that is, they represent somewhat more than might actually take place within any single hour.

Representing the typical therapy session is as tricky as embodying the typical female therapy patient. Some of the fine points that make therapy sessions and people what and who they are are bound to be absent. Despite this, I hope that what emerges will strike many female readers who have been therapy patients as recognizable, and that those who have not been patients will get a taste of what they've been missing.

5

CHAPTER

The Traditional Model:
Polly Patient versus the Doctor

Polly arrives at the doctor's office. Today, as for the past several weeks, Polly's problem is her boss—an executive in an engineering firm in which she is a secretary. Although he is a married man, her boss has been flirting with Polly off and on for months. She has grown accustomed to all the patting and pinching. They are expected aspects of a working girl's life, like making coffee and smiling. But in recent weeks, her boss has been stepping up his flirtations. He has asked Polly to stay after five o'clock, though the work load doesn't seem to warrant her overtime. For the most part, Polly has obliged him, because she is scared that she will lose her job if she doesn't.

Alone with Polly after hours, her boss has been caressing her, and telling her how unhappy he is with his wife. He has implied that he would give her a raise if she slept with him. Frightened of losing her job, but also frightened of his sexual advances, Polly has been playing innocent: pretending not to understand his insinuations, flirting with him just enough to keep him from feeling rejected, but not enough to encourage him too much. This hasn't been easy. Several times, she has managed to get out of staying late by feigning illness. More often, she hasn't needed to pretend: she has been plagued by headaches so severe that they have kept her out of work.

Polly doesn't know what to do about her boss, or how to feel. He is such a nice man, and most of the time he treats her

107

well. She has a decent salary and fringe benefits. But there's no denying it: she's scared of him. Especially when they are alone together after hours. Sometimes, she actually fears he might rape her! But how foolish—he's her boss, not a rapist! There is a vague, confusing sense of being used, which fills Polly with a dumb rage. Sometimes, she wants to strangle him. Her anger frightens her and makes her feel guilty.

She is suspicious of his motives: why does he keep her overtime? It's not really clear it's sex he wants at all. Perhaps he knows she could use the overtime pay and is just being nice. Maybe he's just being friendly and she's making this whole thing up—sexualizing their relationship. Or maybe even provoking his sexual come-ons, as her doctor suggests. Is she being a tease without knowing it? And anyway, what if he really does have a terrible wife and would like to sleep with her? What's so wrong with that? She should be flattered—and actually, she does feel awfully attractive around him. Perhaps she ought to sleep with him and stop being such a prude. (Then she wouldn't have to feel so guilty for refusing him.) Sometimes she finds him sexually attractive. (But this makes her feel guilty too.) It's so hard to sort any of this out: the overwhelming sense of guilt and shame. That sick way she feels in her stomach. Her constant headaches. Her attraction to a man who makes her so mad. She needs her doctor to help her put it all together—by taking it all apart.

For several weeks, the doctor has been questioning her about what she might be doing to provoke her boss's sexual advances. He has this theory that she really, unconsciously, wants to arouse her boss sexually—that her fear of being raped is really the flip side of her unconscious wish to be sexually invaded by an older man. The doctor seems to think that all of this has something to do with her early sexual feelings toward her father. She doesn't remember these feelings because, since they were taboo, she repressed them, along with her anger at her father for loving her mother. All of these feelings (which the doctor calls her "unresolved Oedipal conflicts") are reflected now in her attraction to older, remote, father-like men

—like her boss. She tries to make herself special to the boss, by flirting with him sexually. But at the same time, she avoids any real sexual encounters.

Though Polly has always respected the doctor's wisdom, these sessions have somehow felt all wrong to her. (The doctor calls this her resistance.) Her guilt feelings have been getting stronger and stronger, and she has been feeling more and more depressed. Her dread of therapy is, at times, overwhelming. Often her headaches are worse after a session than before. Sometimes she even wonders if the doctor is really helping her. She feels angry and wants to quit therapy altogether. But other times, she longs wildly for his acceptance. She feels she would do anything to please him—if she only knew what! Does the doctor think she should stop flirting with the boss or have an affair with him? It's so hard to say, since he thinks that both her seductiveness and her fear of a real sexual relationship are neurotic.

At the door of the doctor's office, Polly is filled with a renewed sense of dread. The nauseating guilt that has accompanied her for months is heightened at this moment to a shrill note of self-doubt and fear. Her anger flutters like an insect at the windowpane, dim but persistent. What will the doctor have to say today?

The doctor has been waiting for Polly. He is curious what material she will turn up today. No doubt, she will want to talk about her boss, as she has for the past several weeks. She has been an interesting case, a classic hysteric. Seductiveness, so characteristic of the hysteric, is very much a part of her defensive behavior, masking an underlying fear of real intimacy. The doctor knows this, not only by her diagnosis, but by using his own countertransference feelings as a guide to the patient's pathology. He has seen the coyness with which she enters the office, the movement of her hips, and the shy but sexy smile with which she greets him. His sexual arousal has been a clear indication of her seductiveness. Her unresolved Oedipal strivings toward older, father-like figures is unmistakable. (After all, she has never openly repelled her boss's advances.) Polly has been resisting these interpretations of her feelings and behavior. But this is par for the course. Repressed, unconscious material surfaces only with great difficulty and much resistance.

In thinking about Polly's case at this point, the doctor has ascertained that she is in the middle phase of therapy. In this phase, the patient's transference is at its height. But so too is her transference resistance. It is time for the therapist to interpret that transference explicitly: he must make her aware of her sexual feelings toward himself, the doctor. Exploring Polly's Oedipal fixations with regard to her boss has been important. It has laid the groundwork for the transference work that must be done. Still, interpreting the transference directly always raises the resistance—and it will certainly do so in this case. Polly will probably deny having any sexual feelings toward him. Judging from her persistent anger at her boss, a transference interpretation is likely to make her quite angry at him, the doctor. In all likelihood, this anger will not be expressed directly, but, rather, in the form of passive/aggressive hostility. The doctor is prepared for this.

When Polly enters the office, she smiles as always (*Why do I always feel so nervous?* she thinks) and takes her usual seat. She clears her throat, fumbles with her collar, and crosses her legs. "How are you?" she asks, knowing that she will not really get a response—but how can you just come in and not ask a person how he is?

The doctor nods his greeting.

This is the signal that Polly is to start talking about her problems. Starting is always the hardest part. That terrible, gaping silence at the beginning—better anything than that silence.

"My boss had me work late again last night. There really wasn't much for me to do. He had me take dictation, but it was nothing pressing. He kept telling me how attractive I was, that a girl like me could be a movie starlet instead of just a secretary. That I deserved more than boring office work—or at least higher pay, and all sorts of things like that. He told me that things with his wife were getting worse and worse and he thought they would probably get a divorce. He said if he'd only married someone like me, everything would have been alright because I was so much more kind and sympathetic than his wife. I knew he wasn't for real, but I felt sorry for him."

Polly pauses here and, seeing that the doctor says nothing, knows that she is to continue.

"Anyway, he ended up asking me to go out for dinner and a drink with him. I didn't know what to do, so I ended up going. All through dinner all he talked about was how beautiful I am and how I deserve a man to make me happy. He insisted on driving me home and I let him because it was so late at that point. Then, in front of my house, while we were parked, he kissed me and started to unbutton my blouse. I told him to stop but he wouldn't. I really didn't want to hurt his feelings, so I kept trying to find some nice way to get him to stop, y'know, but he just didn't listen. So finally, I wrenched myself away and yelled at him. First he looked very hurt, and then he got angry. He opened the door and told me to get out."

At this point in her story, Polly, feeling as though she might cry, hesitates—hoping for some kind of response from the doctor.

"Uhm hmn." (*As I thought, the Oedipal feelings have become overwhelming. The characteristic seduce-and-run pattern of the hysteric: her wish for Oedipal gratification, followed by the panic when the fantasied possibility of it becomes more real.*)

Hearing the "uhm hmn," somehow so encouraging and yet so noncommittal, Polly's eyes tear up with a vague anguish and pain. (*If only he would say something,* she thinks.) "I don't know what to do. I'm really scared now that he'll fire me. I feel so depressed." (*It's always safe to say I'm depressed.*)

Still there is silence and, obediently, Polly continues.

"He was so angry with me last night and this morning he was colder than he's ever been toward me. He gave me orders without even a smile. Then this afternoon, he yelled at me in front of the other secretaries over a trifle: I misspelled a word in a letter. He told me I was getting lazy and inefficient and ought to pay more attention to my work. And he threatened to fire me if I didn't." *(I never should have gone out to dinner with him. It's all my fault. I wish the doctor would say something.)*

Polly is silent now. She sits and waits—wanting, but knowing that she will not get, some sympathy from the doctor. The doctor sits and waits too—knowing that Polly's dependency needs are strong and that he must not give in to them. She looks down at her feet. He stares out the window.

It is the familiar, silent war of attrition between doctor and patient: the war Polly almost always loses. In the end, she has less tolerance for the silence than he does. Usually, after a few minutes, the silence pounds in Polly's ears like a drum and she is ready to say anything at all to make it stop. Or the thought of spending sixty dollars to sit in silence spurs an immediate torrent of words.

But today, Polly is feeling more stubborn than usual. She sits and waits. He sits and waits. *(He's cold,* thinks Polly). *(She's resistant,* thinks the doctor.)

They sit and wait. When Polly glances at the clock, she sees that ten minutes have passed. She wonders how much longer this can go on before she submits. She considers saying something, but, seeing the doctor shift his weight, she thinks better of it.

The doctor is impatient today and wants to get on with it. After ten minutes, he has had enough. When he clears his throat, Polly smiles inside *(I won!).* But her joy is short-lived. Hearing his words, she winces.

"Your resistance is obviously at its height today, Polly. But we must continue with this work, even if it is very difficult for you. Tell me, when your boss started to make love to you last night, how did you feel?"

The expression "make love" jolts Polly. It seems to be the wrong word for what happened. A quick image of how the scene in the car must appear to the doctor crosses her mind: a picture of torrid sexuality, of her boss's lust and her own responsiveness. The old shame returns, and she answers the question feeling more like a defendant on trial for some nameless crime than a patient with a doctor.

"I felt confused. I didn't know what to say or how to tell him to leave me alone. But he seemed so forlorn and it's so hard for me to say no. Because I'd accepted his invitation, part of me felt I had no right to turn him down sexually—which made it harder for me to sound convincing when I told him to stop. Then, when he wouldn't, I started to feel scared and angry."

"But did you *really* want him to stop? Weren't you aroused by his touching you?"

A certain lightheadedness, the sensation of losing ground beneath her (a feeling familiar to her in therapy sessions), begins to flood Polly's consciousness at this moment. She talks automatically, the way a drowning woman flails at the water, though she knows she has no chance of survival.

"No—I mean, yes, I did feel a little turned on," she stammers, "but I didn't want him to go on."

"Of course you didn't. You wished to have sexual intercourse with him—but you felt terribly guilty about your wish. Naturally, your guilt was heightened when he started to undress you and you felt sexually aroused. Unconsciously, it was as if your own father were making love to you. So you repressed your wish and became angry instead. Now you are tormented by the fear that he will fire you. Your superego punishes you for your unacceptable libidinal desires."

Polly's eyes are brimming now, with humiliation and anger. She wants to scream "No! That's not it at all!" but she stops herself. (*It's my resistance again.*) She wavers, not knowing what to say. It never helps to contradict the doctor. It only gets her into further trouble. Still, impulsively, she blurts out: "This is all wrong! What happened has nothing to do with my libidinal desires! He just tried to take advantage of me and I ... I let him, but I didn't *want* to let him. . . ." Against her will, she dissolves into hopeless tears.

"It is difficult for you to accept these feelings. You fight me because you would like to banish them. You would like them to remain unconscious."

It is at times like this that Polly would like to kill the doctor. But, having an instinct for self-preservation, she doesn't tell him of her wish. Instead, she feels her body growing numb and all her feelings stop at once. *(What's the use? I was turned on in the car, and I've been feeling guilty ever since. He's probably right.)*

"What are you feeling?" asks the doctor in a gentler, almost fatherly tone. *(She can go either way now—more resistance or, hopefully, catharsis.)*

The kindness in the doctor's voice is disarming, and so unexpected that it triggers a new burst of tears in Polly.

"I don't know. I feel so ashamed," she sobs, "and what you're saying makes me so angry." (Though genuinely upset, there is a corner of Polly thinking, *He likes it when I cry: he always says something nice to me afterwards.*)

Seeing that his kindly tone is having the proper cathartic effect, the doctor continues.

"Of course you feel ashamed and angry, that's natural enough. It is not easy to admit these feelings about your sexuality. But you needn't blame yourself—every little girl experiences sexual feelings toward her father. In fact, these are part of the *normal* feelings of every married woman, too. All of your feelings will be resolved when you find your own mate, someone to love you exclusively and with whom you can desire to be sexually invaded without the accompanying guilt feelings."

This is more than the doctor usually says. He sits back in his armchair, assessing the effect of his interpretation.

Without exactly knowing why, Polly is moved. Her anger has been dissipated and she feels herself softening up. *(At least he's talking to me! Maybe he does care about me.)*

"I guess I just really feel like a bad patient sometimes," she says finally. "I know what you're saying is probably right but it always makes me so angry and upset. And then I feel guilty for being such a bad patient." There is a quiet resignation to her voice now.

"Why don't you let yourself free associate to these feelings?" *(Here, in these "bad girl" feelings, I will be able to make a smooth entry into a transference interpretation.)*

Polly closes her eyes to help herself free associate.

"I get angry at you when you talk about my Oedipal feelings. I want to tell you to shut up. That it doesn't help to hear all that shit. I just want you to comfort me and say something to make me feel better or tell me what to do about my problems. I'm resistant and stubborn. I'm a bad patient. Sometimes, I get scared that you'll get fed up with me and throw me out of therapy."

"What else, how else are you bad?"

"I'm childish. I want your approval all the time. I'm dependent on you."

"Have you ever had sexual feelings toward me?" (said in a clinical tone, but with a trace of suggestiveness about it—a tone the doctor has learned, through experience, helps to bring out the sexual transference).

Polly opens her eyes and blushes. Her blood begins to race with the same feelings of fear, shame, anger, and pleasure that she has when the boss flirts with her. Is the doctor flirting with her too? Abruptly, she remembers a fantasy she once had about making love to him, which she never told him about.

"Well, yes, I once had a fantasy about you." (*I'm lost now. I haven't the slightest idea where this session is going.*)

"Yes?" (*This is going better than I'd hoped!*)

By the tone of the doctor's voice, Polly knows that the doctor thinks that this unreported fantasy is somehow the key to all of her problems. The sense of momentousness is infectious: Polly hears herself telling the fantasy as though she were a third person listening to herself speak.

"Well, it was very short. I came into therapy and you were very cold and distant, which made me very angry. But then you started to make love to me and I felt better."

"How did you feel when I made love to you?"

"It felt good to be close to you, but also scary." (*I know there is something* important *about this fantasy, because I repressed it. But now we'll never get back to talking about what to do about my boss!*)

"It was frightening to feel yourself making love to me? It made you feel guilty?"

"I guess so—because I haven't thought of it since then. I must have repressed it."

"Since when?"

"Let's see. I guess I had the fantasy about three weeks ago, after a session."

"Which session?"

"I guess the first or second time we talked about what was going on at work, my feelings toward my boss. And you told me that you thought I was being sexually provocative toward him unconsciously."

"So you had this fantasy just at the start of our explorations of your unresolved Oedipal feelings. And here, in this sexual fantasy, we have the *very same elements* as in your feelings toward your boss: a desire to have intercourse with an older man; guilt at the fantasy of its gratification; and, in both cases, an expectation of punishment: that your boss will fire you, and that I will throw you out of therapy for being 'bad.' All of the feelings we've been exploring in the last few weeks, and all of the feelings you came in with at the start of this session—your sexual feelings toward your boss, your anger at him, your guilt and your fear of punishment, all of these 'bad girl' feelings toward your boss are *really* feelings you have toward me, aren't they?" *(A very clean transference interpretation.)*

Polly is silent now. She feels as though the curtain has descended on the final act of an exciting play with a depressing ending. She says nothing.

"What are you feeling, Polly?" *(Now for the passive/aggressive hostility. To be expected.)*

The sound of her first name, so rarely used by the doctor, evokes the dim stirrings of longing in her, the same longing as in her fantasy: to feel close to the doctor. But whereas these feelings would have been very sharp a few minutes ago, they are now clouded by a kind of general numbness.

"I don't know." Polly wants to say, "I feel tricked." But she knows this is her resistance talking, and she remains silent. Beneath her numbness, there is a dim rumbling of rage. But like a high cloud on the horizon, it threatens no immediate rain.

"You're angry, aren't you?" asks the doctor. But it is more like a statement than a question.

"No. I'm just thinking about what you said." *(He knows I*

*feel angry—and I've been angry with him for weeks! He al-
ways knows everything! Maybe he's trying to make me feel
angry with what he's saying, so that I can really get in touch
with it.)*

It is close to the end of today's fifty minutes and Polly feels
the onset of another one of her headaches. The dull, empty
numbness is familiar, almost soothing. But why this overwhelming sense of defeat? Perhaps she should explore this
with the doctor next session.

"It is time to end now," says the doctor. "See you next
week."

Polly stands up and slowly murmurs, "Yes, see you next
week," as the doctor accompanies her to the door and lets her
out.

II

Growth Is Not Enough:
THE FAILURE OF
HUMANIST THERAPY

6

CHAPTER

The Growth of
the Growth Therapies

The Father Knows Best model of therapy to which Polly
Patient is treated is the reigning clinical practice in the United
States today, both institutionally and ideologically. But perhaps
you do not see yourself in this picture. If you are accustomed
to thinking of yourself as a client rather than a patient; if your
therapist seems more like a compassionate guide than a rigid
father figure; if your therapy emphasizes human potential and
emotional growth rather than pathology; if it stresses here-and-
now problems rather than childhood trauma; if its focus is on
conscious awareness rather than on insight into unconscious
conflicts—then you are not a patient in traditional therapy. You
are a client in one of the many humanist or growth therapies
currently available.

Since Fritz Perls' popularization of gestalt therapy at the
Esalen Institute in California in the 1960s, a dazzling and often
bewildering array of new growth therapies has exploded on the
market. Gestalt, bioenergetics, transactional analysis, psychodrama, psychosynthesis, encounter, transpersonal therapy, pri-
mal therapy, guided fantasies, Arica training, EST . . . the
number of new therapies and therapy techniques is astonishing. Though enormously varied, all of these therapies of the
human potential movement share a basically humanist perspective. Taken together, they have offered a serious challenge to
the rule of traditional therapy in this country.

Humanist psychology in the United States developed as a maverick offshoot in a field dominated by behaviorist researchers and psychoanalytic practitioners. In the 1950s humanist psychology came to be known as the "third force" in psychology circles. Clinicians like Carl Rogers (one of the founding fathers of humanist psychology) wrote papers and books that were virtually heretical in their orientation to the business of psychotherapy.

Against the traditional emphasis on correct diagnosis and interpretation as major factors in therapy, Rogers insisted that it was the therapeutic *relationship* itself that was crucial. In contrast to the medical stress on individual pathology and its cure, Rogers introduced the idea of personal growth through therapy. He stressed the importance of holding the client responsible for his or her feelings and behavior, rather than viewing them in a crudely deterministic fashion. Consequently, the laborious review of childhood events so central to traditional therapy was considered by Rogers secondary at best. Instead, Rogers insisted that what was primary in the therapy process was that the therapist maintain an attitude of "unconditional positive regard" toward the client in order to foster a relationship maximally conducive to the client's growth.

Rogers refused to accept the complacent and rather self-serving belief on the part of traditional practitioners of therapy that a patient's presenting problems were, no matter how distressing to the patient, not the central concern of therapy, since they were merely symptomatic of the patient's underlying disorder. *

Instead, he believed that it was the client who should decide what she wanted to change about herself, not the doctor. Whereas insight (the goal of traditional therapy) was defined by the therapist, growth (the goal of humanist therapy) was de-

---

* One line of thinking in traditional circles is that it is actually dangerous for the therapist to intervene in a patient's presenting symptoms since they are presumed to be necessary to the patient's functioning. According to this view, to deprive the patient of her symptoms before her underlying unconscious conflicts have been successfully resolved is to risk the patient's decompensation. In other words, helping the patient with the problems she expressly wants to change can lead to her deterioration!

fined by the client. In contrast to traditional therapy, Rogerian therapy was aptly called "client-centered." [1]

The humanist psychology movement has, in some ways, been a progressive force in the psychotherapy world. It has radically shifted both the focus of therapy and its language of discourse. Its major contribution has been a turning away from myth 2 of the traditional system: the myth of the medical model of psychopathology. The growth therapies spawned by humanist psychology and emerging over the past twenty-five years have been founded on the simple belief that many people seek to overcome problems that are not necessarily related to illness and that these people are not served by being viewed as sick. Concomitantly, there has been a humanist modification of myth 3 of the traditional system: the myth of the Expert. The humanist therapist is not the patriarchal omniscient and omnipotent puppeteer who pulls all the strings. Instead, the humanist model of the therapist is that of a compassionate facilitator who helps you get in touch with your feelings so that you can achieve self-fulfillment.*

Some of the dangers of diagnosis and treatment chronicled in chapter one are thus avoided in the humanist therapies. If you are a female patient in humanist therapy, you are far less likely than your counterpart in traditional therapy to see yourself as a neurosis- or disease-ridden helpless patient dependent upon a powerful male authority (and the drugs he dispenses) for your cure. For Woman as Patient, the humanist therapies have offered an alternative.

But the alternative perpetuates some of the old mistakes of the traditional approach, while adding some new dangers of its own. The essential core of the humanist theory and practice of therapy is an unshakeable belief in the individual's capacity to create himself and his life. In contrast to the traditional view of

---

* Certainly one of the most innovative aspects of the new growth therapies is the shift from the attachment of traditional clinicians to individual therapy toward the untapped potential of groups to foster individual change. All-day and weekend workshops, short- and long-term groups are the stock-in-trade of the new growth therapies. This shift to groups entails a considerably reduced view of the importance of a powerful Expert and a greater reliance on the ability of people to help each other.

the self as a bio-social entity driven by its own instinctual impulses, the humanist view of the self is much lighter and freer.
The traditional self was weighted like a stone to its own nature
—and to the repression of its nature. The humanist self can fly.
The idea here is the simple proposition that you are responsible for your own reality—not society, not the environment, not
the past, but you as a person right now. Personal problems are
not seen as products of pathology, as in the traditional system.
But they are still seen exclusively as products of your own
mind.

Despite the enormous difference between the traditional
and humanist views of the individual, both rely on myth 1: the
myth that "it's all in your head." This myth continues to adversely affect clients of humanist therapy who blame themselves for lacking total control over their lives. And it continues
to undermine women with a new set of false promises of power
(see chapter seven).

Traditional therapy demanded a rigorous, disciplined commitment of years of individual analysis in return for a simple
cure of pathology. (Freud once said that curing the individual's
"neurotic misery" freed him to live out the "common unhap-
piness" that healthy people must endure.) The new growth
therapies, on the other hand, ask much less of the individual—
and promise much more. Weekend workshops promise to
change your life forever. Awareness groups offer to alter your
consciousness permanently. The latest growth technique holds
out the tantalizing allure of creating profound changes in your
personality which will bring you everything your heart desires.

The new growth therapies have, in fact, become a multi-
million-dollar industry whose product is nothing less than self-
liberation. One university marketing professor likened the personal growth industry to McDonald's—intending no slur by the
comparison. He was simply referring to the fantastic marketing
success of both growth experiences and hamburgers.*

* See *Boston Globe*, Oct. 16, 1978, article by Susan Trausch, "Mind Merchants at
Work to Help You Find Yourself."

The ultimate commodity on the market today is freedom itself—packaged, distributed, and sold by a number of different competing therapy firms, each with its own gimmick and guarantee of satisfaction, its own ticket to liberation: liberation through body awareness; liberation through expanded consciousness; liberation through assertiveness training; liberation through guided fantasies. Advertisements for growth therapy adventures assure us that it is easy and pleasant to be liberated. For instance, you can even do it while rafting down a river:

> This workshop will bring together two potentially powerful experiences: a gestalt group and a river expedition through the remote and rugged canyons of southeastern Utah. Here's a chance for you to run the river with a group of people who have a common orientation towards growth, a chance to learn about a river and to learn about yourself, and a chance to *utterly remove yourself from the business of the work-a-day world* so that you'll have the time, all the time you want, to find your center, to meditate, and to work with the others in the group. . . . For less than the price of a standard commercial river trip, you get Tag-A-Long's finest services and hospitality, plus the guidance of an experienced gestalt leader.*

The new growth therapies have become the ultimate consumer ride—at the end of which one finds what so many people in our society feel they lack: a self. Far away from the business of the "work-a-day world", you can find your "center": the pristine purity of self unencumbered by its social relations, the self that exists in the natural environment of a Utah river and can be purchased for less than the price of a standard commercial river trip.

Defined in this way, the self need not be concerned with that which is not essential to it: social reality. Growth is defined as the experience of an inner reality in a stress-free environment. Unlike the rewards of traditional insight—which come only after a painstaking and painful analysis of oneself, growth

---

* From a Tag-A-Long Tours brochure, italics my own.

can be won by getting away from it all. If you're feeling desperate, lonely, trapped in your life, you can take a trip—if not down a Utah river then an interior journey, for instance to:

> Nearikaya: visionary world of the Huichol Indians: two-day workshop. Consciousness becomes aware of itself, spewing forth as a playground of energy/light to experience itself, individuating within the experience of separateness, and reawakening to awareness of the timeless self . . . experiencing simultaneous existences, timeless and of all times. . . . Through the archaic tradition of shamanism, we will engage what Jung has called the "two million year old human" being residing in each of us; we do this in order to tap into the mythic roots which feed our awakened consciousness. In this weekend we will re-create a Huichol celebration of life. Costs $90 (includes room and board).*

Individualist escapism is proffered as the gateway to freedom. The more exotic the journey, the more appealing it is. The message is: find yourself by getting as far away as you can from who you are now in the social world.

Liberation through this kind of therapy is thought to depend on the accumulation of more and more growth. Growth becomes another market commodity necessary for our physical and mental well-being. Like a good laxative, growth therapy purges you of the garbage of the past and makes it possible for you to be open to consuming more and more growthful experiences.

In one humanist therapy newsletter, for instance, a therapist documented the use of a journal to monitor his personal growth. He recorded the "learnings" that he found helpful both in his everyday life and in his practice. The more "sensitized" he became to these learnings, the more his "growth curve spurted upwards." In the past year alone, this therapist was proud to assert, he had recorded over a thousand such learnings.

Like any good consumer product, growth can be compiled

* From Associates for Human Resources brochure, Fall–Winter 1976–77.

and accumulated. You can quantify your learnings to reassure yourself that you're okay—you're at least as growth-oriented as the humanist next door. Competition for growth becomes an important factor in the ersatz liberation offered by the growth therapies: the more different kinds of growthful experiences you have, the better off you are. This is not only good for your head, it's also good for the growth therapy business. (After several years of operation, the Erhard Seminars Training, better known as EST, was grossing 16 million dollars per year.)

For an increasing number of people, the freedom-loving optimistic ideology of the humanist orientation is far more attractive than the rather darker view of the unconscious to which traditionalists adhere. But in practice, the liberation of self-awareness that the growth therapist offers ends up looking very much like a solipsistic haven.

Take, for example, the "Gestalt Prayer," written by Fritz Perls, the guru of gestalt therapy:

> I do my thing and you do your thing.
> I am not in this world to live up to your expectations
> And you are not in this world to live up to mine.
> You are you, and I am I,
> and if by chance, we find each other, it's beautiful.
> If not, it can't be helped.[2]

I can think of no finer expression of the humanist view of the self than this little ditty. As in the traditional view, the self is seen as a spinning center with no particular connection to any other spinning center except, perhaps, if one such center should happen—by chance—to collide with another. Should such a meeting take place, so much the better. If not, the self spins off, happily ensconced in its warm cocoon.

The appeal of this prayer is immediate: it offers the reassurance that people are neither politically nor morally nor personally responsible for one another. You needn't feel obliged to change anything or anybody—you needn't feel guilty, so long as you satisfy yourself and "do your own thing." The unspoken assurance is that there is a thing for each one of us to do: you need only find out what it is and do it. "Do your own thing" is humanistic lingo for the great American myth that there are no social constraints on the freedom to fulfill yourself, that the universe is pleased to oblige your wishes and aspirations—so long as you are open to change. One thing is also as good as another—as long as its *yours*. All values are leveled and equated. My thing may be earning money, your thing may be spending it. His thing is being an anti-Semite, hers is getting beaten by the man she loves. Their thing is investing in the stock market. The Pentagon's thing is making nuclear weapons. It's all the same: you do your thing and I do mine.

If you are a client of humanist therapy, you learn not that you are sick, but that you are all-powerful. You and you alone are responsible for your own reality. There is, on the face of it, something very reassuring about this. All remnants of the past are dramatically swept away. So too are all current social influences—including the systematically organized forms of constraint on individual freedom that are built into our society. In the clear light of humanist ideology, you are a product of yourself; sprung free from your own forehead, like Athena from Zeus, you are creator of your own reality, born to win.

It is not difficult to see why the humanist therapies have done so well. The promise of total personal power they offer is rather more alluring than the powerless patient routine of traditional therapy. But the allure soon fades. What starts off as an optimistic assurance of power ends up as a preposterous burden. The Horatio Alger myth has long since been dispelled among the oppressed who know better. For every Horatio Alger there are millions of regular folk who never "make it."

The individual under the sway of humanist thinking is taught to incorporate all forms of social unfreedom within herself, and thereby to lessen their stranglehold. The idea is that you can transcend the social limitations on your life by internalizing them. For the middle-class and upper-class white man, this search for individual freedom represents at least a partial truth: social limitations do not exert the same kind of grip on him as they do on the poor of either sex. It is possible for many middle-class men—and women—to use the privilege they have in the search for "freedom" through growth therapy. They have the money and the leisure to do so. This freedom, of course, ends up looking curiously like an escapist paradise, sheltered from the brutalities of everyday life to which the majority of people in our society are heir. Nevertheless, whether it's a boat trip down a Utah river or a visit to the nearest growth therapy institute, this brand of freedom is something that the less privileged simply cannot afford to buy.

For most women—as well as for the economically and racially oppressed of both sexes—the myth of individual freedom sold by the new growth therapies is yet another betrayal. The impotence of the oppressed individual totally to alter the painful aspects of her existence *by herself* is not only ignored but perpetuated by an ideology that urges people to reject any forms of collective responsibility for one another's pain and to embrace instead absolute individual responsibility for one's own life. Thus the humanist orientation is ultimately useless to the oppressed. It becomes another blame-the-victim hype.

Contrary to the hype, however, consumers of growth therapy do not usually find freedom at the end of the line; often they find merely another ride on yet another therapy train. Growth psychotherapies may pander to the individual's desire to be free. They may thrive on the myth of all-powerful individualism. But, in the end, they often help to create not strong individuals but compulsive therapy consumers: people desperately in search of the new therapy or new pop psychology book or new technique that will finally set them free; people urgently seeking to buy what can be won only through the collective task of transforming the social world.

But if growth therapy clients don't find freedom in their therapists' offices, what do they find? What do the growth therapies actually offer? Most typically, they offer an opportunity for "self-awareness", a term which essentially gets down to awareness of one's feelings. In practice, the growth therapies' answer to how to get your head together is to get in touch with your feelings. Feelings are seen as the great gateway to freedom, and they are the bread and butter of the growth therapist. The assumption is that the more feelings you are aware of and can express, the more successful your therapy. The somewhat intellectual insight prized by the traditional therapist as the final product of successful therapy is, as far as the growth therapist is concerned, not where it's at. The trick is to get past these dead intellectualizations and into the lively business of spontaneous feeling combustions—to help the client get her feelings out.

In fact, the growth therapies have been quite innovative in the development of a variety of techniques designed to help clients get in touch with and express their emotions. Some of these techniques are body-oriented (bioenergetics, movement therapy); others concentrate on consciousness (gestalt); and some combine the two (psychodrama). The growth therapist is skilled in one or more of these techniques and applies them with as much conviction as the traditional therapist applies interpretations. Generally speaking, these techniques tend to be much more successful in helping clients become aware of and express feelings than the traditional "talking cure." An eavesdropper at the door of a traditional therapy session is likely to hear muffled speaking tones—usually of one voice only, while an eavesdropper at the door of a humanist therapy session is more likely to hear groans, shouts, weeping. Emotional catharsis is considered to be an aspect of traditional therapy, but it is not really emphasized, and there are few techniques to encourage it.

A typical growth therapy session, in this sense, can be far more emotionally satisfying to a client than a typical traditional therapy session (compare Polly's experience in chapter five to her experience in chapter eight). Emotional catharsis has a powerful and beneficent effect which, in and of itself, is therapeutic—at least in the short-term. Because such releases are both gratifying and colorful, they are often mistakenly seen by both therapists and clients as the sign of successful therapy. But releasing one's feelings, although an essential part of therapy, can sometimes be nothing more than a kind of "special effects" phenomenon. Like having a good temper tantrum, it can be cleansing—but it doesn't mean that one's feelings have been fully understood or resolved. One of the fatal flaws of the new growth therapies seems to be this confusion between technique and therapy.

This flaw hinges on the erroneous assumption, dear to humanist therapists, that once a feeling is released, understanding and clarity necessarily follow, that self-awareness automatically emerges from this kind of emotional house-cleaning. But as many clients of the new growth therapies know only too well, one can release one's feelings ad nauseam and still remain confused. One can "let it all out" a million times in a variety of ways and still not make any substantive changes in one's personality or life. This is especially likely if the therapist's guidance stops short at the point of emotional release and doesn't extend to helping the client make sense of the feelings she has released in the context of the rest of her life—including her social environment. Therapy that does not help her make these connections often ends up encouraging a brand of "self awareness" that is nothing more than a solipsistic and narcissistic indulgence in one's inner life, an obsessive self-preoccupation that mistakenly passes for self-knowledge. This is precisely why so many growth therapy clients tend to be compulsive therapy consumers: forever becoming more self-aware and forever "going through changes" yet somehow always remaining the same. The experience of emotional release can become addictive, especially if its accumulation is thought to result in profound self-transformation or in liberation that never comes.

In my own therapy practice, I am indebted to the growth therapies for certain active techniques to facilitate the expression of feelings, especially in cases where longstanding feelings have been blocked from consciousness and are interfering with the client's capacity to get on with her life. I might, for instance, suggest that a client use her fists or a tennis racket on a pillow as a means of coming face to face with her anger as a woman. This is simply a part of helping her use that anger in her life rather than repress it and use it against herself. There is a crucial difference between using a technique in this way, as a tool, and using it as an end in itself. The difference has to do with the therapist's view of what feelings are and how they are connected to a person's overall sense of herself and her life. (For a concrete example of the difference between the humanist approach to active techniques and my own, compare the use of pillow punching in Polly's therapy in chapter eight and chapter eleven.)

The therapist in the popular film *An Unmarried Woman* tells her client, the heroine (who has just been unceremoniously dumped by a husband who has been having an affair with a younger woman), that it is okay for her to feel bad. "Feelings," the therapist says, "have no IQ, no morality. They're just feelings. The only thing you can do with them is feel them." All feelings are acceptable, says this therapist—with the exception of guilt. Guilt comes from telling yourself a lot of "shoulds." Shoulds should be done away with. So should guilt. Guilt is the one feeling you should not have. One wonders what this therapist would make of the guilt of the man who systematically undermines his wife's confidence in herself by constantly putting her down? Or the guilt of the rapist? the wife batterer? the Nazi war criminal?

In the humanist view, feelings are fundamentally irrational. They exist in a social vacuum. They are simply to be discharged. There is no relation between feelings and morality, feelings and thinking, feelings and social life. The result, in practice, is that once a feeling is released, it is pacified.

One of the most blatant feelings of the heroine of *An Unmarried Woman* is anger. She is angry not only at her husband's unexpected betrayal, but at men in general, who seem, after her divorce, to be exclusively interested in her new availability as a sexual conquest, rather than as a person with a life of her own. This anger is viewed by her therapist as something to be gotten over rather than understood. The meaning of her anger, its social roots, how it connects to her dependency on men who by and large do not respect her as a person—all this is ignored. So too is the social meaning of the sense of shame she experiences after the divorce. Tracing the relation between these feelings and the sexual politics to which the heroine is subject is not part of her therapy. Instead, the humanist therapist urges her client to get past her anger so that she can "get back into the stream of life"—that is, hook herself up to another man as soon as possible. This is just one example of how the growth orientation to therapy, even with a sympathetic therapist, can end up ensuring that a woman's anger is "blown off" in therapy rather than used to further her own interests.

Therapy of this kind is totally compatible with society as it is. It has little to do with helping clients develop a more comprehensive self awareness—that is, an awareness that includes a sense of the relationship between their feelings and the structure of social life. This is one of the main reasons why attempts to marry the humanist approach to therapy with feminist ideals for women are bound to fail.

7

The Unsuccessful Marriage of Humanist Therapy and Feminism

In contrast to the masculine values of traditional therapy (the search for unconscious conflicts through a rigorous analytic discipline; the obedience to an Expert father-figure; the goal of intellectual insight), the values of humanist therapy are much more feminine: empathy, growth, relationship, emotional release. It would appear that these values can be more easily adapted to the practice of therapy especially suited to women's needs. Indeed, the humanist approach to therapy has found a receptive audience among women—therapists and clients alike.

Humanist beliefs and practices have influenced the development of a feminist approach to therapy for women in some important respects. Certain of these beliefs and practices are clearly more sympathetic to women than the traditional ones. The humanist focus on health rather than pathology is the most significant of these. It is like a breath of fresh air in a room reeking of formaldehyde. The humanist emphasis on therapy as a relationship between more or less equal people, rather than a treatment dispensed by an Expert to a patient, has also been an indispensable aspect of feminist therapy.

It was Carl Rogers who first spoke of "unconditional positive regard," empathy and honest self-disclosure as three qualities of the therapist which are necessary conditions of a successful therapeutic relationship. Without these conditions, said Rogers, clients don't seem to change, and therapy doesn't seem to work.[1] These essential qualities stressed by Rogers are key elements in my own approach to the therapeutic relationship (see chapter ten). But because the humanist approach to therapy fails to see the relationship between the personal psychic lives of clients and the social values and institutions which shape these lives, it ends up severely hampered in its use of the very skills proposed by Rogers. To empathize properly with a woman's story in therapy is not simply to display sympathy or to say "I know how that must feel." It is not enough to "mirror" back the client's feelings, as in Rogerian client-centered therapy. To empathize with a female client and to use that empathy in a therapeutically skillful way, it is first of all necessary that the therapist understand her. And to understand her, the therapist must go well beyond the myth that "it's all in your head" which is so essential to the humanist orientation—to a clear knowledge of the connections between the private and the public, the emotional and social in women's lives. Hence empathy, unconditional positive regard, honest self-disclosure and any of the other humanist therapy skills can go only so far if they do not take place in the context of a therapy that is based on a political understanding of women's problems.

Many feminist therapists have tried to adapt the humanist vision of psychology and therapy to such a political understanding. But, with the best of intentions, they have created a hybrid therapy that is problematic at best. The limitations and dangers of the humanist orientation end up defeating the feminist purposes of the therapy.

In *Notes of a Feminist Therapist*, for instance, Elizabeth Friar Williams puts forth a definition of feminist therapy which, by her own admission, is not different from her definition of any other (humanist) therapy. The goal of feminist therapy, says Williams, is "self-awareness in order to make the most meaningful choices and in order to experience a fully integrated self."[2]

The focus on self-awareness, the promise of meaningful

(free) choices at the end of the therapy road: this is the humanist brand of self-liberation in the feminist mode. The feminist therapist in this mode becomes the champion of woman as a whole person not limited by biology to certain designated sex roles but free to develop into a successful, self-aware, fully integrated individual.

In practice, this ideal of the humanist enterprise applied to women's liberation often ends by equating freedom and power for women with the choice and achievement of professional careers:

> I try to encourage women to stay in therapy until they have found a clear direction in terms of a career and until they know that they can perform and enjoy challenging work. One of my definitions of a "healthy" woman is a woman who is able to support herself in work that is fun for her and gives her a sense of competence. If she cannot do this, I consider her therapy incomplete, for if she is unskilled and inexperienced she cannot feel free from economic dependency (and therefore emotional dependency) on someone else.[3]

Williams' solution to women's oppression is grooming women for male-style careers. In order to achieve this goal, according to Williams, women need only look inside themselves and change their self-imposed limitations:

> I have very little doubt that by and large men's work orientation gives them much more than women's lack of work orientation gives them. The most important advantage among many, of having a serious work commitment, is that it gives people choices. A woman who can do nothing but housekeep . . . must either find a man . . . or live at the poverty level.[4]

The unstated assumptions in Williams' goals for women are that "woman's work" in the family, being unpaid and therefore unseen, is not work at all—only male-style work in the paid labor force is work; that the traditional work of child-rearing cannot be fun or challenging or demand competence; that

people who have careers or work for a wage are free from economic dependency; that financially rewarding, fun, and challenging work is available to anyone who is sufficiently self-
aware; that a woman's proper psychic commitment to such
work determines her economic condition and power in society.

Williams would like therapy to provide for women what
has presumably always been the prerogative of men: satisfying
labor outside the home. She declares that women who do not
succeed in finding such labor are not healthy. Who would not
want to support themselves by performing and enjoying challenging work? Certainly women who have performed the tedi-
ous labor of housework and the socially undervalued labor of
motherhood for free have internalized the low self-esteem that
goes with the job. No doubt many of these women would leap
at the chance to get what Williams wants therapy to offer them.
Many more women than before have come to recognize the
virtues of public, paid work in terms of greater emotional and
financial independence. And there is no doubt that having the
option of such work would greatly improve women's lives. But
does this option depend simply on each individual woman's
"getting her head together" in therapy? The problem with Williams' career goal for women is that, first of all, it is unrealistic
for most women in this society at this time, and, secondly, that
Williams makes women's mental health contingent on this un-
realizable goal!

Williams seems oblivious to the fact that satisfying, fun,
challenging labor—labor that expresses a free play of creative
energy and challenges our sense of competence—is systematically unavailable not only to most women but to most men in
our society. Making it available to a majority of the population
requires a total restructuring of social life, not individual therapy. As society is currently organized, such work exists only for
a privileged few, and it is obviously to this group that Williams
addresses her therapy and her book. But if one considers
women as a whole, it is hardly good reality-testing on the part
of a therapist to groom female clients for a society and an economy that does not yet exist! Nor can this be taken as a particu-

larly sound basis for feminist thinking about women in general or about feminist therapy practice.

Williams' thinking is just one example of the feminist version of myth 1: "It's all in your head." Personal reality is still seen to be totally determined by conscious and unconscious forces within the mind: to change your life change your feelings. Hence in this feminist version of the myth, if you are a woman and you want to avoid poverty, you need only reconstruct your "work orientation" and develop a more "serious work commitment"—the way men do.

Ironically, though Williams' intentions for women's liberation are no doubt sincere, she ends up putting women back in the same old bind: women are not mentally "healthy" unless they feel and act more like men. Through the humanist route, Williams has come full circle back to the traditional view of women.

This brand of feminist therapy can be sung to the tune of "Why can't a woman be more like a man?" And this kind of irony comes from the inability of most therapists—traditional, humanist, or otherwise—to abandon a view of the world as a place primarily determined by feelings.

Elsewhere in her book, for instance, Williams tells us the story of her client Connie, who has a "conflict" between "mothering" and "work." A conflict is a psychological hang-up—as opposed to a real, material-economic dilemma. In this case, the dilemma is one that confronts millions of women daily, the dilemma of the double workday: the paid labor of work and the unpaid labor of mothering. Williams shares the patriarchal bias by which mothering in this society is not seen or defined as work, but as the unraveling of natural female inclination, the bias that "woman's work" is not work at all.

Connie's "resolution" of her conflict (in which Williams takes pride as Connie's therapist) turns out to be rather simple: she hires a live-in maid while she works part time. No more conflict—for Connie. But how about the millions of women who cannot afford to hire a live-in maid or cannot find a suitable part-time job? Moreover, what about Connie's live-in maid?

Does she too have a conflict between work and mothering? If so, she has apparently not resolved it successfully as Connie has, because while the maid works full time washing Connie's baby's diapers, who takes care of the maid's children?

People who work as maids, it goes without saying, cannot afford to have their own. Some women—like Connie—can afford to be served. Others—like Connie's live-in maid—can only afford to be servants. What is most astonishing about Williams' account of her client's conflict resolution is that Williams apparently does not *see* Connie's live-in maid at all, either as a person or as a woman. The maid is merely the instrument of Connie's liberation from psychic conflict. While Connie happily goes off to become a fully integrated person through her part-time career, how will her maid become similarly actualized through the deadening housekeeping that Williams declares insufficient for full mental health and that the culture designates as degrading? Williams' humanist brand of feminist therapy may, in some ways, speak for Connie. But who speaks for Connie's maid?

The goal of satisfying creative labor is certainly something worth striving for—something that would enrich the lives of most men as well as women in our society. Karl Marx saw the human capacity to labor—to create and reproduce the conditions that sustain human life—as the central and essentially human capacity. His critique of capitalism, in fact, is partly based on his analysis of how capitalist society distorts this essential human capacity—makes human labor into a "thing" to be bought and sold on the market for the benefit of the capitalist. The kind of self-integration or actualization that Williams defines as the goal of therapy, according to Marx, can be won only through a revolution in the social organization of labor.

Feminists have since criticized Marx and pointed out that the kind of revolution he foresaw would not really touch the basis of oppression in most women's lives. The feminist critique of patriarchy has included an analysis of how men's "self-fulfillment" through labor in our society has, in fact, been achieved at the expense of the invisible labor of women. Without this free sacrifice of women's domestic work for men and children, male-style self-development as we know it would be virtually impossible. As the saying goes, for every big man there is a little woman at home—on whose back the big man's reputation has been built.

Feminist therapy in the humanist mode runs the risk of attempting to replace more and more big men with more and more big women, placing women like Connie in male-style roles with paid domestic workers to serve as these women's "wives." In this new vision, for every big woman there will still be a little woman at home. Or, alternatively, the big woman will be so big, so powerful, she won't even need the little woman at home. A new race of Superwomen will be born, fully integrated and self-sustaining, fully able to handle any conflicts brought about by the fact that our society is simply not geared to most women's needs.

The danger of a feminist therapy based on a humanist orientation to the self and society is that it ends up creating new myths for women to live by. Humanism replicates the "It's all in your head" myth of traditional theory. Feminist humanism replicates the male myth of self for women—the Horatio Alger myth that only individual merit and perseverance determine success, that people are essentially free, as individuals, to overcome completely the social obstacles in their path. This myth has done much to cripple the psyches of working-class men and can only do the same for women.

The promise of power—defined as a psychological rather than a social condition—is a powerful lure for anyone, but particularly for those who have suffered social subjugation. The message of the humanist therapies is: You can change social reality by transforming yourself; you can transform yourself by being in therapy; you can pull yourself up by your own bootstraps and fly, fly, fly. To those who have not experienced social power, this grandiose promise of personal power that can be reclaimed through therapy is often irresistible. The formidable work of creating a society in which women are socially empowered can hardly compete with the guarantee of getting it all now.

Feminist therapy in the humanist vein is engaged in extending this humanist lure of power to women. Certainly therapy for women can and must help women gain a sense of their own personal power, both as individuals and as members of a community of women. But some of the current feminist ideas about "empowering" women through therapy reflect a confusion about what power is and how women can attain it. There is a difference between an individual woman's psychic sense of her own power, and the social power of women as a group. This difference is obscured by the humanist-feminist ideology that says that a woman can be "empowered" through a strictly intrapsychic process—that is, by liberating her mind and ignoring the systematic and institutionalized lack of power and access to power that is woman's lot in this society. This line of thinking inevitably, if unwittingly, results in educating women to model themselves on male styles of power and success.

In the example from Williams, for instance, we might imagine that Connie felt an increased sense of her own power through her new career. But this sense of power would have nothing to do with an expanded consciousness about what she and her maid have in common as women, or about the power that women of different classes might exert together in the interests of all. On the contrary, judging from Williams' criterion of mental health for women, Connie's new-found sense of power could only increase her sense of division from her maid —her sense of being different and better (more "healthy") than this less "liberated" woman. There is a masculine sense of power involved here, based on hierarchical divisions between individuals, rather than on women overcoming a common social condition together. Is this really the kind of power feminist therapy should be proposing?

I do not mean to minimize the importance of helping women feel confident, competent and powerful enough to do serious work outside of the home. But it is one thing to help a woman find a career and quite another to educate her to believe that because she has done so, she is somehow more "healthy" than women who have not had the same privilege or opportunity; or to educate her to believe that in finding a career for herself she has struck a blow for women's liberation. The "liberated woman" who looks around and sees other women in chains is a contradiction in terms. The humanist-feminist approach to therapy has unwittingly perpetuated this mystification about individual and social power for women. *The ultimate goal of a genuinely feminist therapy must be to help a woman see how her own power as an individual is inextricably bound to the collective power of women as a group.*

The core element in the continued creation of these myths of individual power is a fundamental misunderstanding about the relationship between individual psychology and social structure. Therapists, whose work it is to focus on people's psyches—whether traditional, humanist, or feminist—are especially prone to placing undue weight on the primacy of feelings in determining social reality. Many feminist thinkers have replaced this emphasis on feelings with an emphasis on sex roles and sex-role socialization. The good news, according to this way of thinking, is that the problem of female oppression can be solved by the elimination of sex-role stereotypes. This can be accomplished in a strictly private, individualized way, with couples engaging in nonsexist child-rearing practices, more and more women going out to work, and more and more liberated husbands washing the dishes. Little girls will then be taught that they can be corporation executives, police chiefs, and truck drivers, while little boys will more and more dream of being nurses and kindergarten teachers.

The problem with this analysis is that male and female sex roles are mistakenly seen to stem simply from a sexist socialization process within the family. This is another version of the primacy of feelings expanded to include a conception of sex-role attitudes. Sex roles and attitudes are taken to be the *cause* of female oppression, while the institutionalized structures of patriarchal and class domination which enforce these roles and attitudes are minimized or ignored. In fact, sex roles are not simply born in the family because mommy stays home and daddy goes out to work. Sex roles are based not only on what happens in the family but on what happens outside it, in the paid labor force; based not only on what mommies say and do to little girls but on how daddies exploit mommies—even the best of daddies. Sex roles are based, to some extent, on the fact that women's labor within the home is systematically exploited for male and overall societal use—whether or not the particular mommy also has a career, or the particular daddy does housework. Sex roles are based on the fact that women in a society such as ours—patriarchal capitalism—constitute a kind of "sex class" which economically and psychologically benefits men as a whole, and men in the capitalist class in particular.[5]

How the overall economic condition of women affects female personality structure and the development of a particularly female style of "symptoms" is the subject of chapter nine, section 3. For now, I want to stress that sex-role socialization is only an aspect of the total picture of the oppression of women. It helps to generate the psychic structures necessary for women to accept their specific economic position as a "sex class" in patriarchal capitalism. Certainly changing sex roles within the family is an important part of women's liberation. But it can only be accomplished in full if women are actually structurally equal to men in the society as a whole. Our society has a long way to go before this becomes the case.

In short, female socialization happens for important economic reasons and has crucial economic underpinnings. The humanist-feminist myth is that in changing female sex-role socialization we can create real power for women. But if therapists train women to have different attitudes about their power as women and do not simultaneously work (and help their clients to work) to alter the institutionally built-in socioeconomic oppression in the society that awaits them, then therapists will end up merely creating a different kind of blame-the-victim myth: that if a woman doesn't make it, doesn't succeed, doesn't integrate herself, it is because she is not Superwoman enough, not liberated enough to do so. (This myth is already adversely affecting women in the generation that grew up with the women's movement as an accomplished fact.)

A feminist therapy that is truly in the interests of all women cannot be built on an exclusively humanist base, or it will end up applauding Connie and ignoring her maid.

There is nothing wrong with humanist ideals for men and women except that they cannot be actualized in this society as it now stands. For this time and this place, they remain pipe dreams unless actualized through a process of profound social, institutional change that cannot be won through getting in touch with one's feelings in therapy—though there is no doubt that therapy can help.

There has yet to be a working model of such a therapy: a therapy geared to the interests of women as a group, not merely as individuals; a therapy geared to the kind of personal change that both acknowledges and confronts the social world; a therapy in which self and social reality are seen together, and how one influences the other is part of the process as well as the goal; a therapy in which the goal is personal/social power for women rather than the mythic freedom song of humanism.

Such therapy must throw out myth 1's "It's all in your head" stranglehold once and for all. It must start with a firm grounding in the socioeconomic facts of women's condition in this society. It must attempt to make the connections between what is *inside* women's heads—the common features of female psychology—and what is *outside* women's heads—the socioeconomic structuring of women's lives. Finally, it must map out some strategies for working with women in such a way that these connections can be made therapeutically useful to them. The development of such a way of thinking about female psychology and about feminist therapy practice is the subject of chapters nine and ten, respectively.

But first let's see what happens to Polly Patient when she encounters the growth therapist.

8

The Humanist Model: Polly Encounters the Growth Therapist

As Polly enters the waiting room, she is greeted with the sound of soft, pleasant music. She is tired and tense from a day's work and beginning to feel one of her headaches coming on. The sound of the music relaxes her. She becomes aware of the tension in her neck and shoulders and wonders if Dick, her therapist, will pick up on it. Suddenly, she feels like crying, but she's not sure why. *This mess with my boss is really getting to me,* she thinks. *I can see that I still have a lot of work to do on it.*

Dick is taking a rest in between clients. He takes a long, deep breath, filling his lungs and then slowly letting the air out as he rolls his head around on his shoulders. He is aware that working with Polly, for some reason, makes him tense. He finds her likable enough; but she seems to vent her emotions without really getting anywhere. Recently, she's been working on feelings that come up around her boss. She has a lot of anger, guilt, and resentment, and often ends up depressed about her job. Dick has pushed her to get into her issues around sexuality, anger, and relationships with men. But Polly puts up a lot of defenses. It is hard to get near her sometimes. He finds himself getting more and more bored in the sessions. The problem, he thinks, is that Polly is holding onto a lot of stored up anger at men, unfinished business from the past which keeps her from being fully centered in the present. She finds it hard to take responsibility for herself in relationships, including this one with her boss. Letting go and really trusting herself and others seems to be one of her major issues. But how to get past the impasse in their sessions?

Dick does some stretches as he continues his train of thought. *Perhaps I should try some more consistent bodywork to help Polly fully release and get past the anger she's holding onto,* he thinks. He takes one last deep breath, focusing on releasing his tension as he exhales. Feeling more relaxed and centered, he is now ready to work with Polly.

As he opens the door to the office, Dick sees Polly sitting in the waiting room, absorbed in a magazine, "Hi, Polly!" he says with a broad smile. "Come on in."

Polly looks a little flustered but pleased to see him. As she gets up, she feels the knot of tension in her neck and shoulders. At the door to the office, Polly and Dick hug one another. Once inside, she takes a seat on a floor cushion in the corner of the room. Dick sits down opposite her, close enough to touch her.

"Hi," says Polly, smiling at Dick.

"Hi," says Dick, smiling at Polly. "How are you doing?" he asks as he looks warmly into her brown eyes.

Polly squirms a little in her corner, wondering why Dick's gaze always makes her feel a little uncomfortable. She likes his warmth and intensity, so why should his looking at her make her squirm? *Must be my fear of intimacy,* she thinks.

"Oh, I'm okay I guess . . . well, not really. Actually I feel rotten! I have a headache and feel tense and depressed. I hope you don't mind, but I really need to talk about my boss again today." (*I must be boring him to death with this by now.*)

"Why should I mind?" asks Dick.

"I don't know. . . . I guess I'm just feeling a little bit insecure because I've gotten the feeling that you think I ought to be done with this issue by now?"

Polly's statement is really a disguised question. (*Why do I always need Dick's approval?* she thinks. *It's so uncentered!*)

"Hey listen, Polly—" Dick smiles. "If that's what you need to do, that's fine. This is *your* hour to do with as you wish."

"Thanks, Dick." Polly's relief at Dick's approval instantly turns into anxiety about how to start. She hesitates a few moments, then launches into her story.

"Well," she sighs, "my boss had me work late last night even though there wasn't very much work to do. Then he invited me out to dinner. I don't know exactly why, but I accepted. We had a candlelight dinner at this fancy restaurant while he told me all about what a wonderful secretary and great gal I was, and how much he wished he were free to have a serious relationship with me, all that kind of stuff. . . . I mostly listened, and felt kind of . . . you know . . . weird about him." (*I wonder what Dick really thinks about all this,* Polly thinks nervously.)

"What do you mean, you felt 'weird'?" asks Dick. His voice is inquisitive, supportive, and nonjudgmental. It gives Polly the courage to go on.

"Well . . . mostly guilty I guess, wondering if his wife knows what a flirt he is. The way he tells it, she pays no attention to him at all. I guess I felt kind of sorry for him when he asked me to have dinner with him, so I said yes. But once in the restaurant I felt so guilty about being there, I just wanted to run away. Sometimes I think he's really sincere, you know, but mostly I feel he's just after my ass and is putting me on so that I'll have sex with him."

"What makes you think he's putting you on?"

"Well, I guess I know a line when I hear one. I mean, he's my boss, for godsakes! I don't exactly trust him, you know? All this time he's been flirting with me I've had the feeling that he just wants to get me into bed and that if I don't do it, he may fire me. And as of today, I think I may be right."

"What do you mean?"

"Well, to make a long story short, it got pretty late at the restaurant and he insisted that he drive me home. I was nervous about that, but I said okay. Then, while we were parked in front of my house, he . . . well . . . he started pawing me. At first I just nicely told him that I really didn't want to do that with him, but he just wouldn't take no for an answer." Polly is feeling more and more agitated as she speaks. The knot in her shoulders feels very tight and there is a growing ball of anxiety in her stomach. She forces herself to go on.

"Finally, I couldn't help it . . . I just lost my cool completely and got very angry. I guess I blew it because he kind of ordered me out of the car. And then, this morning, he said I was slacking off in my secretarial duties, just because I made a mistake in a letter! He said that if I didn't get with it, he would fire me!"

The knot in Polly's stomach feels like it's about to explode. As she looks at Dick, her lip begins to tremble.

"What's that tremble in your lip about, Polly?" *(If I go after the physical feelings here, maybe I can help Polly past her intellectualization.)*

"Oh, I don't know, I guess I just feel like crying and I'm not sure why."

"Let it out, Polly, it's okay."

Polly begins to cry a little but can't really get up a good sob. She feels too self-conscious.

"I guess this whole thing with my boss is really getting to me because I have one of my terrible headaches right now," she sniffs.

Dick is uncertain whether he should go after this headache through gestalt or encourage Polly to do some bodywork, as he had previously decided. Which technique would work best? While thinking about this, he asks, "What feelings are trapped in your headache, Polly?"

Polly represses a smile. Dick has asked her this question before. He is very sharp about going after the feelings that come out in her various bodily gestures and aches and pains.

"Oh, it's probably my anger at my boss again!" *(So what else is new?)*

"Yes. Your shoulders look very tense today. You look like you're holding a lot of anger in them. Do you want to work with that anger, Polly?"

"I guess so," says Polly, somewhat reluctantly. She is amazed at how easily Dick picks up the tension in her body. But the prospect of bodywork always fills her with dread.

As they both rise from the floor, Dick suggests that if Polly would like to take her clothes off to do the bodywork, she should feel free. As usual, Polly declines. "I'm not ready to be that open," she says to Dick apologetically.

Dick looks into her eyes. "That's okay, Polly. You'll let go of your defenses when you're ready to." His voice is supportive and makes Polly feel a little less guilty. But at the same time, she finds herself inexplicably resenting him.

There is a stool in the corner of the room which Dick is now carrying into the center. It is a bioenergetics tool. Polly has learned how to breathe deeply while bending backwards over it. Dick has explained to her that this is a technique for helping her get in touch with and let go of the feelings that are locked up in her body. The idea is that feelings are bound up in the body "armor" that we all carry around with us: places that we hold the tense energy from past emotions. The deep breathing helps Polly release some of the tension and the openness of the stance helps her to get in touch with her center. Ultimately, the goal is to let go of feelings from the past so that she can be free to live in the present moment.

Polly has done these exercises before. She has mixed feelings about them: she always feels awkward, self-conscious, and silly while doing them, but she does feel better afterwards. Also, though Dick has always been totally supportive, she knows that being physically open in front of him makes her feel vulnerable and anxious.

"Just relax and let yourself go," says Dick in his most soothing voice. "Let yourself really *feel* the feelings in your body."

As Polly exhales and bends backward over the stool, she tries to focus her mind on how her body feels. The pounding in her head has gotten worse, and her neck and shoulders are painful. "I guess there's a lot of anger in my body," she says as she straightens and stands up. She feels somewhat faint.

"Okay, Polly, why don't you continue the deep breathing while you just let yourself really experience that anger in your head, neck, and shoulders. Get into it. What do you feel like your anger is saying?"

Polly closes her eyes and projects herself into her head and shoulders. She imagines herself a little dot in the back of her head that radiates out until it reaches her shoulders. As she does so, she begins to feel more and more angry. Her breathing gets heavier and she feels that she could scream.

"I feel like screaming," she says in a quiet voice.

"Why don't you?" Dick urges. "Why don't you scream? Really let yourself get into it!"

Polly swallows. She finds this very hard. For some reason, whenever Dick encourages her to get angry, she feels like retreating and forgetting the whole thing. She knows this is her defensiveness, but she finds it hard to get past it. "I don't know what to say," she stammers.

"Don't try to say anything. Just let whatever comes, come," Dick says. His voice is calm and reassuring. Polly says nothing and there is a brief silence.

"Don't lose the moment. It's all there right now. Feel what your shoulders want to do. Feel what your head wants to say." Dick is looking into her eyes, as usual, but there is a note of slight urgency in his voice now. He is directing her toward the pillow, encouraging her to use her arms on it.

Polly closes her eyes again and the rising anger is still there, though somewhat more muted because of her increasing self-consciousness. She starts to say the words that have been in her head all day:

"Why don't you get off my back, you goddamn prick! I'm sick and tired of all your sexual come-ons. Why don't you just leave me alone and let me work in peace! You just confuse me and give me headaches." Polly is pounding the pillow with her fists as she yells, but there is a rote quality to it.

"Try it with fewer words, Polly," Dick suggests. "Let it come from your guts."

"Damn you damn you damn you damn you damn you," Polly repeats. Her face is flushed and her voice is getting stronger. She can begin to feel some release. Her arms, however, are getting very tired. Finally, she stops and slumps back onto the floor.

"So," Dick says. "What's going on?" (*It's time to process*

the feelings that came up for Polly in this exercise. Hopefully, Polly will come to understand her anger and let go of it.)

"I guess I still have a lot of anger in me," she offers with a weak smile. *(This is embarrassing. I wonder if I'll ever get past this stuff.)*

"Sure looks that way," says Dick, smiling back. *(There's so much of it, and no matter how much bodywork we do, there's always more.)* "What's it all about?"

"Well, I'm not sure. I think I'm just angry at my boss for coming on to me when I'm working and for threatening to fire me . . . I don't know, for making me feel vulnerable, I guess." *(These feelings are so confusing.)*

"What about that vulnerability—what's hard about that?" *(Now we're getting someplace, thinks Dick. If only Polly could get into this feeling, she could learn how to stop being so angry at men.)*

"Well, I just feel that I'm obliged to put out or else I'll get fired . . . and that makes me feel really vulnerable."

Dick looks at her steadily. For some reason, whenever he looks at her this way, Polly feels she has given the wrong answer. The silence between them grows larger until Polly blurts out: "Well, what do you think?"

"What do I think about what, Polly?"

"What do you think about my feeling of vulnerability?"

"Well, I don't know, Polly. Only you can really answer that question. But, I pick up that there's a trust issue involved here —an issue of how much you trust your boss, how much you trust men."

Polly considers what Dick has said, feeling a mixture of irritation and respect. Certainly there is something to what he's saying, but for some reason it makes her resent him.

"Sure, there's a trust issue—I mean I *don't* trust my boss, that's for sure. I feel that he's trying to use me and that he has an unfair advantage in the situation. I feel like he's playing with me."

"If that's how you really feel, Polly, why don't you just tell him to stop?"

"I *have* tried to tell him to stop! I have hinted that I don't really appreciate his come-ons, and once I even told him that I thought we should have a more professional realtionship. But he just went right on doing what he was doing. I think he thought it was cute that I got a little mad. But it didn't stop him."

(*Polly has a way of always blaming others,* thinks Dick.)

"Perhaps, Polly, I don't know . . . this is just a hunch . . . but perhaps he didn't stop because he was getting a mixed message from you. I mean, you say you *hinted* that he should stop, but did you come right out and say so? Not until last night in the car. And you *did* go out with him, so he had some reason to believe that you're interested in him sexually. Maybe you need to take some responsibility for your part of the interaction with him. And if you really don't want him to come on to you, if you can let him know in a firm but friendly way, perhaps he won't keep responding to your mixed signals, know what I mean?"

Polly tries to take in what Dick has said. The guilt and shame she has been feeling all along with her boss are triggered by his words. She knows he's right. There *has* been a part of her that has been returning her boss's flirtations. But even so, despite herself, Polly has the inclination to argue with Dick now. While this internal warfare goes on inside her, she sits in silence.

"What's going on, Polly?" Dick asks gently. (*Here it comes —the same old impasse. Why does she always seem to get stuck on this issue?*)

"Well, I don't know . . . I guess I feel some anger at you for what you're saying, even though I know you're right."

"Do you want to get that anger out, Polly?"

"I don't know." Despite herself, Polly feels like being stubborn and not doing anything.

"How about having a gestalt conversation between you and your boss and seeing where that goes?"

Polly can feel her stubbornness growing. More and more she feels like fighting with Dick, even though she knows that he's only doing his job as her therapist. Impulsively, she finds herself blurting out: "Well, okay, maybe I *do* have an issue around trusting men, but what about the fact that my boss threatened to fire me? What about that?"

"What about it, Polly?" (Dick takes a deep breath. It's hard to keep himself centered when Polly goes after him in this way. He reminds himself that her trust issue is *her* problem and that he shouldn't take it personally.)

"Well . . . I don't know . . . it doesn't seem like you're really taking that seriously." Polly averts her eyes. Challenging Dick always makes her anxious, especially when she knows, deep down inside her, that he's right. She feels trembly all over, as though she could burst into tears any minute, but she holds back, not wanting to give him the satisfaction of her feelings.

"Do you think your boss was serious when he threatened to fire you, Polly?"

"Serious? Well . . . yes, I guess he was. Why? What do you mean?" *(I'm getting more and more confused about all this.)*

"Well, I don't know, but maybe he was just sounding off today because he felt rejected by you. I mean, from what I know, you're a really good secretary. Why should he want to fire you? But if you really think there's a serious threat there, why don't you talk it over with him?"

"Well—I don't know," Polly stammers. "That's the problem. I don't know *what* to do about anything he does!" Polly feels herself beginning to cry now. "I know you're right that I feed into this thing in some way by letting him flirt with me, but I honestly don't know what to do besides what I have done. My headaches just keep getting worse and worse."

Polly is crying in earnest now, letting the sobs come out in great heaps of sound the way she has learned to do. As she does so, she feels a release in her body. But her confusion remains.

"It's okay, Polly, it's okay," says Dick, taking Polly's hand as she cries. This makes them both feel better. Polly looks up to see Dick's clear blue eyes gazing at her with compassion. Her resentment begins to fade.

"I guess this anger of mine is always getting in the way of everything," she says.

Dick softens up as Polly says this. He wants to find a way of supporting her while getting her to confront her issues with men.

"Look," he says, "if you really want to stop your boss's actions, why not tell him you'd like to talk to him about your feelings about his behavior towards you?"

"Because I'm afraid that that would only make him *more* angry at me, or that he'd even use my talking to him about his behavior as a reason to get rid of me. I'm scared to confront him."

"What's the fear about?"

"I told you—I'm scared of losing my job!"

"Yes, I know that, Polly. But let's look at the facts, okay? You're a good secretary, right? You do all your work well, right? You have no *real* reason to fear that he'll dismiss you. So what's your fear of vulnerability *really* about? What's really going on in your *guts*?"

Polly thinks a minute. "Well, I'm not really sure, but I know that something about him makes me feel sorry for him and then, later on, after I've responded to him, I end up feeling guilty and resentful and scared and vulnerable."

"Yes," says Dick reassuringly, "can you let yourself really *feel* that vulnerability and look at it?"

"Well, I don't know . . . I just . . . feel vulnerable." Polly feels stuck now and is beginning to feel guilty that Dick is trying so hard to help her and yet she can't seem to get anywhere with this one.

"Have you felt that vulnerability before, in other relationships with men?"

"Well, yes, in a way, I guess I have. I find it hard to trust men sometimes, to trust their motivations, or to trust that they really care about me, that they're not just after me sexually, or just playing with me in some way. Sometimes I even set up tests for them to pass to prove that they love me."

"What kind of tests?"

"Oh, like not having sex with them for a while, to see if they will still be there anyway."

"So your boss's sexual interest really brings up this distrust, doesn't it?"

"Well, Dick, he *is* a married man!"

"Right! He probably has some patterns of his own that he's playing out with you. But that's not the point. The point is to look at *your* patterns in relation to him. You can't change him, but you can change the way you behave with him. He's a married man who wants to have sex with you. Okay, that's *his* trip! You don't have to say yes and you don't have to say no. You can do what you want to do—*if* you stay centered in yourself."

"Yes, but how do I do that? I mean, I lose my center very easily with my boss because he . . . he intimidates me."

"Well, we need to understand more about what it is that intimidates you but, for starters, does your boss have a name?"

"Why sure . . . of course he does. His name is John Dudley, why?"

"Well, it just might help for you to start calling him by his name, instead of always referring to him as 'my boss.' I mean, underneath his role, he's just a person like you or me. Perhaps calling him by his name would help you begin to relate to him as a person instead of as an authority figure. You know what I mean?"

"I hadn't thought of that. I always do call him 'my boss,' don't I? I guess I sort of set him up as an authority and then end up feeling intimidated by him." (*Leave it to Dick to point out something so simple and obvious!*)

Polly is pleased with this idea of calling her boss John. It gives her something to do and makes her feel less hopeless. Dick, seeing that his suggestion has had some effect, decides to push further.

"Once you feel a little less scared, perhaps you can find a way to open yourself up to John and tell him what's really on your mind so that you can get past what's hanging you up with him. But to do that, I think we're going to need to look further into that fear of vulnerability. It seems like some unfinished business from the past that keeps getting in the way of your staying centered in the present."

"What do you think it is?" Polly asks excitedly. For a moment, she finds herself hoping that Dick has the answer that can free her from this mess with her boss. But as soon as the words are out of her mouth, she realizes that this is just a wish. She's been in therapy long enough to know that only she has the answers to her problems.

"Only *you* know the answer to that one." Dick smiles. "It's all inside you, if only you look deeply enough."

Dick is glancing at the clock and they both can see that the hour is just about up.

"Well, I *do* feel better," Polly says as she starts to gather her things. "I guess it really helped to get some of that anger out. I know I have a lot of issues in relationships with men. Making myself vulnerable to men does scare me. In fact, I sometimes feel that way with you too. As we've been working on this issue of my relationship with my boss . . . I mean with John . . . I've been having all sorts of feelings toward you: distrust, anger, fear, the whole bit."

As Polly admits this, she feels a flush rising in her face. She is embarrassed but pleased with herself for having the nerve to tell these feelings to her therapist.

"Well, it's only natural that your issues around intimacy with men would come up in here with me. Maybe we can take a closer look at those feelings next time. But we've got to stop now." *(Great! Polly's really made some movement in this session!)*

They both rise from the floor. Polly feels grateful to Dick for his help, glad that he pushed her to do the exercises she finds so difficult. She feels much more relaxed now than when she came in. Her body feels about ten pounds lighter. But her headache is still there. In the back of her mind, a small voice is anxiously asking, *"But what about my boss? How will calling him by his name get him to stop bothering me?"* But thinking of how good she feels right now, Polly manages to make the voice go away.

Dick too is feeling glad, relieved that Polly has been able to get past the feelings that were holding her back in therapy. He has a sense that now that Polly is less angry, she can move on. As they reach the door, Dick smiles his most engaging smile and Polly returns it. There's a shared sense of excitement at the progress Polly's made this session.

They give each other a big hug till next time.

III

A New Approach to
Women and Therapy

9

New Ways of Thinking About Women

1. Woman as Body

AMY'S STORY: THE TERROR OF BEING SEEN ■ Over the past ten years of working with women in therapy I have heard the same stories repeated over and over again: stories of women who are chronically depressed; of women who lack self-esteem—or a sense of self at all; of women who are sexually unresponsive; of women who feel lost without men; of women who live with men who abuse them but whom they love too much to leave; of women who live with men they no longer love but are terrified to leave; of women who want to be in a stable relationship with a man but cannot sustain one; of women who feel empty and lost and don't know what they want—except to feel better.

It becomes obvious that the major features of these apparently "individual" ordeals, are, in fact, part of a pervasive social phenomenon. Furthermore, one hears similar tales told by women who are not in therapy. Certainly, the working-class woman who has been hospitalized for depression and given a set of electroshock treatments has had a very different experience of depression than the middle-class woman who manages to function (though often only with the help of a daily fix of Elavil or Valium). But every woman—housewife or career woman, working-class or middle-class—knows what it is to be depressed.

In this chapter, my purpose is to examine, from a female perspective, some of the major themes in female psychology in our society. I believe that the stories that follow embody these themes and reflect the problems of women in general, not just the problems of women in therapy. My attempt has been to address the question of how the "outer" becomes "inner" in women's lives—how social values and social structures become embedded in individual female psychology. Certainly, the recent widespread attempts of women to define ourselves from our own point of view have cut into the pervasiveness of the problems that follow. But years of psychosocial gender conditioning and the continued oppression of women put a considerable brake on these attempts to radically alter female consciousness.

I hope that female readers will recognize themselves in some, if not all, of the stories of chapters nine and ten. The problems of female identity in these stories are not to be interpreted to women's discredit. Nor do they belie the commitment of millions of women to free themselves psychologically and socially. Rather, the stories are evidence of how our society continues to affect women's psyches adversely and how women carry on despite these effects.

Amy was the first patient I took on as a pyschology intern. Her chief complaint was a bizarre and disturbing physical symptom: an uncontrollable facial twitch around her mouth. Her face was most likely to twitch at work when she was being looked at by her male superiors. The twitch made her feel terrified of being seen by men, at the same time that it made her more visible to them.

The twitch was getting worse and worse, so much so that Amy began to feel that she was "going crazy." Recently, it had started up in the presence of a man who was looking at her in the subway. Unable to contain her panic, she fled from the subway at the next stop and took a bus home. She now found herself calling in sick at work on certain days in order to avoid being looked at. She was morbidly self-conscious in social situations, frequently turning away from men in an effort to avert their gaze. She lived in dread of being noticed.

To understand Amy and her twitch, we must understand the dilemmas of what I call Woman as Body. After a general discussion of Woman as Body, we will return to the specifics of Amy's symptoms.

As we have seen in chapter three, the achievement of an adult feminine identity in this society is a double-bind dilemma: since personhood is culturally defined in male terms, being feminine and being a person appear to be mutually exclusive. One aspect of this double bind is the fact that to develop herself as a person, woman must develop herself as a body for men. In this context, it is hardly surprising that women develop conflicts about being seen, or that a woman's visibility to men is fraught with great ambiguity.

On the one hand, the feminine woman is everywhere conspicuously visible *as a body*. On the other hand, woman as a person with all the rights and prerogatives of men is still a concept and a reality to be attained. On the one hand: woman as beautiful object, pampered and adored by the worshipful male world. On the other hand: rape as an everday fact of life in America, countless women beaten daily in their own homes by their own husbands. The patriarchal subjugation of women requires that women be made to suffer a kind of overexposure of physical visibility as bodies, combined with a profound disregard for women as people.

Under a system of male rule, a woman's body is the source of her power. The high-class call girl makes more money with less effort than the executive secretary ever dreamed of. What prostitutes sell directly, most women barter in exchange for money, security, status, and protection from the random violence of men. The more beautiful a woman's body, the more power she has—either to win fame and fortune on her own, or to lure a man into marriage and win his fame and fortune vicariously.

Most of us will never be showgirls, actresses, or models. But we still have to make do with the raw material of our power: our bodies. Hence, woman's preoccupation with cosmetics and fashion. Women are fashion crazy not because we are frivolous but because we know that our bodies are our only power and we take them as seriously as men take their work. Cosmetics and clothes are the female tools of the trade—the weapons women need in the battle for survival. Think of the way that men talk about "ugly" women: they are dogs, hags, old bags, losers, zeros. Every woman learns that the ugly woman has nothing to hope for. But the beautiful woman can work her way up. She can stop a man in his tracks and turn his head. There is an old Yiddish saying, "When the cock stands up, the head is buried in the ground." Women's bodies have the power to make men lose their heads. Since men pride themselves on their rationality, this is no insignificant loss.

The important point is that *woman in contemporary patriarchal society is fundamentally identified with her body. Her body is her power.* Men are their brains; women are their bodies. Man is culture; woman is nature. Woman is Woman as Body.

In the history of western society up until fairly recently, a large part of the power of a woman's body was thought to reside in its capacity to bear children. Legal, patriarchally sponsored motherhood was thus the most powerful and prestigious position most women could hope to attain. "Illegitimate" motherhood—maternity in which the offspring was not the legal property of a particular man—was, conversely, the lowliest lot a woman could suffer. Of course, the hidden side of this public worship of Woman as Mother was a secret obsession with Woman as Sex.

In the last half century, and particularly since the so-called sexual revolution of the 1960s, this secret male preoccupation has gone public and respectable. Woman as Body has come out of the closet and onto the newsstands and TV. The publicly identified power of a woman's body has undergone a gradual shift: from its capacity to reproduce, to its capacity to provide sexual gratification for men. The Vamp, the Sexual Seductress, the High Priestess of Sexual Titillation, have replaced the Mother as the image of female power.

A woman was once supposed to drape her body in robes that concealed its beauty while at the same time displaying it

—offering secrets that only the man who owned her could know. Now, female "sex appeal" in the form of unclad or scantily clad female bodies is used to sell everything from Ajax to Cadillacs. Even female pubic hair, formerly airbrushed away in *Playboy* magazine, now stares at us from the newsstand. Pornography—both soft- and hard-core—is enjoying a heretofore unprecedented period of public acceptance. The brown paper wrappers are off. No longer is it considered seedy to ogle women's bare bodies. At no time in history has Woman as Body been more overtly visible than in the United States today.

But the positive images of female sexuality turn (un)easily into their opposites: the Vamp becomes the Castrating Bitch; the Sexual Seductress becomes the Nymphomaniac; the High Priestress of Sexual Titillation becomes the Tease. The dark underside of the male worship of female sexual power is men's terror of the power of female sexuality to maim and destroy them.

This male terror of the "Vagina with Teeth" is one of the most deeply entrenched myths of patriarchal culture. Around for centuries prior to the recent sexual revolution, it found its most fanatical expression in the medieval persecution of the Witch. For medieval man, the ungodly power of the Witch lay in her carnality. The sexual power of her body was immense. It was the epitome of evil. The Witch was responsible for consorting with the devil, rendering men impotent, castrating men and pickling their penises in jars(!). The Witch was considered the cause of the Plague. The immense negative power attributed to female sexuality can be gauged by the enormity of the attempts to destroy it: an estimated 8 million witches burned at the stake in medieval Europe.[1] The flip side of male adoration of the female body is, and always has been, male fear and hatred of the female body.

If a woman's body is her only real asset, it is thus also her greatest liability: a guarantee of her inevitable defeat at the hands of men. The female body grows old, ceases to reproduce, loses its beauty, and fades in its power.

However visible Woman as Body may be, her power must

not be confused with the institutionalized power of men in a society run by men. It must not be confused with anything like genuine freedom or autonomy, the power of a woman to run her own life. If a woman's power is centered in her body, so ultimately, is her powerlessness. Because in patriarchal society a woman's body does not belong to her—it is appropriated by and for men. It is defined as an object for men's use. Whether in providing heirs or sexual service for men, the power of a woman's body is ultimately subservient to male needs and interests. It is the prerogative of men to make use of a woman's body with or without her consent. This privilege is reflected in everything from the legal power of the state and medical profession to control a woman's sexual and reproductive life, to the legal right of a husband to rape his wife, to the widescale rape and battering of women endemic to patriarchal society.

Rape and the threat of rape, as Susan Brownmiller has argued, is the bottom line of male domination. The fear of rape serves to keep women in our proper place.[2] Rape is the ultimate show of male force, the final act of male dominance. It gets Woman as Body in the only source of power she has and thus confirms her essential helplessness and vulnerability to men. Rape is, as many feminists have pointed out, merely the furthest extension of the "normal" relation between the sexes in patriarchal society. The old adage about lying back and enjoying it epitomizes the general message that women get everywhere else: that we are bodies for the use of men, and that we are to exult in our submission. Woman as Body is really Woman as Victim.

Before the advent of capitalism, the division between Woman as Body and woman as a person could not properly be said to exist at all. For the most part, women in feudal society were so bound by the patriarchal rule of husbands and fathers that they did not really have the choice to be persons, in the modern (male) sense. Under feudalism, the basic value of a woman's body lay in its capacity to work and have babies. In the upper class, men needed women to bring forth male babies in order to perpetuate patriarchal lineage. In the peasantry, men needed women to bring forth offspring to help with the essential toil necessary to survival. To succeed in these allotted tasks, feudal women had to have strong bodies. Consequently the strong, rotund body of feudal woman was considered beautiful.

Capitalism "freed" women to sell their labor for a wage, as men did—thus allowing women a measure of freedom and autonomy they had never enjoyed before. But just as capitalism made woman as a person more of a possibility, it spawned Woman as Body in her recognizable modern form: as an ornamental appendage to man, an incontrovertible sign of his wealth and power. The strong, utilitarian, and corpulent female body came to be seen as fat and ugly. It was succeeded by the fragility and weakness that have been the hallmark of Woman as Body ever since—until very recently.

From the pear shape of the Rubens beauty, to the hourglass figure of the Victorian lady, to the stick-figure flatness of Twiggy, the fashion in female body type has shown much variation. But the exact location of our curves and whether we are allowed to exhibit them at all have always been the prerogative of men to determine. Women have had to shape not only our clothing but our bodies to suit men. The woman who doesn't conform to the prescribed image of Woman as Body loses her status as a feminine being. But on the other hand, the woman who makes her body into the male image of what a woman should be, loses her body altogether—loses it as something that belongs to her—as opposed to something that belongs to men. Ultimately, Woman as Body cannot be a full person. How can a woman be a person if her body is not her own?

With the arrival of the women's liberation movement in the last decade, women have struggled to make our bodies our own and to become persons in our own right. Slogans like "Our Bodies Are Ourselves" have appeared—seemingly strange and tautological, unless one understands the oppression of Woman as Body. In the 1970s Woman as Body started to revolt. She clamored for her rights to safe and free contraception and abortion. She learned how to defend herself on the streets. She demanded to be let into competitive sports. She examined her own cervix and took her health into her own hands. She dressed as she pleased. She made love to women and publicly declared her pride in being a lesbian. She struggled to reclaim her sexuality, her body, herself as a person.

There are some who claim that in the post-women's liberation era, women have overcome the social conditions of Woman as Body. Certainly, there is no doubt that, as a result of the women's movement, women are freer now than ever before to define our bodies and our selves in our own terms. But the rise in woman's status as a person since the contemporary women's movement has been followed by a further retrenchment to the old patriarchal norm—that woman is still, whatever else she may be, primarily a beautiful body. As women develop our bodies through self-defense and sports and begin to think of our bodies on our own terms, liberation from the bondage of being a body for male use and on male terms is simply co-opted by the consumer industries that thrive on this bondage. Fashion's retort to the progressive development of women's bodies for ourselves has been the spike heels and hooker skirts of the 1980s. To add insult to injury, we are now told that we have come such a long way baby that we can afford to wear "ultrafeminine" fashions with no threat to our newly found sense of "independence." By this maddening species of doublethink, the Liberated Woman becomes the latest in the long line of female images made for men. Woman as Body dies hard.

Furthermore, as Woman as Body has tried to break her chains, the crimes of violence against her have begun to climb. In the last few years, the bodies of mutilated, battered, and victimized women have become more visible than ever before —on record albums and in the movies as well as in reality. According to one study, more than half of all married women in the U.S., Canada and Britain are beaten by their husbands.* Pornography (one of the male industries that most directly cash in on Woman as Body) has been openly sadistic toward women.

* See Boston Globe, "Wife Abuse Common," June 6, 1982.

"Snuff" movies have emerged, encouraging men to keep uppity women in their place through sexual domination and death. The rape and even murder of women have been played up as sexy. And the incidence of rape and sexual harrassment in general has soared to new heights. Women are paying for our emergence as persons—paying with our bodies.

The final retaliation against women's attempt to reclaim our bodies has been the rapid rise of the New Right, with its fanatical campaign to wipe out the gains that women have made in the area of contraception and abortion. What the New Right wants is to return Woman as Body to her pre–sexual revolution place: as the living incubator of children whose rights are guaranteed even at the expense of the woman's life.

Woman as Body—whether the body beautiful or the body battered—is in an impossible situation, socially and psychically. That which is defined as most thoroughly her own—her body—is also defined as most thoroughly not her own—an object for male use. To be seen as a body is woman's power: the source of her attraction as a person. It is therefore a psychic necessity for a woman's sense of self. At the same time, it is just this way of being seen that puts a woman most in jeopardy as a person. To be seen as a body means that neither a woman's body nor her self are her own. It means that, ultimately, a woman has nothing of her own—that her body and her self do not belong to her. To be invisible, not to be seen, appears to be the only way to be safe as a person. Yet for a woman to be invisible is to be lost, to lose her power and sense of self. Either way, visible or invisible, Exhibitionist or Wallflower, woman suffers from a gnawing sense of self-loss and a profound hunger to be *seen* in the authentic sense, to be recognized as a person.

With this as background, let us return to Amy's story. Amy's particular symptom, as we shall see, reflected the conditions of Woman as Body in a unique and compelling way. Yet psychiatry understood her symptom totally divorced from its social context. In fact, it only contributed to her condition as Woman as Body.

For instance, even before I met Amy, I learned from her

medical record that she was physically unattractive. I had picked up her record from a waiting list pile in the outpatient clinic. The first line of Amy's medical record had read: "Amy is a 34-year-old divorced, white, unattractive female." This was standard form for first lines of medical records. The patient's looks were considered as essential a vital statistic as her age, sex, race, and marital status—but only if she was female. Never, in my two years of training, did I see this routine "medical" notation of the patient's physical attractiveness on a male patient's record.

Female patients were rated on a scale from "attractive" to "moderately attractive" to "unattractive." The rating was a kind of signal flare sent up by the evaluating doctor for the benefit of his male colleague who was shopping around for a patient. An ingenious male-bonding system of communication was at work here, one psychiatric 'old boy' taking care of another. Because aspiring male therapists, like males in general, preferred beautiful women to plain ones, the female patient with an "attractive" rating on her record was guaranteed little or no delay on the notoriously long waiting lists for therapy in the outpatient clinic. The "moderately attractive" or "unattractive" patient, by contrast, often waited for months. In the clinic, as outside, woman was Woman as Body.

Amy had been diagnosed by this same psychiatrist as an inadequate personality. This was defined as "a behavior pattern . . . characterized by ineffectual responses to emotional, social, intellectual, and physical demands. While the patient seems neither physically nor mentally deficient, he [sic] does manifest inadaptability, ineptness, poor judgment, social instability, and lack of physical and emotional stamina."[3]

This diagnosis was based on the evaluating doctor's assessment of Amy's presumably "ineffectual" responses to the hardships of her life. Amy had withstood a terrifying and brutal marriage to a man who threatened, battered, and raped her with increasing ferocity. (Toward the end of their marriage, her husband had held a knife to her throat and threatened to hurt both her and their son unless she submitted to him sexually.) She had mustered the strength to divorce herself from this man and to raise her son on her own with no financial support from her husband. Though she considered herself an artist, she had been unable to paint for months. She worked a dead-end job as a low-level, underpaid secretary in an insurance firm—a job she despised but in which she felt trapped. She was lonely, depressed, and anxious a good deal of the time.

The expert psychiatric opinion on all this was that Amy was a characterological failure. By some inherent flaw in her character structure, she was incapable of coping with her life. From the prevailing psychiatric point of view, she was a collection of lacks—lacking in emotional strength, social stability, and judgment, inept at adapting to the stresses of marriage, motherhood, and work. It was that simple.

The psychiatric diagnosis of Amy's problem simply blamed her for her social oppression as wife, mother, and worker. This male-centered, blame-the-victim approach to Amy's problems was shared by Amy herself. Had she been told her diagnosis, it would have confirmed, with a final, scientific ring, her profound despair and self-blame. Long before her psychiatric evaluation, Amy had already internalized the society's—and the doctor's—view of her as an inadequate person. Her psychiatric label, with its baldly stated value judgment, was clearly more an expression of psychiatry's contempt for her than a contribution to understanding her.

Amy experienced her facial twitch most often in the presence of men—especially men who had direct power over her life. The process started with a slow, burning sensation in her stomach. Her heart would beat rapidly and her adrenalin start to flow, as though her body were preparing for flight. She would begin to sweat, her jaw to stiffen. Then she would sense her facial muscles twitching. She felt, she said, like a "monster."

She first noticed her twitch after an angry interchange with her roommate, in which she felt accused of being an inadequate mother. She then became increasingly aware of it following two episodes at work. First, a female co-worker (a woman whom Amy admired for her competence and assertiveness) had asked for a raise. This woman had been abruptly and inexplicably fired. Shortly after this, Amy was reprimanded by her boss for making too many mistakes in her secretarial tasks. Both of these events made Amy very angry. Since then, she often felt her face twitching when being looked at by her male superiors on the job. She also noticed her twitch when being looked at by men in social situations.

As a therapist-in-training, I was instructed by my supervisors to *ignore the specific relation of social context to Amy's inner life.* The entire constellation of her response to powerful men at work was relegated to the category of "precipitating circumstances"—events that somehow triggered the deeper cause behind her bizarre facial behavior. This deeper cause was thought to lie in long buried and unexpressed feelings residing in the depths of Amy's unconscious, feelings that were being indirectly expressed through the symptom—the facial tic. My job was to understand Amy's symptom *dynamically*— that is, to interpret its unconscious psychological motivation in repressed, underlying affect.

Old feelings toward her parents were indeed involved in Amy's facial twitch. By her own description, when her face twitched, she felt as though it were hardening into that of her mother. Amy did not like her mother and, like most women I've ever known or worked with, she was terrified of being like her. She described her mother as "crazy, out of control, and panicked"—a woman whose considerable talent and energy were wasted because of her dependent attachment to an overbearing and cruel husband. Often, her father accused his wife of being a bad mother. They fought frequently. Her mother complained bitterly to the children about her husband, and threatened to leave him. Yet despite several attempts to separate while Amy was growing up, her mother had never succeeded in divorcing. Though Amy described her father as "cruel, tyrannical, and blind" to others, she blamed her mother for her parents' marital troubles. It seemed to Amy that the burden of responsibility was on her mother for being too "dependent" rather than on her father for being abusive. His cruelty was, somehow, more excusable than her mother's dependence.

Of the four children in the family, Amy's father had pre-ferred the two girls because they were "sweet," unlike his wife, who was too angry to be sweet. The two boys were not sweet either. They were defiant of their father's authority. Conse-quently, Amy's father had expelled one of them from the house when he was an adolescent. Though Amy had once dreamed of being a dancer or a swimmer, her father forbade both ambi-tions. Later, when she decided to be an artist, her father refused to pay for her education, insisting that she change her major. Amy refused. Her defiance, she was convinced, had lost her his love.

Amy had unconsciously learned that being sweet—com-pliant and passive—was the way to win her father's love and approval. Being assertive/aggressive/angry (Amy used these words interchangeably) was dangerous; it meant risking her father's abuse or the loss of his love. Yet despite her superficial sweetness, deep inside Amy harbored a profound rage at her father's cruelty and blindness to her needs and ambitions.

The dynamic interpretation of Amy's facial tic was that this repressed anger at her father was the underlying cause of her symptom. In all three precipitating circumstances (Amy's ar-gument with her roommate, the firing of her female co-worker, and her being scolded by the boss), Amy was angry. From the psychiatric point of view, her anger in all three instances was inordinate—disproportional to the "real" events. In the argu-ment with her roommate, she felt accused of being a bad mother. This infuriated her, just as it had infuriated her mother twenty years earlier. Clearly, Amy unconsciously identified with her mother. Like her mother, she feared she was bad at mothering. Like her mother, she felt that she had talent that was going to waste. Like her mother, she felt trapped. Like her mother, she felt dependent on men—first on her husband, and now on her boss. Like her mother, she was very angry with her father.

The two events at work restimulated this ancient anger at her father. Like her brother who had been thrown out of his home, Amy's co-worker was banished from her place of work for being aggressive. The description that Amy used for her father—"cruel, tyrannical, and blind"—might well stand for how she felt about her boss, whom she could not forgive for being blind to her co-worker's competence. Her boss unconsciously reminded Amy of her own father.

In psychiatric terms, one would say that Amy's ancient rage at her father was triggered by her current anger at her boss. The long-buried anger emerged, displaced and somatized, in the form of a facial twitch. The sense that she could not control her facial muscles was the immediate reason for Amy's search for a therapist. But dynamically, it was Amy's fear of losing control of her repressed rage that motivated her. It was this rage that made her feel like a "monster" when her face twitched. The twitch was a signal that there was more to Amy than sweetness. Her fear of having her facial twitch noticed by others was really her fear of being found out in all her monstrous anger. She turned away from men who looked at her because she was terrified lest her father see that, underneath her sweetness, she was a seething cauldron of buried rage.

The intricacy and cleverness of this psychiatric view of Amy's inner life is undeniable. As an explanation of her facial twitch, it is enormously appealing. It has a sleek symmetry and is rich with many insights. It is true that Amy unconsciously identified with her mother and that her boss unconsciously reminded her of her father. It is true that she had a great deal of repressed anger at her father. It is true that this old anger was stirred up in the present, when she got angry at her boss. But it is *not* true that *only* the past anger at her father was the cause of her facial tic, or the cause of her anger at her boss, or the cause of her current emotional distress. Emotions are not simply interior, irrational events symbolically evoked by current events but actually caused by earlier experiences. Reality is not merely something that happened in one's early childhood and keeps recurring in the present through the recapitulation of unconscious feelings. Both emotions and social reality are much more complex than this.

Amy was angry at her father for his arbitrary and cruel power. She was also angry at her boss for his arbitrary and cruel power. In psychodynamic theory, the two figures—father and boss—are understood to be related only symbolically (within Amy's unconscious) rather than in reality. The anger at her boss is subsumed within the anger at her father, and only the latter is taken to be causally determining. In this way, the nature and origins of both angers and their relation to one another are not merely simplified but misunderstood. In this way, it is also possible to circumvent the question of the legitimacy of Amy's anger—both at her boss and at her father. Anger (like all affect) is seen as a purely intrapsychic affair: by definition irrational. In mistaking one aspect of Amy's reality (her anger at her father) for the totality, psychiatry misdefines both the nature of Amy's problem and its solution.

What gets overlooked in all this is that both father and boss are not merely male authority figures within Amy's unconscious, but also *real men, who occupy real positions of power within a real social system.* Father and boss are linked not only unconsciously but institutionally by the two symmetrical social arrangements of male dominance in which they rule: the nuclear family and the capitalist workplace, respectively. Amy's anger at both men must be understood within these two related social contexts.

Amy's anger at her father begins in a situation aptly described by Amy herself: a family with a mother who is dependent upon and subservient to a father who is emotionally distant and physically overpowering. From a social point of view, it is obvious that the essential elements of Amy's family dynamics mirror the familiar, recognizable features of nuclear family life in America. Yet psychiatry goes about understanding Amy's family dynamics as though there were no other families in the world but Amy's.

Psychiatry chooses to ignore that within the family as an institution, all men rule the roost systematically, through a combination of physical force and economic superiority—just as Amy's father did. Psychiatry chooses to ignore that, within the family as an institution, wives not only feel but *are* dependent and powerless—just as Amy's mother was. A wife may be free, as an individual, to divorce a particular husband. But she is not free, as an individual, to escape the exploitation of female labor institutionally upheld by the nuclear family. Amy's anger at her father, and her mother's anger too, are part of a potentially subversive and therefore culturally repressed social reality: millions of women who are burning with anger (repressed and otherwise) at their husbands and fathers. And with good reason.

Similarly, psychiatry goes about understanding Amy's anger at the two displays of male managerial power at work as though Amy's boss were merely the latest in a series of unconscious authority figures rather than a person with real power over her life. Yet the essential elements of Amy's emotional predicament at work—her economic dependence upon a manager with the power to fire, pay, and scold her—are also the recognizable features of wage labor under capitalism. Amy, like all workers in a capitalist society, not only feels but *is* trapped by economic necessity. She may be free as an individual to search for another job, just as the wife is free to search for another husband, but in so doing she merely exchanges one master for another. She doesn't escape the system by which her labor is exploited, nor her female caste status within this system. Amy's anger at her boss is a small part of another potentially subversive and therefore culturally repressed social reality: millions of workers in factories and offices throughout the country who, like Amy, hate their bosses. And with good reason.

In psychodynamic theory, all of the symmetries in Amy's experience—between her past and her present anger; between her father and her boss; between herself and her mother; between the nuclear family and the workplace; between her mother's dependence upon her father and her own dependence upon her boss—are reduced to one thing: Amy's unconscious symbolic association of her father and her boss. But the symmetries in Amy's experience are actually based on the real symmetries in the social arrangements and relations that structure her economic, social, and psychic life. Amy identifies with her mother not only because she has been psychosocially conditioned to do so within the family, but because she shares the same conditions of oppression. The nuclear family and the capitalist workplace, the two social contexts of Amy's anger, are social arrangements that, in different but related ways, institutionalize male dominance and female socioeconomic dependence.[4] In both her family and at work, Amy is actually as well as unconsciously a dependent being. In both situations, she is ruled, in different ways, by men. In fact, it *is the rule of the father in Amy's family and the rule of the boss in Amy's workplace that, taken together, provide the social basis for Amy's unconscious symbolic association of the two male authority figures.* It is not Amy's anger at her father that is the underlying cause of her current distress. Rather, the social arrangements of male dominance are the underlying cause of her anger—both at her father and at her boss. Her anger at both men is the intelligible response of a powerless female in two different but related situations of male rule.

But why should this anger appear, as it does, in so unconscious and indirect a form as an involuntary spasm of Amy's facial muscles? The answer, in psychodynamic theory, is that Amy was taught to repress her anger in order to keep her father's love and that this repressed anger reemerges in the form of a somatic symptom. This answer, while true, is insufficient.

Most women, like Amy, learn to repress their anger at men —beginning with their father—in order to survive. The lessons learned by Amy in her family are the very same lessons learned by most girls in most families. Be sweet—passive, compliant, and obedient. Never be angry, aggressive, or assertive. Respect male authority and power. Turn all anger inward, against yourself.* The repression of female rage at being ruled by men and its redirection inward, toward the self, is then construed by

* These are similar to the messages that workers in relation to bosses and blacks in relation to whites must internalize in order to play successfully by the rules of our social institutions. One important function of the nuclear family is precisely to produce people who have correctly learned these lessons. Our social system needs certain types of people in order to perpetuate itself: aggressive, dominant males (Amy's father, her boss, her husband, et al.) who will nevertheless respect the power of those above them in the class/sex/race hierarchy; and passive, subservient females (Amy's mother, Amy, et al.) to serve these males.

psychologists as the female individual's successful adaptation to society. The social sanctions against women who do not succeed in this adaptation range from subtle forms of social coercion and ostracism, to battering and psychiatric hospitalization.

Not surprisingly, repressed rage in women may often take indirect and unconscious forms—like Amy's peculiar and bothersome facial twitch, experienced in the presence of powerful males. When Amy's face hardens into that of her mother, she becomes, like her mother before her, a woman caught in the powerful grip of masculine domination, trapped in the poisonous well of her unexpressed hatred of all men. Years of legitimate rage are shut tight within Amy's facial muscles. Under the penetrating glance of her boss, the muscles start to give way. When he looks at her, her mouth twitches in defiance—a feeble, unconscious revolt against his power, and the power of all men to control her life. A twitch instead of a scream.

Furthermore, the most obvious element of Amy's facial symptom was that when men looked at Amy, she literally flinched away from them. Amy was a woman who suffered from a terror of being seen by men, especially by powerful men in high places. In Amy, this fear was heightened to alarming proportions. The unexpected firing of Amy's co-worker, whom Amy admired for her assertiveness, provoked these feelings of terror and vulnerability. In Amy's mind, it was because this woman was assertive—that is, because she was unabashedly *visible* to her boss—that she was fired. The firing somehow proved Amy's unconscious conviction that a woman's visibility to a powerful man means certain harm. Amy's aversion from the gaze of men was, in part, a desperate attempt to avoid that harm.

On the other hand, her symptom made Amy even more conspicuous, more visible to others. Like many female symptoms, it embodied contradictory impulses. Amy was not only terrified of being seen, she also wildly longed for it. Her early desires, squelched by her father, were to be a dancer or competitive swimmer. Both are center-stage activities in which an onlooking audience is necessary to the performance. Amy had numerous exhibitionist fantasies: to be seen while performing, dancing, making love. In her art, she painted many self-portraits. Essentially, Amy's repressed rage at her father had to do with her never having felt truly seen by him. "Cruel, tyrannical, and *blind*," her father was unwilling or unable to give Amy the recognition she craved. He was unable to see and bless her ambitions, to respond to her need for approval, to understand who she was or what she wanted. Amy's twitch embodied her wish to be seen as much as her fear of it.

Since working with Amy, I have worked with dozens of women who share, in one form or another, Amy's ambivalent wish/fear of being seen. One of these women, Kate, described her fear this way: sometimes, while being looked at, she experienced herself as "an animal frozen in the headlights of an oncoming car." Yet, on the other hand, Kate was a poet and teacher. She enjoyed the attentions of her captive audience and often gave poetry readings in which she exposed her most intimate and private emotions.

Similarly, Pat spoke of her fear of being "noticed." In therapy, she remembered that as a child she left the house by walking along the side of the driveway rather than straight down the middle of the road, where she was more likely to be conspicuous. As an adult, she still walked down the street "hugging the walls." Yet again, Pat was a very talented teacher and an actress; center stage was her element. Many other women who would not necessarily be able to articulate these feelings so clearly nevertheless share them. In milder form, these feelings appear as the fear of self-assertion common among women.

The fearful self-consciousness contained in Amy's facial tic and shared by Kate and Pat is merely an exaggerated extension of the general experience of Woman as Body. Though men too can be self-conscious, women are self-conscious in a different way. The self-consciousness of Woman as Body is that of the woman who lowers her head walking down the street, painfully aware that she is being visually dissected by the men who look at her. It is the self-consciousness of the woman who gets edgy when a strange man on the subway looks her in the eye. Woman as Body learns that to meet the eye of a strange man is to "invite" trouble. The only acceptable recourse for sensible girls is to look away and feign blindness. Pretend you don't see that you're being looked at. Avoid, at all costs, reciprocal recognition. To look a man straight in the eye while he's looking at you is considered provocative—and makes a woman even more vulnerable to sexual harassment than she is ordinarily. Woman as Body learns that to be looked at by a man can be dangerous.

At the same time, to be looked at by a man is what Woman as Body is groomed to expect, solicit, and revel in. The more we are looked at by men, the more "beautiful" we are. Beauty is the quintessentially feminine virtue. Women learn that to be looked at favorably by a man is the highest compliment a woman can get.

It is just this social contradiction of Woman as Body that is embodied in Amy's facial twitch. The contradiction is internalized as a psychic conflict between two warring internal selves: one fighting to be visible, the other demanding to remain invisible, the Exhibitionist versus the Wallflower.

Amy's twitch was the indirect physical expression of Woman as Body's anger at being in a social double bind: a situation in which being seen as a woman is both mandatory and dangerous. Her symptom was not the manifestation of an underlying character pathology. It was an adaptation to the unhealthy psychopolitical predicament of being Woman as Body, of being dominated by a group upon which she was also dependent; of being ruled by men and yet socialized to repress anger against that rule; of having no socially permissible outlet for that rage. The contradictions inherent in this social predicament give rise, in turn, to certain psychic contradictions which, experienced individually and privately, are called "conflicts" or "symptoms." Amy's conflict about anger—her inability to express her anger directly and its subsequent manifestation in hidden form within her symptom—is just one example of characteristic feminine symptomatology. (For a further analysis of characteristic female symptoms of femininity, see the next section of this chapter.)

While Amy's specific symptom may be unique, her problem as a woman is not. Her twitch is unusual because it embodies the dilemmas of Woman as Body so clearly.

There is no running away from this problem. In the last century, doctors called it housewife neurasthenia and recommended lots of bed rest. Sheila Rowbotham has called it the problem of being "oppressed by an overwhelming sense of not being there."[5] Betty Friedan saw it in the tired, empty women of the Feminine Mystique—and called it "the problem that has no name." It is the problem of Woman as Body: of suffering from an overexposure of physical visibility as a body combined with an impoverishment of genuine recognition as a person. As long as woman is essentially defined by her body and as long as her body is appropriated by men, she will always have a problem of feminine identity.

Whatever one calls this problem of feminine identity, it is the stuff of which female symptomatology, nervous breakdowns, and madness are made. It is reflected in the countless women who come to therapy complaining that they have no selves or that they feel empty inside. It is reflected in the characteristically feminine project of trying to achieve self-affirmation through self-negation; for example: the woman who feels worthy by denying herself, or the woman who feels sexual by giving up her sexuality to men, or the woman who feels feminine by effacing herself as a person, or the woman who (like millions of others in this country) is a compulsive eater and dieter, forever trying to make herself simultaneously more and less visible.

Amy understood the powerlessness of Woman as Body intimately. As a child she had been overpowered by her father. As a wife, she had been (legally) raped by her husband. As a worker, she had been (legally) dominated by men on the job. As a patient looking for emotional help, she had been deemed ugly as a body and inadequate as a personality—condemned to be a nobody by a psychiatric judgment that both reflected and contributed to her problem.

Amy's problem is every woman's problem. As long as patriarchal society is, like Amy's father, "cruel, tyrannical, and blind" to women, there will always be women like Amy. And there will always be a problem.

2. *Victim Psychology and the Symptoms of Femininity*

LINDA'S STORY: DEPRESSION AS A WAY OF LIFE ■ Without a conscious repudiation of the femininity of Woman as Body, women are bound to experience a host of conflicts that are traditionally labeled symptomatic of pathology. Without rebelling against the condition of female social powerlessness, women will inevitably suffer the symptoms of this condition. Without breaking her double-bind chains, Woman as Body is bound to become Woman as Patient.

But acts of overt defiance are forbidden to women who wish to be considered feminine, and the social sanctions against them are abundant. Simply to be called "unfeminine" is often enough to make a woman shrink back into her proper place. A woman's sense of identity as a person is so early on linked to her identity as a feminine being, that to be called unfeminine is tantamount to having her core sense of identity invalidated. Any woman who was part of the social revolt of Woman as Body in the early days of the contemporary woman's movement knows what it's like to be called butch, dyke, castrating bitch, dominating female, ballbuster, witch. These male responses to women in the movement were ways of saying that women who fought for themselves were unfeminine. The use of such terms was often effective in crippling women's attempts to rebel.

As we have seen in chapter three, it is still true today that women who defy the cultural conventions of normal femininity are not socially accepted as women. These women are culturally and psychiatrically viewed as emotionally abnormal or even mentally ill. But the rules forbidding female uprisings against normal femininity are not simply psychological in nature. The weapons are often quite real and material. Psychiatric treatment for rebellious women who are labeled "violence-prone" is involuntary incarceration, the suspension of civil rights, the use of forced drugging. Recently, the psychiatric prescription of psychosurgery for such women has been viewed with increasing favor. Many women who have not been psychiatrically hospitalized still know that to rebel against their proper place is to risk getting battered by husbands or lovers. Thus the complete array of acceptable social sanctions against female insubordination ranges from subtle forms of social unacceptance to violence and the threat of violence.

Not surprisingly, women who rebel against their lot as Woman as Body, who revolt against femininity as culturally defined (particularly in the absence of a social movement by which such rebellions can be channeled and legitimated) are often thrown back on essentially isolated and indirect forms of protest: subversive private uprisings which are often unconscious. This was the dynamic involved in Amy's facial twitch. Amy's symptom was her way of saying No. Feminine women are supposed to smile, not twitch.

It is also the dynamic involved in the secretary who loses important papers and spills coffee on the files; the middle-aged housewife who develops chronic lower back pain so incapacitating that she can no longer do housework; the so-called frigid woman who is sexually invulnerable to men; the closet lesbian who goes out with men but won't let them touch her; the psychotherapy patient who refuses to develop insight. These are just the kind of behaviors that are likely to be picked up by a psychiatric Expert as symptomatic of an underlying neurosis or character disorder. But given the proper conditions of support for doing so, most women would register a smile of recognition at these kinds of behavior. From the point of view of someone who identifies with women, rather than someone who wants to cure them, such behaviors can be seen as the unconscious recourse of persons who are angry and have no legitimate, socially sanctioned outlets for their anger. They are ways of registering protest without taking too great a social risk. The secretary who tells her boss to get his own coffee can lose her job. The middle-aged housewife who openly refuses to do housework for her husband risks being abused or beaten. The so-called frigid woman who claims her sexual autonomy by renouncing her sexual attachment to men risks being seen as a sexual deviant. The closet lesbian who comes out as a lover of women risks serious economic and social losses. The psychotherapy patient who openly defies her psychiatrist may risk enforced tranquilization or hospitalization. Consequently, women learn to express anger and resistance passively, indirectly, and largely against ourselves—the feminine way.

Psychiatrists call such behavior patterns passive aggressive. Indeed they are. But psychiatrists, as we have seen, are blind to the ways in which such patterns are inevitable responses of women caught in the double bind of feminine consciousness. Many women do, in fact, develop passive and indirect ways of fighting back against the code of acceptable feminine behavior. We do so because we are afraid to exert more direct forms of anger and power. And we are afraid not only because of the social conditioning which trains women to be passive and avoid conflict, but also because it is often objectively dangerous for women to strike back openly.

In *Women and Madness,* Phyllis Chesler documents the different patterns of symptomatology that develop among men and women. She cites studies of childhood behavior problems which indicate that boys are most often referred to child guidance clinics for aggressive, destructive, antisocial, and competitive behavior, whereas girls are referred for personality problems such as excessive fears and worries, shyness, lack of self-confidence, and feelings of inferiority. These masculine and feminine patterns of symptomatology persist in adults, says Chesler. Men's symptoms are more likely to display a destructive hostility toward others, as reflected in behavior patterns such as robbery, rape, alcoholism, and drug addiction. Women's symptoms are more likely to express a harsh, self-critical, and self-destructive set of attitudes as reflected in patterns of behavior such as depression, frigidity, paranoia, suicide attempts, and anxiety.[6]

Chesler was not the first to point out that many of the symptoms that women bring to therapy reflect passive forms of feminine revolt against femininity. In *The Myth of Mental Illness,*

Thomas Szasz explained chronic fatigue states and other symptoms prevalent in women as expressions of "patients who are
unconsciously 'on strike' against persons (actual or internal) to
whom they relate with subservience and against whom they
wage an unending and unsuccessful covert rebellion."[7]

Persons victimized by a social system will develop the consciousness of a Victim. Victim psychology—the psychology of
women and other oppressed groups—is characterized by the
hidden protest. Indirect communication, indirect use of power
in the passive/aggressive mode, internalized anger that
emerges in acts of unconscious hostility: these are all Victim
traits. If we drop the dominant (male) point of view which tells
us that these are symptoms of individual neurosis or of mental
disorders, it becomes clear that these symptoms are to a large
extent socially produced. From the submerged, dominated (female) point of view, feminine symptoms are often ways of coping with the double binds of constructing a feminine identity
in a man's world. They are both a manifestation of this double
bind and a desperate attempt to retrieve oneself from its grip.
Looked at closely, each symptom, like Amy's twitch, can be
seen as an unconscious strategy of both adaptation to and rebellion against the condition of female powerlessness known
as femininity.

The single most common characteristically feminine symptom is depression. Depression is a condition endemic to
women as a group. Women are three times as frequently depressed as men and try to kill themselves twice as often. Ask
any therapist for the most popular diagnosis of his or her female
patients and the answer is likely to be some form of depression.
Depression is more common in married than single women. It
is temporarily chased away by Valium and wine. But it persists.
Depression is the feminine symptom to end all symptoms.

Depression was Linda's problem.

Single and in her thirties, Linda came to see me after a
brief stay in a private hospital, recommended by her former
therapist. She had been diagnosed in the hospital as manic-
depressive and treated with lithium and individual therapy.

Neither the lithium nor the hospitalization nor any of her previous therapy experiences had cured Linda of her depressions. She had been depressed, off and on, since early adolescence.

When asked to describe her depression, Linda talked about overwhelming feelings of hopelessness, helplessness, worthlessness, and terror. Uncontrollable crying jags alternated with an abiding numbness, as though her entire body and mind were anesthetized. She felt as though nothing really mattered. She slept too much, ate too much (or sometimes not at all), and had no interest in doing anything. Through an effort of supreme will, she managed to crawl out of bed each morning and go to work. The worst moment of every day was coming home from work and facing her lonely apartment. Sometimes Linda would compulsively organize her life so that she was constantly busy, in an effort to avoid this moment. But whenever she returned to her house, her depression would hit hard. Then it was all she could do to keep herself going until the next day.

Linda's terror of being alone was profound. It was in flight from this feeling that she often indulged her fantasies of doing away with herself. (We further explore this common female affliction in the third section of this chapter.) Linda dreamed of being with a man to take her away from all this. Her most intense feeling was a wretched self-hatred.

What Linda wanted from therapy was deceptively simple: she wanted to be "happy." She wanted to stop being depressed. She wanted to feel good about herself. My subjective estimate is that at least 75 percent of all women in therapy want the same things.

The way that Linda explained her depression to herself was that she lacked self-esteem and was too dependent on men. In an autobiography composed for me, she wrote:

> Since high school my life has been the story of one man after another. There has never been any *me* except hurt, loss and rejection since then. . . . The only times I've remembered feeling okay in the last fifteen years or so was when I had a man with me, and then I was always afraid he'd leave because he always did in the end. . . . I am right now a sum

total of all these years—too afraid to get involved with a man again and too afraid not to. Having nothing of my own. Knowing that there must be life in me, but feeling that without a man to love me I am nothing and might as well die.

Linda was a man-junkie. She lived for the moment of her next fix of male approval and love, and then lived in terror of the moment when the fix would wear off—as it inevitably did. Ultimately, except for the brief time that such fixes lasted, she never felt good about herself—with or without a man.

Central to Linda's experience of depression was the feeling that had plagued her throughout her adult life: the feeling that she did not really have a "self" at all, that she was a collection of other people's (especially men's) desires and expectations. She often said, "I don't know who I am or what I want." Linda called this lack of a sense of identity her "dependency." It was the part of herself she most hated.

On the one hand, Linda felt that if she could keep a man bound to her, she would feel better about herself as a person. But on the other hand, this belief only furthered her depression because she thought that wanting to be with a man in order to raise her self-esteem was only another sign of her hated dependency. Consequently, her depressions were vicious cycles with the viciousness directed at herself.

As our sessions progressed, it became increasingly apparent that Linda was actually ambivalent about achieving self-esteem. The more self-love she felt, the more she experienced an odd, inexplicable pull toward the old habit of self-hate. An ancient part of Linda believed that women were simply not supposed to be people who valued themselves. They were people who valued other people—particularly men. A sense of competence and completeness as a person was not something she felt she *should* possess as a woman. It was something that belonged to men only.

It was, in fact, precisely the kind of self-possession and self-confidence that Linda wanted for herself that she found so attractive in men. What Linda called her dependency was largely the attempt to get some of this feeling of self-worth through her association with a man—as though it could be gotten through osmosis. In a man, self-confidence was something to be admired, envied, and sought after. But in a woman, it appeared to Linda as a deformity: the monstrous dragon of conceit. In a profound way, the self-esteem she longed for appeared to be a betrayal of her core sense of femininity.

Her femininity, in turn, was the part of Linda that was geared to other people's—particularly men's—expectations, rather than her own. The part of herself that Linda most hated —her dependency—was also the part she felt made her feminine, made her a woman. It was this woman in herself that she hated. But it was also the woman in herself that she wanted to preserve. Self-esteem was something she desperately wanted and most strongly resisted.

What Linda wanted from therapy was to conquer her depression and learn to feel good about herself. My problem as a therapist was to help her overcome her resistances to her own wish.

Linda had had countless relationships with men, all of which ended disastrously. In therapy, Linda repeatedly faced the ways in which she had been victimized by the men in her life: men who used her sexually; men who were emotionally dishonest or emotionally cruel; men who had no respect for what she felt or thought; men who abused her verbally and, at times, physically; men who wielded power over her body and mind in a variety of ways both subtle and harsh. Linda complained bitterly about how badly these men had treated her and sometimes blamed them for her depressions. But at bottom, she was convinced that she got what she deserved from them.

The Victim in Linda viewed all of her feelings of sadness, hurt, fear, and anger at the men who had variously abused their power over her as proof of her inherent worthlessness. Some internal tape in Linda's head told her over and over again: "You *feel* bad because you *are* bad." And even more unconscious, "You are bad *because you are a woman*." *The worthlessness itself was somehow felt to be an essential part of her feminine*

self. Emotional invulnerability, emotional violence, and
aggression were all aspects of masculinity as culturally defined.
Woman's acceptance and embracing of these male attributes
was essential to femininity as culturally defined. Hence the
Victim in Linda unwittingly complied with the way men
treated her. In doing so, Linda was unconsciously attempting to
be "in synch" with the internalized social definition of herself
as a woman.

Like most women in therapy and out, Linda preferred to
think of herself as a patient with a personal problem rather than
as a woman with a social problem which had been deeply internalized. She preferred to think that the problem was all in her
head rather than to think that there was a larger problem of how
men were trained to treat women in patriarchal society, and
how women were trained to accept such treatment. Like most
women, she believed that men would be nicer if she chose the
"right" ones. Her problem, she thought, was her pattern of
choosing the "wrong" ones. She never thought to ask herself
why there was such an apparent abundance of wrong men to
choose from! What superficially appeared to be Linda's insight
into her own compliance with men's oppression was, on closer
inspection, the sophisticated workings of her Victim self-blame.

For Linda, playing the Victim was preferable to the alternative: recognizing, expressing, and finally letting go of the
tremendous rage that she had toward men. She fantasized about
men who would rescue her from her ordeal of self-hatred and
depression, and then repressed the contempt and rage that she
felt at all the men she'd ever known who hadn't accomplished
this rescue mission. In therapy, she transferred this craving for
rescue to me, playing the Patient whose therapist would set her
free.

It took months of therapy for her to begin to see that while
she dreamed of Prince Charming, she was far more ambivalent
about his coming than she thought. Between her and the love
of her life was a mountain of anger. Linda assumed, both consciously and unconsciously, that this mountain had no business
being there. She habitually tried to get around it by leveling it

into a valley of depression. In virtually every relationship she'd ever had with a man, she had tried her best to tailor herself to her man's specifications and swallow her anger. But the strategy didn't work. In every case, she ended up losing the man and feeling ripped off.

In therapy as in her life, the more Linda came face to face with her anger at men, the more she wanted to flee. She felt that anger, more than any other emotion, was a sure sign of her ugliness as a person. No matter how much she wanted to hear from me that her anger was valid, she could not get herself really to believe it. If she weren't so angry, Linda thought, then she could make it with a man. She believed that it was her anger, more than anything else, that pushed men away. Linda's tendency at these points in the therapy was to dampen the flames of her rage—and to deepen her depression. Rather than risk a rage that threatened to engulf her, she retreated to the habitual ground of self-hate. Depression was almost comfortable, something she could wrap herself in when she was frightened of her anger.

Clearly, Linda's depression was connected to an unexamined, unconscious, and unresolved source of anger. Indeed, traditional experts in chronic depression do recognize that the major dynamic here is anger which has been displaced from its original "aim" and instead directed at the self. This original aim, as we have seen in the case of Amy, is almost always viewed as a single "significant other" in the patient's past, rather than as an entire social configuration which has been internalized. We have occasion to examine the central role of unconscious and unresolved anger in women's lives in the next chapter.

The point I am making here is that such displaced and internalized anger is, in fact, an inevitable aspect of female identity in patriarchal society. In this sense, depression in women is bound to be common.

In Linda's case it was clear that her depression had everything to do with her desire both to preserve and to eradicate her dependency on men. Dependency was a term Linda had learned from the male-dominated culture. It was the name she gave to her way of giving herself away in relationships with men, and then feeling used up and empty. But abandoning herself in this way was exactly what she—and the culture—saw as the feminine way to be. Dependency, as we may recall, is one of the hallmarks of normal femininity as defined by Freud. Fundamentally, this culture sees femininity as powerlessness and self-loss. Being a man-junkie (whether in the form of living from one man to another as Linda did, or in the form of a stable addiction to one man only) is the logical extension of this cultural definition.

For Linda, and for many women, this feminine powerlessness had its moments of ecstasy: at the start of an exciting new love affair or, sometimes, in sex. But for the most part, femininity was a curse from which Linda could not escape—because she wanted it as much as she hated it.

The seemingly personal knot in which Linda was bound clearly turned on her deeply ingrained, core sense of female identity—of herself as a feminine person. She wanted to be self-confident and self-possessed. She wanted to belong to herself. In a male-dominated society, the model for this kind of person is masculine. Feminine persons, on the other hand, are supposed to be persons who belong to someone else: particularly to men. Becoming a person who prizes herself means, in this sense, becoming a male person. The problem for Linda was that conquering her depressions and raising her self-esteem were bound up with extricating herself from a complex double bind: she wanted to be whole in a way that threatened to destroy her as a woman.

To see Linda's conflictual knot as simply a "clinical" problem in therapy is to avoid the obvious: that in a woman-hating culture, it is normal for women to hate themselves. Depression is, for one thing, a survival strategy adopted by women in a society that devalues women while demanding and idolizing femininity. Linda's conflicts about feeling good about herself are a simple reflection of this social double bind. No matter which way a woman turns, she is bound by the law of the double bind itself to end up devaluing herself as the culture does.

This is obvious if one thinks about the problematic relationship of femininity to self-esteem historically. Traditionally, women in this society were taught that self-esteem is to be won by satisfying what male society defined as the "biological" demands of femininity. Hence the Freudian norm for healthy women: marrying and having babies, preferably male. But the happiness supposedly guaranteed by the culture for these feminine pursuits often turned out to be a false promise. The "Feminine Mystique," as Betty Friedan called it, led to a widespread malaise afflicting women who, on the surface of it, had everything their feminine hearts were supposed to desire. The Feminine Mystique did not end up making women feel good about themselves. It ended up as housewife neurasthenia: an overwhelming listlessness, emptiness, and sense of not having a self—Linda's problem in epidemic proportions! It ended up as female addiction to liquor and tranquilizers, as female sexual problems and suicide. The name of "the problem that has no name" is chronic depression. Everything that was supposed to make women feel good about themselves ended up making them feel depressed.

It is tempting to think that this ended with the decline of the Feminine Mystique in the 1960s. But a closer look at the last twenty years reveals the same social fact: *femininity is depressing*. With the so-called sexual revolution of the 1960s, women were supposed to feel good about themselves by having sex with men. With the widespread use of the Pill, female sexuality enjoyed a new birth. An end to sexual repression and the double standard for sexuality, women were told, would liberate women to be as free as men were sexually. Rather than (or in addition to) marriage and babies, it was now being a "good fuck" (by male standards) that promised to make women glow with self-esteem.

But it is hard to make a career out of being a good fuck. When you got right down to it, the sexual counterculture still saw women (and women still saw themselves) as yet another version of Woman as Body—this time, Glorified Cunt. It is difficult to build up anything that resembles genuine self-respect on this shaky pedestal. The Marilyn Monroe road to depression may be more glamorous but it is the same dead end for women. Most women, in any case, weren't eligible for the glamour: they were just eligible for the depression.

With the advent of the women's movement, the subject of how women could feel good about themselves became more and more confusing. Self-esteem could no longer mean satisfying a man through reproduction or sex. It had to mean satisfying oneself. But how? The resounding answer from the media's version of "Women's Lib," and from a good many feminists themselves, was: get a career, but without necessarily sacrificing the old feminine ideals either. More and more, feeling good about oneself for a woman came to mean being Superwoman: having it all and doing it all with style. Not many women can carry this off, especially since the society is still a long way from satisfying even the most minimal socioeconomic needs of most women. A fancy male-style career was something that, all things considered, most women did not have access to. Another false promise. Another road to depression.

The conclusion is inescapable: oppression is depressing. Something inherent in being feminine in a male-dominated society (despite minor modifications in how femininity is defined over the years) inevitably leads to depression for women.

The major ingredients of depression—the feelings of hopelessness, helplessness, worthlessness, futility, and suppressed rage—are the affective components of the objective social condition of female powerlessness in male society. Traditionally, such feelings, when "extreme," are seen as pathological. But *feeling* helpless is in some sense a rational adaptation to the social fact of *being* powerless. As such, depression is quite normal, acceptable feminine behavior, a way of getting cared for or protected by men who have power over women—husbands, lovers, bosses, and therapists.

As long as men as a group have power over women as a group, the power to institutionalize the ways in which women are defined, treated, and mistreated as persons, large numbers of women will be depressed. People without power, people who look around at the world and do not see themselves reflected in it, learn to feel marginal, unimportant. People for whom the social order shows contempt learn to hate themselves. Powerlessness breeds depression.

Feeling good about oneself has something to do with power, with having power and feeling powerful; with being rooted in one's body and believing in one's sense of *agency*—that is, one's capacity to exert power. Psychically speaking, women's oppression consists largely in being deprived of a sense of agency. How can a woman believe in her power in a thoroughly male society in which all the major institutions are run by men, and in which culture itself is male? A deep-seated conviction of powerlessness and suppressed rage is what is commonly called depression. Depression is just the clinical name for one of the individual effects male domination has on women.

Coming to love oneself as a woman has everything to do with getting very angry about this state of affairs. But here is where the double bind of femininity exerts its most insidiously powerful tug: for it is precisely the inability to get angry directly that most characterizes depression. Women are depressed, to simplify, because they cannot, or do not feel able to, get angry. Without an authentic sense of one's capacity to feel and express anger, there is no fuel to burn, nothing to get a genuine sense of power going. Eventually, to experience one's personal power, it is necessary to give up one's attachment to permanent, unconscious anger. But this process cannot happen if the anger is not recognized in the first place. The result is the passive/aggressive hostility so characteristic of the depressed.

Women are afraid not only of anger, but of power—of the feeling of power, as well as the institutionalized ways of exerting it. Everything in a woman's social experience teaches her that power is masculine and powerlessness is feminine; that anger is masculine and depression is feminine. Women tend to associate feeling and being powerful not with feeling good, but with social isolation and no longer being protected by men. Since women are trained to get whatever we can through this protection and, in fact (given the violence of male society), often appear to need it, the specter of giving up feminine powerlessness with no guarantee of anything tangible to replace it is truly terrifying. For many women, power is associated with abuse—because the two have been connected in women's experience of male power. Many women quite rightly resist becoming "masculine" in this sense. Yet there are few nonmasculine models of power for women to envision; for the genuine power in women is, like everything else female in male society, devalued.

Virtually every woman I've ever worked with in therapy comes up against this knot. Feeling good means feeling powerful. But feeling powerful, for women, is closely associated with not feeling womanly, which is a fundamental threat to identity. Feeling good then becomes feeling bad. Almost every breakthrough for women in therapy is thus accompanied or followed by what I call a "backlash of the feminine," a pull toward the old, familiar powerless feelings of the Victim. Often, women in therapy take this backlash as a sign that they are getting nowhere—but the backlash is often strongest just when women are breaking through the most entrenched patterns of powerless behavior.

Ultimately, all of the features of Linda's depression were aspects of what I have called Victim psychology. Institutionalized powerlessness makes the Victim see herself as the powerless prey of others. The Victim thus develops strategies of indirect anger and indirect power that psychologists label manipulative or passive/aggressive. Depression is probably the most typical of such strategies among women. It is an unconscious attempt to retrieve oneself from a society which makes it practically impossible for women to feel authentically powerful and feminine at the same time.

Depression allowed Linda to feel at one with her social definition as a female, while at the same time exerting an indi-

rectly powerful tug on others. Anyone who has ever tried to
cheer up a severely depressed person knows just how powerful
such a person can be. The hidden protest in depression, the
submerged message of resistance is: "I'm determined to be
miserable and mean and depressed, no matter what you say or
do. You're not good or wise or strong enough to help me, try as
you will." There is an unmistakable though extremely indirect
challenge to authority in depression. Strategically, it allows the
Woman as Victim to make herself feel more powerful, by making the other feel less powerful. The Victim manipulates in
such a way as to make the helper feel as powerless as she does.
This is the Victim's way of protesting without taking a risk; of
bidding for and resisting care at the same time; of submitting
to and challenging the reality of being dominated; of being
feminine and struggling against femininity at the same time.

In one sense, depression works for women. Linda's depression had elicited some of the only emotional nurturance she
had ever gotten from her lovers. It had gotten her former psychiatrist to prescribe pills for her and to increase her sessions
to twice a week. A direct appeal for emotional nurturance and
support might not have gotten Linda this far with her lovers—
and certainly would not have with her psychiatrist. The Victim
exerts her power indirectly not only because she is limited in
her experience of power and has been taught to shun such
experiences, but also because *indirect power exerted on men
often works* where direct power will not—as any woman
knows, who has ever cried (rather than argued) to get her way.

Ultimately, however, depression does not work for women.
It is a strategy of desperation and defeat, ineffectual and self-
destructive. Like other strategies of the oppressed, designed to
strike back indirectly and to help the powerless gain some measure of the feeling of power, it fails. The kind of power a woman
feels in depression is inauthentic and self-defeating. Depression is unhealthy not because it is pathological but because it
weakens a woman's capacities to develop her power authentically. Like other unconscious strategies of the oppressed, it
represents an accommodation to a social reality which, like the
reality itself, is not in the interests of women.

In the symptomatology of femininity, depression rates number one. Typically, feminine symptoms are clumped together in certain constellations. Depression is quite often seen together with two other common female symptoms: so-called frigidity and psychosomatic pain. In Linda's case, despite her numerous involvements with men, she had only very rarely experienced orgasm. She suffered from recurrent headaches and stomach pain which were clearly related to her emotional distress.

A close look at female frigidity and psychosomatic pain reveals a dynamic similar to that of depression. On the one hand, frigidity in women can be seen as an adaptation to a society in which female sexuality in and for itself has been repressed and distorted to suit male interests. Centuries of such repression has resulted in the emergence of a feminine style of sexuality that Freudian psychologists label masochistic. This feminine style of sexuality is the most intimate expression of women's lot in other areas of life. In sex, as in life, the feminine style is modeled on that of the slave serving herself up to her master. (This is why *The Story of O,* a book that exploits female sexual masochism in great detail, continues to be one of the most popular books of pornography among women.) We should not mistake the recent sexual revolution for a genuine reversal of this inauthentic form of female sexuality. The sexual ethos typified by *Playboy* magazine merely expands the slavish tricks in the female repertoire to include aggression, sadomasochism, lesbianism, etc. What hasn't changed is that the sexual terms are still defined by and for men. (The genuinely exciting and progressive changes in female sexuality have been the result of the women's movement's attempts to redefine female sexuality from a woman's point of view.)

The very word "frigidity" has a masculinist ring: it assumes that a woman who refuses, consciously or otherwise, to be sexual with men is "cold." But the frigid woman is, in essence, Woman as Body on (unconscious) strike. She unconsciously refuses to produce her sexuality, or her orgasm, for the use of men. This does not mean that she is incapable of sexual satisfaction or of sexual giving.

On the one hand, female frigidity is inevitable in a society that has for centuries repressed female sexuality. On the other hand, frigidity is also an unconscious strategy of revolt. It is an unconscious protest against male standards for female sexuality. It is an unconscious (and at times conscious) way of saying: "I will not give my sexuality over to you," or "I will not come for you." In the long battle between the sexes and the consequent power struggle called making love, this is the woman's way of not allowing the man to win. It is her way of refusing to grant him the pleasure of producing her orgasm and thereby enhancing his own virility, the source of his power over her. In this sense, frigidity, like depression, has its own rationality or logic. It represents the woman's refusal to make herself sexually vulnerable to the power of masculinity, her refusal to adopt the feminine norm of masochistic sexuality. It is another indirect means of exerting power—a way of making a man feel denigrated and helpless by denying him sexual access. Women who fake orgasm (a widespread phenomenon which women have only recently begun to air publicly) are engaged in a similar pattern of indirect refusal to succumb to male power. In this case, the refusal is both unconscious and conscious—the woman *knows* that she hasn't come, but she fakes it for the sake of the man. Technically, she lets him win his satisfaction in her orgasm, but only at the expense of a secret poisonous contempt for him and how easily he is fooled by her playacting.

Similarly, psychosomatic pain in women (chronic headaches, menstrual pain, lower back pain, etc.) is often related to the unconscious struggle both to adapt to and rebel against femininity. On the one hand, it is still, despite the era of the New Woman, quite feminine to be sick or in pain.[8] There is a cultural acceptance of "female troubles," for instance, during menstruation, the monthly "reminder" of femininity. It is interesting to note that in psychiatric circles, the woman who suffers from psychosomatic symptoms is often held in contempt and considered to be a pain in the neck (in psychiatric slang, she is called a "crock"). Nevertheless, she never loses her femininity; consequently, she tends to arouse the most paternalistic impulses in her male medical benefactors. I remember one psychiatrist in my training, the resident expert in hypochondriacal disorders in women, recommending that the therapist exert a firm but gentle hand with female hypochondriacs. He called this a "fatherly approach." The combination of contempt and benign paternalism in his attitude typifies the culture's response to women in pain: a woman on her back in pain may be irritating, but she is still a woman.

What is feminine about the female hypochondriac is that she does not get angry; she complains. She does not fight; she whines. She tends to confine herself to the range of emotions considered appropriate for females: sadness, fear, neediness, despair. She is unlikely to exhibit any feelings along the more culturally defined masculine spectrum: anger, rage, aggression, or direct hostility. The feminine range of emotions is largely restricted to those characterized by passivity and impotence, unlike masculine emotions, which are more outwardly directed. Women cry, men fight. Both may be suffering from similar unmet needs and repressed wishes, but the man gets his feelings out on the other, while the woman wallows in herself. Thus these repressed needs and wishes in women are likely to appear in the form of physical pains in the head, stomach, genitals, back, etc. Woman as Body literally "em-bodies" her repressed emotions.

It is often only through such "displacement" and "somatization" (as psychiatrists call it) that her emotions are considered socially acceptable. The woman who lashes out and attacks her husband, for instance, is quite likely to be considered severely disturbed and even hospitalized for the terrible error of adopting a masculine style of expressing emotions. (Think of how often this takes place the other way around; yet men who beat their wives are hardly ever considered mentally disturbed or hospitalized for that reason.)

On the other hand, psychosomatic symptoms are often ways of going on strike against expected feminine cultural tasks such as domestic service. The most frequently psychosomatic woman is what I call the burnt-out housewife: the woman who has served her family all of her life and develops her symptoms in middle age, often after her children have left home and she is faced with her only remaining feminine tasks: housework and sexual service. Her psychosomatic symptoms are her way of refusing to do these tasks without taking the risk of doing so consciously and directly. It is a way of saying "I will no longer do the shitwork for you." In saying so directly a woman often risks getting beaten or deserted financially or emotionally. In fact, these women are often dragged into mental hospitals by irate and worried husbands who want them to be "fixed" so that they will return to their normal feminine labors. Unfortunately, the hospital is there to fix them. As with depression and frigidity, these psychosomatic rebellions against femininity are a lost cause.

In the end, symptoms like depression, frigidity, and psychosomatic pain are counterproductive and self-destructive. The woman does to herself what has been done to her. Patriarchal society has contempt for women; so the depressed woman hates herself. Patriarchal society represses the development of an autonomous form of female sexuality; so the "frigid" woman robs herself of the capacity for sexual pleasure. Patriarchal society views a woman's body as an object for men and makes it difficult for her to experience her body as her own; so the psychosomatic woman develops pains that cripple her body.

This kind of *internalization* is one of the most prominent features of Victim psychology. Internalization is the process by which what was initially an externally imposed dictate is transformed into an internally imposed command. The Victim takes in the societal expectation in an attempt to transform necessity into a felt free choice. Thus the social message that women are worth less than men is converted through internalization into feelings of worthlessness. The social condition of female powerlessness in relation to the institutionalized male control over women's bodies in reproduction and sexuality is converted through internalization into feelings of physical shame, disgust, and frigidity. Rather than feeling angry at being at the mercy of male society, we become angry at ourselves, putting ourselves at our own mercy.

This internalization, of course, does not work. Women are not more free for internalizing their social condition. On the contrary, freedom becomes even less attainable through this internal crippling. Internalization further debilitates women and renders us even more vulnerable to further victimization. Once Woman as Victim's symptoms have emerged, they become proof that all of her problems are of her own making. In this way, she holds herself exclusively responsible for a suffering in which there are, to say the least, other parties involved.

Having done this much, the Victim-Patient is trapped in the powerlessness of her own consciousness. She becomes easily overwhelmed by the magnitude of her problems; they seem awesome and impossible to change. She never quite feels up to the responsibility she has imposed upon herself: self-perfection. Most women suffer from this compulsive perfectionism of the oppressed. In striving to be perfect, the Victim attempts to pacify the forces she cannot control in the world. As a child, I used to feel that if only I were *good* enough, the overwhelming sorrow that my parents suffered as victims of the Holocaust would disappear. This was more than an internalization of my parents' hope that their children would somehow redeem their agony. It was also my way of wishing, as a child, that I could have personally spared my parents that agony: that I could be all-powerful enough to have wiped the Nazis off the face of the earth—even though I was not yet born at the time that the Nazis destroyed my parents' universe. It was my parents' overwhelming, excruciating helplessness in the face of oppression that I attempted magically to wish away by my grandiose fantasies of self-perfection. Unconsciously, I felt that if only I were good enough, the Holocaust would never have happened.

For the victim of social oppression, the self at least appears to be under one's individual control, whereas the social world most certainly doesn't. The psychic struggle for self-perfection is thus an attempt to feel in control, rather than to feel helpless. In trying to act on this impossible self-imposed demand of perfection and this grandiose sense of personal power, the Victim ends up losing a more realistic sense of responsibility for herself. She then takes refuge in yet another unconscious process.

Having internalized her oppression, she now *externalizes* the very real personal problems that result, feeling that the power she needs to solve them must come from outside of herself. The Victim becomes the Patient, turning her problems into "issues" that exist independently of her. Such issues are presumably worked on until they disappear. (In psychiatric lingo, the issue is "worked through".) But for the professional Patient, old issues never die, they only fade away . . . and are replaced by new issues.

The net result is either interminable therapy—the mating of a patient and a therapist for life—or what might be called therapy-itis: a psychological disorder consisting in the continual, compulsive search for the therapy just around the corner which will offer what the last therapy did not.

In short, the unconscious mechanisms of internalization and externalization operate together in the consciousness of the Victim-Patient. Internalization produces a grandiose, unrealistic sense of power which one cannot possibly act upon. This, in turn, results in constant self-deprecation and profound feelings of powerlessness. The powerlessness then cycles into the need to externalize. The net result is the Victim-Patient's characteristic posture of eternal expectation of external cure, and eternal disappointment. The Victim-Patient is always blaming herself and/or others. She is constantly complaining. Her life is ravaged by a constant fire of bitterness and helplessness which can never be extinguished. (I am reminded of Woody Allen in the movie *Annie Hall* saying, "Excuse me, it's time for me to go to therapy and start whining.") Her anger at herself and others is not a feeling of power which cleanses and moves her forward. It is an endlessly internally recycled miasma of self-pity and envy. It is an anger that has only been indirectly expressed through symptoms and which is therefore never quite released. Often, it has been piled up for so many years that the Victim-Patient is deathly afraid of touching it for fear it will be totally destructive. Instead, the Victim-Patient holds on to her repressed anger, her symptoms, and her issues. She does not know how to let go of being a Victim. The bottom line of Victim consciousness is this perennial feeling of being trapped or powerless.

The symptoms that women bring to therapy are the individual manifestations of what is essentially a collective problem for all women. The cure for this problem must be collective as well. Feeling powerful for women cannot simply be an isolated emotion, unconnected to social reality. The antidote to female social powerlessness is female power, not only as a psychological state of mind but as a social fact. This is not something that women can achieve in the therapy room.

Nevertheless, women like Linda enter therapists' offices every day, asking for help in overcoming their depressions and learning how to love themselves. How can therapy help such women?

Therapy cannot end women's oppression. But it can help women understand our oppression and minimize the ways in which we internalize and comply with it. It can help make explicit the indirect anger that underlies unconscious Victim strategies. And it can help women develop more overt and direct means of using our anger and exerting our power on our own behalf. The essential task of any therapy geared to the interests of women as a whole has to do with helping women redefine and reexperience our authentic power as people. This means helping women redefine and internalize a women-identified, rather than male-identified, sense of femininity. It means helping transform the Victim in women into the Fighter.

Helping a woman undo the Victim in herself must, however, go beyond helping her get angry about her powerlessness. It must help her see the power that she already does possess—both individually and collectively. No woman is simply her oppression or simply her response to it. She is also a unique being with her own will to live, to express, to grow, to love, and to be powerful. No woman is simply the Victim.

The peculiar social powerlessness of women stems not only from the fact that women have traditionally been denied access to the public spheres of power, but equally from the fact that the domain to which we have been assigned—the private sphere of home and family—is not seen to be important to the ongoing work of society. Despite the fact that women are superficially revered for the feminine functions of child rearing and housekeeping, these activities are not seen as meaningful or powerful *in male terms*. (Many feminists have adopted these same terms in their view of feminine labor as less important than masculine work, hence their idealization of women who manage to imitate men successfully.)

But it is not only the "exceptional" woman—the one who has managed, despite the odds, to make a dent in the public sphere of male culture—who is powerful. Ordinary women who have never been named in books have been powerful throughout history in precisely the feminine ways that society expects but devalues. Women as a group have kept the thread of human society going through the feminine work of raising and nurturing children, loving and sustaining families: the very work that has been so devalued and exploited in patriarchal society.

The power of femininity, as a source of nurturance, love, and connectedness to others, can be reappropriated from the male distortions that have arisen from the fact that femininity has been compelled to be subservient to male interests. The power of femininity can be used to further our interests as women. It is a matter, to start with, of seeing ourselves as persons through our own eyes, and thereby undoing the lie of patriarchal society: that all things masculine are of greater value than all things feminine, including that male sources of power are superior to female sources of power. In redefining our femininity in our own terms, we can begin to come into our full potential for power.

My goals for helping Linda overcome her depression and value herself as a person were thus very different from those set by her former psychiatrist. He wanted to keep her on an even keel, to prevent her chemically from getting too "high" or too "low." I wanted to help her develop her potential to exert her own power in such a way that her unconscious depressive rebellion would be converted to conscious, joyous warfare against the conditions that depressed her.

On the one hand, this task involved the very simple process of listening to her story—and helping her see both her depression and herself as a feminine person with eyes that are neither the eyes of male society nor the eyes of the Victim. On the other hand, it necessarily included helping Linda to see the connections between the self-transformation she sought and the transformation of the social reality for women as a whole, which she preferred to ignore.

Ultimately, helping women like Linda value themselves as persons entails helping them realize that the power of self-esteem women long for cannot be separated from the power for women that comes from fighting for ourselves and each other. For it is in the fighting itself that the Victim is overthrown, and the power in women that has been there all along begins to emerge in a new light.

3. Women and the Labor of Relatedness

DIANE'S STORY: THE FEAR OF BEING ALONE ■ One of the basic premises of this book is the belief that the socioeconomic condition of any group of people necessarily structures the psychic life of that group. Society and psychology mutually influence one another in complex ways. The task of a feminist psychology of women is to draw the connections between the common features of women's psychic lives and the common socioeconomic backdrop that women share.

Women develop Victim psychologies in a context of socioeconomic subordination. It is true that we are freer now from some of the limitations of strict gender identification, freer to see ourselves as persons, rather than women. But it is also true that these changes in self-image are not greeted by significant advances in the socioeconomic opportunities available to the majority of women. The economic class that dominates all other classes in this society is still a class of men. A few more token women enter this predominantly male preserve; but the major-

ity of women are poorer now than they were twenty years ago.
More girls than ever before are growing up to believe that they
can do anything a man can do; but the society still won't let
them do it. More women than ever before are entering the
public work force; but the majority of women who work are in
the lowest-paying, most dead-end clerical, service, or blue-col-
lar jobs—the dregs of available paid labor. More husbands than
ever before wash dishes and play with and care for their children; but women retain primary responsibility for the realm of
the family and, within this realm, they continue to perform
unpaid labor for men.

In a series of articles written for the *Boston Globe* in De-
cember 1980, Dianne Dumanoski documented the increasingly
poor economic condition of women in the economy, a phenomenon she called the "feminization of poverty." Her research
shows that women have been increasingly segregated into
lower-paying jobs over the past twenty years (with as many as
78 percent of women who work in the paid economy doing the
lowest-paying work); and that, as a group, women are persis-
tently poorer than men and have less chance of working themselves out of poverty. At a time when a rapidly increasing
number of women find themselves the family breadwinner,
their access to the kinds of jobs and salaries that will allow them
to support their families at the same level as their male coun-
terparts is diminishing. Dumanoski quotes a 1978 US Commission on Civil Rights report investigating the economic
condition of women and other "minorities" (hardly an appropriate term for women). This report concludes that:

• The median per capita income in households headed by
women has been declining since 1959 relative to white male
households. In 1959, the income in a white female household
was 75 percent of that in a white male household. In 1975 it
was only 59 percent.
• The poorest of the poor, people with incomes one-half
of the official poverty level, are largely women.
• In 1975, white females with the same employment char-

acteristics as white males could be expected to earn only 57 percent of what these men earned.

● Women have increasingly been segregated into lower-paying jobs since 1960, and despite the rise of the women's movement in the 1970s, this segregation continued to increase from 1970 to 1976.

● The chance that a woman would end up poor was greater in 1975 than in 1969.

This same article quotes economist Barbara Bergmann of the University of Maryland as saying that despite the growing number of women in the work force, the structure of the workplace remains virtually unchanged. "Women and children still make all the accommodations," she says. Women heads of households are especially penalized because they work in a situation that implicitly assumes that workers have wives at home. These women must then combine the functions of both mother and father in the family, with inadequate resources in both realms of work: mothering and working in the paid labor force. Child care, for example, is still both expensive and almost impossible to find. Child-care assistance is minimal. Such women, says Bergmann, "suffer from unceasing toil and responsibility and inadequate rest." If this is not a setup for depression and emotional problems of all kinds, I don't know what is.

This article clearly demonstrates that from childhood to retirement, the culture and the economic system continue to work against women on their own—whether it is the working woman who joins the pink-collar ghetto to do a job for a minimum wage that offers virtually no chance of mobility; or the single mother who labors in a workplace not geared to the needs of single mothers and faces a hopeless child-care situation; or the widowed or retired woman who encounters discrimination in the pension system and ends up without a penny; or the divorced woman who has no way to guarantee her husband's alimony and child-care payments. The woman who seeks to actualize the feminist ideals of today confronts an economic system unwilling to make the changes that would allow for a greater accommodation between the workplace and the family and continues to make women pay the cost.

Women who are increasingly convinced that we can make it without a man—because feminist ideology says we can—are, in fact, no more likely than ever before to do so economically —because our economic condition as women guarantees that we can't. What exactly is this economic condition? That is, what, specifically, is the socioeconomic function of women in a society organized along patriarchal and capitalist lines? Under capitalism, the public and private spheres of labor have been divided from one another, with women as a group consigned to do the work of the private, or family, sphere. This work, performed without a wage, consists of the emotional, physical, and sexual labor required to keep husbands going, and the emotional and physical labor required to reproduce and to raise children. While providing a necessary social function, woman's work in the family sphere has been hidden from view by the ideology that has defined housework and child rearing as the natural labor of femininity—and therefore nonremunerative by definition. Because woman's work is considered a labor of love, it is not seen as *work*. Because it is not seen as work, it is performed without a wage; and because women's work is wageless, it is not seen as work. Thus patriarchy and capitalism work together in defining women's economic position.

In describing this economic position, I prefer a term coined by Ann Ferguson: women are a "sex class" whose wageless work in the family benefits both men as a group and capitalism as a whole.[9] In performing the tasks involved in this family labor, women constitute the unpaid workers in an unseen economy in which husbands reap the benefit and women are the exploited class. The work done in this economy is crucial to that performed in what gets called the "economy"—the sphere in which men (and increasingly women) perform the tasks of wage labor.

There is no doubt that the organization of work in the paid workplace would have to undergo vast changes in order to accommodate the needs of women (for example, workplace child-care centers, paid maternity and paternity leaves, etc.). Alternatively, changes such as paying women for their work in the home would also cost capitalism a pretty penny. As we have seen from the *Boston Globe* article, these are changes patriarchal capitalism would prefer not to make. Consequently, women's economic position as a sex class remains hidden, and women's "class" position is, instead, defined as the class of their husbands and fathers—a definition consistent with the general invisibility of women as persons in patriarchy.

Though not all women are housewives and mothers, and though many women do other work besides family work, women as a group constitute this sex class, doing the family work of patriarchal capitalism for free.* Women's psychology today continues to be structured within this overall socioeconomic context. How does this socioeconomic position of women affect female psychology? To answer this question, let us turn to Diane's story.

Diane first came to therapy because she wanted help in sorting out the tangles of a primary relationship with a woman

---

* The fact that women are recently increasingly entering the labor force on the lowest rungs of the labor hierarchy is an illustration of another economic function of women in patriarchal capitalism: women serve as a reservoir of cheap labor that capitalism can hire when necessary. As a group of lesser-skilled, low-paid, and unorganized workers outside the home, women can be shuttled in and out of the work force at will and used to keep wages down for the work force as a whole. The most dramatic example of patriarchal capitalism's manipulative use of women in the labor force was the fate of women workers after World War II. During the war years, 'Rosy the Riveter' became a familiar face on billboards and other media advertisements which sought to induce women to take up the jobs that the men had left behind. Rosy was sweet and feminine but a patriotic hard worker—every bit as good as a man. Under the guiding light of this new imagery of femininity, women entered the male labor force by the thousands, learning the masculine skills of riveting, soldering, electronics, and heavy industrial work of all kinds. When the war was over and the boys came home, patriarchal capitalism had to convince these newly trained women that the work they were doing was no longer for them, that their job was now to move over and let the men take over again. Femininity was now redefined as a matter of having shiny homes and new babies; and the years of the Feminine Mystique began. Rosy the Riveter was replaced by the 1950s wife and mother. Katharine Hepburn fighting for women's rights in *Adam's Rib* was replaced by Doris Day acting cute with a mop and pail in *Pillow Talk*. In this way, thousands of women returned to their primary work as household laborers.

whom she both loved and wanted to leave. She described herself as "married" for ten years to the woman who shared her
home. From the start, this relationship had been marked by
intense ambivalence and numerous problems. Foremost among
these was the fact that the sexual relationship between Diane
and her spouse was virtually nonexistent. Diane considered
herself someone with a fairly strong sexual drive and this absence of sex was a source of deep resentment and frustration.
She had tried to get the sex to work but it never had. Consequently, she had spent years ruminating about leaving her partner. Despite her stated desire to do so, she felt trapped in the
relationship. Whenever she so much as thought about splitting
up, she was overcome by her terrible fear of being alone. She
ended up convincing herself that living alone was out of the
question—she was incapable of it.

As a lesbian for fifteen years, Diane was long accustomed
to supporting herself; there was never any question that a man
would do it for her. She was a highly competent social worker
whose work entailed a great deal of responsibility. She was a
caring, sensitive, nurturant person and in many respects a mature woman. Yet, her fear of being alone was often so intense
that it effectively reduced her to the psychic level of a small
child. When I first saw her, Diane was too frightened to sleep
alone in her own home; someone she trusted had to be there or
she would remain awake most of the night.

On the other hand, even in her own room with the doors
closed, she found it difficult to experience herself as alone if
there was anyone else in the house. There was always, for her,
a sense of the other person's presence which kept her from
feeling the freedom of her own space. As much as she was
frightened of it, she also sometimes hungered to be alone and
felt deprived of her privacy.

As long as Diane's spouse was in the house with her, Diane
could feel her need to be alone. But without the presence of
this other person, Diane's need was instantly transformed to a
fear so acute that she experienced it as a sense of her own
disintegration. Diane was eloquent in describing this experi-

ence (which psychologists refer to as a "loss of ego boundaries"): she spoke of being "disconnected" from herself, as
though all of her energy were leaving her, or of feeling "out of
herself," driven by a desperate need to "get back into herself."
For Diane, the colloquial expression "falling apart" had a vivid,
terrifying, almost literal meaning.

Prior to therapy, when Diane felt herself falling apart in
this way, one method she used to get herself back together was
to wrap herself in her living-room drapes until she felt better.
This creative drape-therapy seemed to provide her with a stur-
dier sense of her own physical limits, of where she started and
where she left off. It provided temporary, symptomatic relief
for her intense fear of being alone, but no long-standing solution. The problem remained: in the absence of the other, Diane
felt that she had no self.

Diane's fear of being alone was matched by an equally
intense fear of being close to someone. Just as she was unable
to sleep without her partner in the house, so she was often
unable to sleep with her partner in her bed. In the latter case,
she would be overwhelmed by a fear of being swallowed up, of
getting lost in the other. From one side, Diane feared disintegration; from the other, engulfment. In both cases, she was left
with a terrifying sense of self-loss.

Diane's long-standing, unconscious attempt to resolve her
dilemmas of intimacy and aloneness was to keep herself in the
middle of a protracted love triangle. She lived with a woman
with whom she could not have sex, and had sex with a woman
with whom she could not live. With her spouse, Diane could
feel the comfort of commitment to someone with whom she
shared the intimate facts of daily life but with whom she could
feel neither sexually nor emotionally open. With her lover, she
could allow herself to feel sexually and emotionally open,
given the understanding that they would never actually live
together. Many such love triangles (whether homosexual or
heterosexual) are designed to ward off the twin terrors of intimacy and aloneness: of losing oneself in someone else or falling apart by oneself.

Threatened on both sides with immanent self-loss, Diane lodged herself in this triangle relationship. Her word for it was her "sandwich." The word revealed her ambivalent feelings of being both comforted and confined in her position in the triangle. Wedged comfortably in her sandwich, she could, at times, ward off the devastation of self that she feared. On the other hand, being wedged in, she sometimes suffered from an overwhelming sense of being trapped. She lived in constant terror of being abandoned by one or the other side of the sandwich —of being left alone. In short, the triangle defense did not really work.

Diane's fears were immediate, concrete, and intense. As a lesbian, she did not experience the fear of being alone the way that many heterosexual women do—that is, a fear of being without a man. Nevertheless, her fear of being alone contains many of the same elements that pertain to heterosexual women's fear. It has been my repeated experience as a therapist that the most apparently extreme instances of a phenomenon often serve to illuminate the commonplace instances. Certainly, many women who do not share Diane's particular terrors *do* experience crises of self-loss both alone and with others.

All too frequently expressed in therapy, the fear of being alone heads the list of female terrors. We may remember from Linda's story the centrality of the fear of being alone in her experience of depression. Many women, like Linda, tend to explain their need for a man and their overall anxiety in living by saying that they are scared to be alone. This fear may range from a mild to an extreme anxiety and dread. I have seen it take many forms. The housewife whose husband leaves for work and children leave for school is left with a void that no amount of activity can fill. The busy career woman schedules every minute of her waking day because she enjoys being busy. But beneath the enjoyment lurks a terror of experiencing her own consciousness apart from other people. The "busyness" is, in part, an avoidance of being alone. There is the woman who complains endlessly about an unsatisfying or dead-end relationship which she cannot leave—because she is frightened of being alone. The most extreme case is the woman left alone through divorce, death, separation, or abandonment, and who feels that the only recourse is suicide. To this woman, self-extinction seems preferable to a life in which she has to face her own solitude.

Whether in its mildest or most extreme forms, the fear of being alone is familiar territory for women.

Men and women tend to experience being alone in different ways. Unlike men, who often think of being alone as a welcome relief or as a prelude to adventure, women view aloneness as deprivation and abandonment. Aloneness and loneliness are seen as synonymous. Furthermore, men and women alike tend to think of women "alone" in a different way than they think of men "alone." A woman alone is to be pitied. A man alone is to be admired. A woman alone is a spinster (the very word evokes black spiders in a corner weaving webs for no one). But a man alone is a great artist, or a brave adventurer, a mind unshackled by convention, a free spirit. Solitude is a male virtue, a female affliction.

Consider, for example, the following two scenarios:

In the first, two women are sitting in a bar, drinking and talking with one another. Two men enter and, seeing the women, saunter over to their table, sit down beside them, and ask, in an apparently friendly way, "What are you two girls doing here *alone?*"

In the second scenario, a woman is sitting in a sidewalk cafe, reading a book. Though alone, she is perceived by male bystanders as waiting for someone to join her.

The first scenario illustrates the shared consensus of the meaning of the term "alone" when applied to women: for a woman, "alone" means *unaccompanied by a man.* In the situation of the two women at the bar, a real occurrence, my response to the male interlopers was simply, "We are not alone; we're with each other." The two men were clearly baffled by my words. My simple assertion—a mere statement of what was obvious to anyone's perceptions—was taken to mean that my friend and I were lesbians. Women in relation to other women are both culturally understood and actually perceived as being alone unless they have chosen what is still predominantly viewed as an "unnatural" relation to one another—lesbianism. This is simply another manifestation of what we have already seen in chapter three: that in this culture, only men are actually conceived and perceived as persons in the full sense.

Women internalize this social definition; in the company of women and children, we often experience ourselves as alone. Only with a man are we not alone.*

Given the social definitions of male and female identity, it is not surprising that the men in the bar would consider it their prerogative to intrude, and would interpret my relationship to my female friend as a lesbian affair. One of the most radical aspects of lesbianism, and the most threatening aspect for men, is that lesbians choose one another as *primary persons*—in defiance of the cultural message that women are not persons (in the male sense) at all.

In the scenario of the woman in the cafe, though in fact alone, she is actually perceived by the men who walk by as waiting for someone; that is, she is perceived in relation to an *absent other*. Again, the internalization of this cultural set-up often leads the woman to experience herself in this way, even if she knows that she is not really waiting for anyone. She experiences herself in relation to the presence of an absence. Sometimes, she may actually pretend that she *is* waiting for someone, for this allows her to feel less alone, and therefore less frightened. This bit of psychic make-believe is also an unconscious attempt magically to ward off the unwanted atten-

---

* In this regard, I am reminded of certain Saturday nights with girlfriends during the so-called sexual revolution of my college days. Those nights, we shared what were actually deep and warm relationships with female friends. Yet we experienced ourselves as alone. Despite what was often an unacknowledged passion in these relationships with other women, there was an unstated but universally understood code: that our relationships with each other were secondary to those we might have with men. If a male suitor called to ask us out on a date, even if we'd already planned to spend the evening with each other, there was never any question but that the date took priority. Though we might share a joke about what a creep the guy was (reflecting the unconscious contempt we felt for men), we nevertheless abandoned each other to our dates without any overt feelings of betrayal. In those days, that was simply the way it was.

tions of male onlookers, for a woman knows that as long as she belongs to one man, another man will not try to claim her. In a way, a woman seated alone in a cafe is not really alone in the way a man is. She is openly and even verbally surveyed, scrutinized, visually undressed, and approached by the male world around her ("What's that book you're reading?" "Smile!" "Waiting for someone?"). A woman's privacy, in the sense that men know it, is not really her own.

These paradoxes of aloneness underline the ways in which being alone and being with others may be experienced very differently by women than by men. For a woman, it is as though in the experience of her aloneness, even the things she most enjoys or values seem to lose their meaning and their purpose. The varied colors of existence seem to drain and turn gray. Indeed, without the presence of some other in a woman's life, she is often overwhelmed by a sense of her own self-disintegration. The absence of the other is experienced as a loss of self. This is not true in the same way for men. Why should it be this way for women?

The traditional psychiatric explanation lies in the psychological concept of "ego boundaries." Traditional psychologists would label Diane's experience of self-loss as a severe and pathological loss of ego boundaries. According to the psychoanalytic literature from which this term is derived, ego boundaries are the borderlines between self and nonself which are presumed to develop in the first years of life and first arise as a consequence of the absence of mother. The latter absence, particularly the withdrawal of mother's breast, is said to occasion the child's first experience of separation of its own drives and wishes from their object. This is the beginning of the ego's individuation, the process by which the self develops an identity separate from the other.

Traditionally, women's ego boundaries have been considered to be more "fluid" or "loose" than male ego boundaries, which are described as more "rigid." In the case of female ego boundaries, one imagines an amoeba, slithering along and merging indiscriminately with other amoebas. By contrast, the imagery of male ego boundaries conjures up the solid stone walls of a fortress. Given what we have learned about the double standard for mental health, it is not surprising that the more rigid ego boundaries of the male are presumed to be the healthy norm.

To explain Diane's fear of being alone, the traditional psychologist would say that because her ego boundaries are pathologically loose, the integrity of Diane's ego is threatened both when she is alone and when she is in relationship to others. Ordinarily, the traditional psychologist would turn to Diane's relationship with her mother, expecting to see evidence of what is called a "symbiotic" bond between them—one in which the ego boundaries of mother and daughter merge.

Indeed, Diane often spoke of her mother's inability to separate herself from her daughter. Diane described her mother as a "vacuum." What is a vacuum but a powerful, unbounded space which sucks other entities into it? Diane experienced her relationship to her mother as an intense physical and emotional bond in which the separate identities of mother and daughter were lost.

Therapists have noticed that symbiotic ties such as those between Diane and her mother appear to be more common between mothers and daughters than between mothers and sons. Why do women seem to lose their ego boundaries more easily than men? In answering this, traditional theory relies on its Freudian roots. The answer lies in what is taken to be the biological fact of mothering. That is, it is women who perform the tasks of motherhood and not men. A woman-mother is bound to develop stronger bonds of identification with her girl child than with her boy child because of the sameness that mother and daughter share. Boys differentiate themselves in contrast to a mother figure who is "other"; while girls differentiate themselves from a mother who is the "same." Consequently, according to this view, symbiotic bonds and an impaired capacity to keep one's ego boundaries intact are more characteristic of females than of males.

The traditional view, in short, concludes that females have

inherently weaker egos than males. Once again, we are up against the unfortunate but inevitable result of the male theoretical bias, which runs like a bad thread throughout traditional psychoanalytic theory—that is, the belief that it is male development that represents the norm and female development the deviation. The traditional psychologist stops here, thinking that in Diane's symbiotic relationship with her mother he has found the cause and explanation for her "pathological" fears of being alone and with others.

But it is just where the traditional psychologist leaves off that we must begin. It is hardly adequate to theorize that because mother and daughter share the same kind of genitalia, women grow up to have weaker egos than men. There are major difficulties with the traditional account of ego boundaries. The psychoanalytic theory of ego development takes for granted, rather than explains, the all-pervasive social fact of child rearing as the exclusive province of a single, biological mother, who is the only "significant other" from whom the infant ego must individuate. Imagine a society in which not a single female figure but a group of women were all called "mother," and all performed the tasks of motherhood. Or imagine a society in which several figures, both male and female, were equally considered "mother." Clearly, the genital similarity between mother and daughter in these latter societies would have a meaning very different from the one it has in the single-mother patriarchal nuclear family of our society. The entire process of ego individuation would be quite a different story from the one described by traditional theory.

The point is that different societies require different types of egos, structured in different ways, in order to function smoothly and perpetuate themselves. Historically, because all societies have been male-dominated, they have required that men and women be psychically structured along gender lines: lines that clearly demarcate the types of personalities that will perform certain specific tasks in the division of labor. Our current social structure, patriarchal capitalism, needs men who are competitive, individualistic, hierarchically oriented, and emotionally defended: people who will work for a wage, manage a business, join the army, because these are considered masculine endeavors. And it needs women who are nurturant, altruistic, emotionally connected to others in subservient ways, people who will voluntarily work as unpaid laborers in the family because this work is seen as a function of femininity.

The male style of rigid ego boundaries described by traditional psychology is adaptive for men in our society, because capitalism requires that men develop in such a way that they see their own individual needs and interests as against, or in competition with, those of others. The development of a rigid division between self and others, and its corollary, the development of a ruthless pursuit of the needs, wishes, ambitions of the self as against all those who compete with it for the same "objects" (money, fame, women, jobs, etc.) is appropriate in a society in which such attributes of ego are prerequisites for male mastery and success. The so-called healthy male thus develops a rigidly aggressive, individualist stance toward the world: "If I want it, I'll have to go out and get it for myself and, if need be, grab it from all those others who have it or want it too." This attitude of "I'll compete with those on my level, obey those above me, and dominate those below me" is the standard model of ego for the normal man in our society. It is as an adaptation to capitalist male culture that men develop this attitude.

There is, however, an important qualification here; the adaptive success assured by the rigid ego boundaries of aggressive male individualism is limited quite clearly by class. The working-class man who has adopted this ego style and finds himself, nevertheless, in a hopeless situation of inescapable poverty has come up against the contradictions into which he was born by class and for which he has not been adequately prepared by his psychic structuring. He has been taught that anyone can "get ahead," as long as he is ambitious and talented enough; so he ends up blaming himself for his poverty. This self-blame is hardly adaptive for him, but it serves the dominant economic class by diverting a legitimate rage into a debilitating self-contempt.

In short, the development of a male style of "healthy," normal rigid ego boundaries is not without its inherent problems, even for men who successfully adapt; for the adaptation itself is to a society that demands such personality types in the interest of an elite class of economically dominant men. One can, with some imagination, picture a society that does not economically, socially, and psychically structure its male individuals in this way. In an egalitarian society based on cooperation rather than on competition, the preservation of rigid ego boundaries might be seen as a hangover from the past which interferes with the ongoing work of society. In such a society the more loose ego boundaries of women would be a distinct advantage. The norm of male and female ego boundaries would be reversed: the female style would appear to be more healthy than the male (we have, of course, yet to see such a society).

As an explanation of Diane's fear of being alone, the concept of loose ego boundaries derived from psychoanalytic theory is clearly problematic at best. Jean Baker Miller has made this point very well in her book *Toward a New Psychology of Women*. In her discussion of female ego development, she suggests that the terms "ego" and "ego boundaries," as conventionally used, may not apply to women at all. Her analysis of this subject is worth quoting in full:

> Prevailing psychoanalytic theories about women's weaker ego or super-ego may well reflect the fact that women have no ego or super-ego at all as these terms are used now. Women do not come into this picture in the way men do. They do not have the right or the requirement to be full-fledged representatives of the culture. Nor have they been granted the right to act and to judge their own actions in terms of the direct benefit to themselves. Both of these rights seem essential to the development of ego and super-ego. This does not mean that women do not have organizing principles or relate to "a reality" in a particular way. But women's reality *is* rooted in the encouragement to "form" themselves into the person who will be of benefit to others. They thus see their own actions only as these actions are mediated through others. This experience begins at birth

and continues through life. Out of it, women develop a psychic structuring for which the term ego, as ordinarily used, may not apply.

We are suggesting then that the organizing principle in women's lives is not a *direct* relation to reality—as reality is culturally defined. Nor is it the mediation between one's own "drives" and that reality (which is the source of the development of ego). Instead, women have been involved in a more complex mediation—the attempt to transform their drives into the service of another's drives; and the mediation is not directly with reality but with and through *the other person's purposes* in that reality. This selfhood was supposed to hinge ultimately on the other person's perceptions and evaluations, rather than one's own.[10]

Miller's claim is that the term "ego" itself is a male-defined concept derived from male experience. She attempts to define the specifically *female* form of ego structuring in our society from a feminist standpoint, by pointing to the centrality of what she calls "affiliation" in female psychic structuring. By this she means the self's capacity and need to form relationships with others. Self and other, says Miller, are constituted very differently for men and women in this culture. Females do not learn what it means to be an individual in the same way that males do. We learn to develop and value a kind of other-directed selfhood: that is, to recognize and value our own actions and purposes only insofar as these are in the service of others. We learn, not to work and compete overtly for our own ends, but to subject our aims to a process of what Miller calls "mediation" through the aims of others.

The mediation that Miller is talking about has two distinct but related meanings: First, we learn that our needs, actions, and purposes are *secondary* to those of others. Second, and perhaps more important, we learn to feel that it is only *through* the aims of others that our needs, actions, and purposes appear valid at all. Female identity is structured according to the demand, externally imposed and deeply internalized, that a woman is a person only insofar as she is in relation to an "other."

The centrality of relating to others in the development of a distinctly female sense of self starts, of course, with a girl's relationship to her mother. Miller, however, does not subscribe to the psychoanalytic idea that the female's loose ego boundaries result simply from the fact that girls are more biologically similar to mothers than boys are. She instead emphasizes the ways in which females are supposed to form themselves as persons in a society which is dominated by a male group.

Miller's analysis of female ego development is refreshing and illuminating, particularly her emphasis on the fact that what has always been considered a deficiency in female ego structure (the looseness of female ego boundaries) can be regarded as the strength of "affiliation"—the capacity to nourish and sustain relationships with other human beings. While devalued by the dominant culture, the fact that a woman's sense of self is organized around being able to make and maintain affiliations with others, says Miller, "contains the possibilities for an entirely different (and more advanced) approach to living and functioning . . . it allows for the emergence of the truth: that for everyone—men as well as women—individual development proceeds *only* by means of affiliation."[11]

This can become the case, however, only if the dominant culture begins to value affiliation as highly as, or more highly than, the male ego style of self-enhancement. Unfortunately, this is not the case, nor is it likely to be, without enormous social changes. In the meantime, as Miller puts it, the only forms of affiliation that are available to women are "subservient affiliations." One result is the creation of emotional problems for women which are then labeled neuroses.

The fear of being alone, like depression, is one of the most conspicuous of these problems. For women, the fear of being alone *with oneself* is fundamentally (given the conditions of female psychic structuring described by Miller) a fear of being *without oneself.*

Miller's analysis helps explain Diane's experience in a

much fuller way than traditional theory. But I wish to take this analysis one step further: to establish the links between the type of female psychic structuring that Miller describes and the socioeconomic position of women I referred to earlier.

We have seen how women function as a sex class of wage-less household workers in the family. The very nature of women's work is that it is designed to meet the needs of others: to feed, clothe, nurture, and maintain husbands and children. It is *through* this activity that woman's identity is constituted.

The economic backdrop for female ego development in our society is the fact that women's labor is the *labor of relatedness*. The fact that a woman's sense of self is centered around her relations to others is an outgrowth of the fact that women are responsible for the emotional/physical work of maintaining relationships in the family.

As a sex class, women serve a dual function. First, as homemakers, women provide emotional, nurturant, sexual, and physical maintenance services directly to their husbands. Second, as homemakers and child rearers, women produce the labor power that is necessary to the ongoing work of capitalism—that is, women maintain the present and future labor force. In the first case, women's labor is exploited *directly* by husbands who benefit from it. (Single men, for instance, must pay a salary to a hired domestic to get even a fraction of the services provided by a wife.) In the second case, women's labor is exploited *indirectly* by the dominant capitalist class of males, which gets the benefit of women's socially productive labor at no cost. (Again, think of what a housewife could earn if she were paid a salary for all of the tasks she performs which are comparably done in the paid labor force: cook, domestic worker, child-care worker, sexual provider, social worker, governess, etc. Housewives would be wealthy women!)

Women's economic functions require that women learn to accept, both consciously and unconsciously, a fundamentally *indirect* relationship to their own identities. Thus a woman is encouraged, from infancy on, to develop her sense of self only through her relation to others. Economically organized to work for families directly and for the capitalist economic class indirectly, women are simultaneously psychically organized to be and act for others, often at our own expense.

The position of women as a sex class thus provides the economic basis for Miller's formulation of the organizing principle in female psychic structuring. Miller defines the psychic aspect of women's economic position. In short, a woman's ego structuring and her economic position in our society are mutually reinforcing and interdependent. Because a woman has to perform certain economic functions, she becomes the kind of person who will willingly serve others. Because she becomes this kind of person, her economic position is psychically reinforced.

Women's place in society, and not the fact that mothers and daughters both have vaginas, is the crucial cause of the ways in which mothers influence their daughters' (and sons') development.

It is true, as traditional theory holds, that mothers are bound to identify with their daughters in a more pronounced way than with their sons. But again, depending on social structures and values, this identification can come to mean any number of things for both mother and child. In our society, it does not mean that mothers feel closer to girl children. It means that mothers transfer to their female children, from the very earliest day of infancy, their own feelings about what it means to be female. One research study shows that male children are generally allowed, if not encouraged, to wander much greater distances away from their mothers than are little girls, who are required to stay closer to mother.[12] The implications for the sex-differentiated development of ego boundaries, even from this little bit of information, are enormous. Mothers seem to separate themselves from their male children more easily than they do from their female children. In demanding, consciously or otherwise, that her daughter not stray too far from her side, a mother is already educating her girl in how to narrow her range of experience. This conditioning process is one that will continue throughout the girl's educational and social life, and one that the mother herself has already undergone.

This study points to the ways in which, generally speaking, boys are sooner and more often immersed than girls in a world in which they are left to their own devices, free to learn, through trial and error, what psychologists call "mastery skills": the skills involved in both self-control and control of the environment. Girls are schooled in an omnipresent *relatedness* to others, which begins with the continuous scrutiny of mother's eyes. They are immersed in a world in which the verbal and nonverbal skills of communication and service to others attain an overriding importance.

Women learn through their mothers how to be the kind of female persons that the society needs: persons skilled in what Miller calls subservient affiliations. One result is the lasting hostility between mothers and daughters characteristic of women in our time. It is almost uncanny how many times I have heard women utter virtually the same sentence: "I'm afraid of being like my mother." Alternatively, one hears heated denunciations such as "I hope I'm never like my mother," or "Thank God, I'm not like my mother." Apart from the vivid and heartrending display of the misogyny women have inherited from the culture—the conviction that the worst, craziest, stupidest, or most evil lot that could befall a woman is to be like Mom—these statements reveal a profound bond of identification that exists between mothers and daughters. More often than not, this bond is characterized by an apparently endless hostility—a phenomenon that psychologists dub "hostile dependence."

Women who say that they do not want to be like their mothers, most often consciously mean that they do not wish to be housewives, or that they do not wish to be emotionally and economically subservient to husbands. But these women's statements also include the desire not to invest their lives in their children the way their own mothers did. The formation of women's egos around a principle of relatedness to others has been most insidious in the case of mothers who derive a sense of self exclusively through the activities and personalities of their children. Since this mothering capacity has traditionally been the one "expertise" allowed women, it is not surprising that mothers have desperately clung to it. One result, sad for both mothers and children alike, has been the permanent hostility of children who feel "smothered" by mother. Women who develop a repulsion toward their mothers often see only their mothers' weaknesses as mothers, not their strengths. Such women tend to have far less compassion for their mothers than for their fathers, missing the social oppression which their mothers have had to face and instead blaming Mom for everything wrong with them—a pastime reinforced by most traditional psychiatrists. The "boomerang" effect, by which mothers who have become the kind of persons required by society end up with children who hate them for it, is one of the most poignant aspects of the cultural double binds of femininity.

To combat the tendency of mothers to lose their identities in their children requires not only some radical changes in the ideology of motherhood, but also some radical economic changes. Mothers paid for their labor would come to develop and value mothering as work in a very different way than they do now. The economic autonomy this would provide could only positively affect the relationship between mothers and (especially female) children.

There are some who will find this economic analysis of women unpalatable. We are not used to thinking of women's capacity to affiliate to others in economic terms. In most circles today, it is as unthinkable that a woman should receive a wage for her labor in the home, or for raising children, as it once was for people to consider abolishing slavery. The medical science of the nineteenth century diagnosed the disease of "drapetomania" among black slaves: a disease that consisted in the repeated attempts of the slave to run away. (The cure for drapetomania was whipping.) Similarly, psychiatric science today

speaks of the disease of depression in housewives who are symbolically running away from home by not doing their house
chores. In the dominant culture of the day, slaves were thought
to be made for the work of slavery. And in the dominant culture
of patriarchy, women are thought to be made for the work of
relatedness.

There are few things more certain in the popular wisdom
than the belief that "love is a woman's whole life." The essential definition and value of womanhood is still thought to reside
in a woman's relationship to others. Certainly, as Miller has
pointed out, there is a wisdom and value that women have
developed with regard to the life-sustaining activities involved in relatedness to others. Nurture, empathy, compassion,
loving warmth and support are all aspects of women's wisdom
in relatedness, a wisdom that has hardly been tapped, given its
widespread devaluation. But we have also seen that, in a social
context of inequality and domination, the female capacity for
nurture, empathy, and relationship takes on a more oppressive
cast. For in patriarchal societies, the female capacity for the
work of relatedness is not seen as a reciprocal responsibility of
men and women toward each other. In such a context, the labor
of relatedness is demanded of women and not of men; it becomes an insidious kind of oppression. Both the value of wom-
en's expertise in nurture—in knowing how to recognize,
understand, respect, and meet the needs of others—and the
exploited nature of this work of women have been obscured by
the ideology that defines such work as the unravelings of female inclination.

Women are made for love. Women's work, we are told, is a
labor of love. Our labor *is* to love—to love others, often at the
expense of ourselves; to love ourselves only in and through our
capacity as the primary caretakers of others; to see ourselves as
belonging to others.

One of the most painful results of this labor of love for
women is the widespread and frequent ways in which women
experience a sense of self-loss, whether in connection to others,
or alone. The dramatic experience of self-loss in Diane's story

is only one example. Other examples abound: the identity loss
of mothers in their children; the identity loss of women like
Linda in their relationships with men. These are ordinary experiences for women even now.

But the fear of being alone does not take only these more
familiar forms. It is often a matter of a woman's fear of being
separate or autonomous in the way that men are. The self-di-
rected activity routinely pursued by men in the attempt to advance their careers is often very difficult for women precisely
because it entails a distinctly male sense of separateness from
others, a sense of separateness that is often a severe threat to
female identity. Ambition as we know it is an attribute belonging to a male sense of self. Ambitious women often fear that
their pursuit of self-enhancement will cost them their relationships with others—whether it be family or friends. Or they fear
never being married in a way that men do not. Or they fear,
most of all, being isolated, in a way that men do not. And isolation, as we have seen, is tantamount to self-loss for women.*

Women by the thousands are consulting therapists every
day to help them with the conflicts engendered by seeking to
become independent in the way that has been a routine prerogative of men. There is no doubt that the problems in female
identity that center around issues of autonomy and dependence
are foremost among those that women today are bringing to
therapy. (We have further occasion to examine them in section four of the next chapter.)

The problems in female identity that grow out of women's
economic position as workers in the family labor of relatedness

---

* The risk of social isolation is unfortunately reality-based. Historically, exceptional women who have pursued careers in the male style have been isolated from both
men and women alike. They have never quite been one of the boys, and they have lost
their status as one of the girls. Men have not been asked to make the choice between
work and relationship that women have. On the contrary, the pursuit of a career is a
requisite of masculinity and provides men with a sense of shared purpose and community, albeit a competitive one. The terror of being alone in women is perhaps compa-
rable to what men go through if deprived of the opportunity to work. The latter situation
is as threatening to masculine selfhood as the deprivation of relationship is to female
selfhood. Think, for example, of the identity crises undergone by most men when they
become unemployed or reach retirement age.

are not, then, problems that pertain only to women who "choose" to be housewives and mothers. (The latter choice is hardly made under noncoercive economic and emotional conditions; in any case, it accounts for most women in our society and in the world.) *The work of relatedness is every woman's work.* In patriarchal societies, women are economically and psychically organized to carry the responsibility for relationships, just as men are economically and psychically organized to carry the responsibility for work. The very use of the words "relationships" and "work" in the previous sentence contains one of the major facts of life in current patriarchal capitalist society: namely, the total separation of relationships and work into two mutually exclusive, polarized realms. In this way, the nature of both realms is mystified. Only the work of men in the paid economy is recognized as work; the labor of women as emotional givers remains unseen.

Men take care of business, women take care of life. The fact of the total disjuncture between the two is a facet of late monopoly capitalism: the separation of the public and private realms of existence, work versus love, labor versus relationships, the workplace versus the family.[13] In our society, work is estranged from the world of human emotion, love, and relatedness. And the realm of human emotion, love, and relatedness is seen as independent of human labor. What gets lost is the fact that "work" is not simply some place you go to get paid, but a social relation, organized in certain ways in certain societies, and therefore amenable to change. What gets lost is that love and relatedness take work—at present, a work exclusively reserved for women. What gets lost is the fact that men could not take care of business at all if they did not have women servicing them at home; and that women's life-giving functions as nurturers, sexual servers, homemakers, childbearers, and child rearers take place against a backdrop of exploitation of women's invisible labor.

The separation of business and life in the above ways is not always recognized by the players in the play. Yet everything, from the most apparently trivial details of how men and women conduct themselves to the great facts of life as we know them, reveals this dichotomy.

Take, for example, the different ways in which men and women make telephone calls. The man dials, names himself, and states his business: "Frank, Larry here. About the electron microscope." Women dial and make what gets called "small talk." Women chat, apparently aimlessly, before getting to the point. Indeed often there is no point—in the way that men define it—to women's conversations at all. The point is the process itself, a way of connecting to someone; *the point is relatedness*. If there is some specific objective information we wish to relay to each other, it often waits till last. I have always felt a little guilty when relaying a bit of business information immediately to a friend I've telephoned, instead of asking first how her life is going—as though I've betrayed her and myself by taking so cold and callous a stance. I am quite certain that men do not experience this kind of guilt.

On the contrary, men often find the way women talk on the phone rather silly. The woman who spends a lot of time on the phone speaking to girl friends is the butt of the male comic's humor. Her relationships to other women are thoroughly trivialized. Here, as elsewhere in the culture, the female mode is devalued and its inherent strength is missed. In the example of the two men talking on the phone both may be furious at one another but neither acknowledges the emotions between them. Instead, they funnel their rage into a political debate. The wives of both of these men may see through their husbands' conversation. But their expertise in the field of relatedness goes unnoticed. Instead, they are held in contempt for being ignorant of politics.

The primacy of relatedness in women's lives is not simply an intrapsychic or interpersonal matter, any more than work is simply a technological matter. There is a danger in seeing women's strength in the area of relatedness divorced from its material context. Often women talk about all of their relationships (including to their bosses) as purely personal events which have nothing to do with the world of power and work.

In this way, women tend to miss the importance of the material conditions of their lives.

Sometimes women also fall prey to the myth that if only we find the right relationship, all will be well. In so doing, we attempt to choose as our own the domain to which we have been driven by necessity—the realm of responsibility for human relatedness. We try to persuade ourselves that, though everything else in our lives may be uncertain, dangerous, and overwhelming, relationships, at least, are totally under our control. In this way we attempt to substitute an activity that appears to be under our control for an activity that appears to be overwhelmingly out of our control—namely a massive overhaul of the institutionalized power relationships that structure women's and men's lives in our society.

But in the end, women's escape into this haven of relatedness is not miraculously exempt from the social forces we choose to ignore. Women remain subject to those forces in the public world which, until we seize control over them, indeed remain out of our control. We may, for instance, find the "perfect" man or woman, only to discover that our relationship with this person is profoundly constrained and influenced by such public factors as unemployment.

Women's work, when viewed as an isolated and perfectable realm apart from the outside world, is doomed to failure. As Sheila Rowbotham says about the family, the institution that is supposed to be this haven of relatedness:

> The family under capitalism carries an intolerable weight: all the rags and bones and bits of old iron the capitalist commodity system can't use. Within the family women are carrying the preposterous contradiction of love in a loveless world.[14]

We can no more create a loving world by working on our relationships apart from the public world of work and power than we can create a loving world by perfecting the technological control over production while ignoring our relations to one another.

There is another danger for women trained in the labor of relatedness: in throwing off our shackles, we may try to become persons in the way that men are, perceiving ourselves as totally separate from and not emotionally responsible for anyone else. But this would only be a loss of the genuine value of women's particular mode of psychic structuring: the recognition of our mutual interdependence and the consequent need to be responsible for and to care for one another.

The task of feminist therapy is not to encourage women to develop a male style of ego based on the model of competitive and aggressive individualism. Rather, it is to help women develop their own female style of self without the subservience that it has always entailed. This is a matter of helping women take ourselves seriously as primary persons—and thus to overcome the ways in which we tend to lose ourselves to and for others. To do so is not to abandon our psychic structuring in favor of men's. It is to use the positive aspects of our own identity structures on our own behalf and in our own interest—which, I believe, are truly the interests of all human beings. This perspective is one of the essential cornerstones of my approach to women in therapy. As such, it is the basis for the entire next chapter.

The capacities to form relationships with others, to empathize, to put oneself in another's place and cooperate with someone else, to "lose our ego boundaries"—all of these are strengths that grow out of women's psychic structuring. The recognition of these strengths can be the basis for an entirely new approach to working with women in therapy, as well as a new approach to what is valuable about women in our society. To exercise these capacities, rather than rigidly to defend our own turf in the male style, can be a source of great wisdom and power. Women can use this wisdom not only for ourselves as individuals, but in the collective struggles that still need to be fought to restructure this society in a way that favors female—and human—freedom.

10

Changing Women's Stories/
Feminist Therapy in Action

1. Introduction

As a therapist, one of my operating assumptions is that any woman's experience, no matter how apparently remote or different from my own, can teach me something about myself, if I am willing to look and listen. I learned this lesson along with thousands of other women who participated in the consciousness-raising groups of the late 1960s and early 1970s.

Consciousness-raising was a tool for understanding personal and political reality in a new way. Its method was to search out the commonalities in women's apparently personal, individual experiences and to trace their political roots in the social organization of women's lives in male-dominated society. I remember resisting a friend's suggestion that I join a C-R group in 1969. "What's consciousness-raising but a bunch of women doing therapy together?" I asked flippantly. My friend was amused. Her retort was: "So what's wrong with that?" I had no answer—or none that I could rationally defend. So I joined the group.

In the process, like millions of other women, I learned that consciousness-raising was an extraordinary and exhilarating method of understanding politics in a new way—one that did not leave women out of the picture. And it was *also* women doing therapy together—as it had never been done before.

232

Without a male or female leader, guide, or expert, the simple process of women sitting and listening to each others' stories respectfully and with an ear to the shared strengths as well as the shared ordeals had some very powerful therapeutic effects. Our relationship to everything—our bodies, our work, our sexuality, the men and women and children in our lives—emerged in a thoroughly new light. Together, we saw that the old terms used to describe politics, relationships, sexuality, power, and language itself were an outgrowth of male experience and had to be reinvented from our own point of view as women. For many of us, the overwhelming sense was of seeing the world through our own eyes for the very first time. Through this process, thousands of women were able to explore, understand, and change painful aspects of their lives that had never even been named before.

"The personal is political," the leading slogan of the women's movement, is the basis of my approach to women and therapy. The traditional therapist listens for pathology. The humanist therapist listens for self-awareness. The feminist therapist listens for the connections between the personal and political in women's stories. In my own work, I have tried to combine the strengths of the traditional and humanist approach with the strengths of a political approach to women in therapy. The outstanding contribution of the psychoanalytic tradition to therapeutic work has been the knowledge of the importance of working with transference and other unconscious operations. The outstanding contribution of the humanist tradition has been the emphasis on the importance of the therapeutic relationship to the success of therapy. Both of these contributions have been limited in scope and impact precisely because they are not combined with a comprehensive understanding of people's psyches in relation to their social environment. The traditional therapy goal of resolving unconscious conflicts and the humanist therapy goal of emotional growth are not ignored by feminist therapy. Rather, these goals are included within the ultimate goal of helping women develop a sense of our personal and political power.

Whether one speaks of "treatment" or "growth-enhancing experience" or "feminist therapy," or whatever, it is crucial not to lose sight of the fundamental fact that whatever else it may be, *therapy is always a relationship between persons.* In this relationship, the combined energies of both the person called client and the person called therapist account for whatever change takes place.*

From the client end of this relationship, the most important factor in such change is what psychologists call motivation, and what is more generally known as will. Without the patient's will to change, nothing is possible. The therapist, in turn, must help the client nurture her will to change. In the therapy relationship that ensues, the therapist's major and essential tool is not the manipulation of transference or the use of any number of techniques in her therapeutic bag of tricks, no matter how valuable these may be. *The therapist's most essential tool is herself as a person.* It is the creative use of oneself to further the interests of another that constitutes the therapist's work. Just as the dancer must develop her body, so the therapist must develop herself as a person who can be useful to others.

A genuinely new, woman-oriented approach to therapy must enhance rather than shun the connection between people in the therapeutic relationship. It must say good-by to the Expert-Patient model of therapy in favor of a more equalized relationship between women working together. It must stress caring cooperation, rather than rigid, hierarchical distance.

A concrete way to distinguish this new approach to therapy from the traditional approach is to compare the psychiatric diagnostic interview (which we have seen in chapter two) with what happens in my own practice with women. We may recall that much of what the patient can expect from traditional therapy is painfully evident in the first interview: the therapist formulates an elaborate analysis of the patient's family and so-

---

* For lack of a better word, and in the interests of clarity, I am using the word "client" to designate the subject of therapy. It is an improvement on "patient" because it lacks the medical connotations. It will have to suffice until someone comes up with a better word.

cial history, psychodynamics, diagnosis, mental status, prognosis, and treatment plan, all of which are intentionally withheld from the patient.

By contrast to this Evaluation of the Patient, I consider the first interview a meeting with a person. I do not work by diagnosis. Instead, I explain at the outset that our first meeting is an opportunity for her to tell me why she is seeking therapy and what she wants from it, as well as for me to reveal what kind of therapy I do and what kind of therapist I am. In this way, we can come to a mutual decision about whether we want to work together.

In this initial session, I encourage the client to ask questions of me, just as I do of her. It is not unusual for clients to ask what kind of role I take in therapy, what skills I possess, what feminist therapy means, what my sexual orientation is, and how I think I can help them. I see these questions neither as invasions of my privacy nor as clues to the client's pathology. They are the legitimate concerns of any person who is considering investing time, money, and increasing vulnerability in a total stranger. In fact, I believe it is the responsible thing for any prospective client to do. Often, the most difficult part of this process is helping the therapy seeker (who has already been trained in subservient Patienthood) exercise her right to examine the therapist before she chooses to work with her.

In order to provide the therapy seeker with a clear idea of what she's in for, I give her a concrete example of how I work in this introductory session. For instance, if her problem is depression, I ask her to tell me about her experience of it. Then I explain both how I think about her depression and what kind of work we would do to overcome it (see section five of this chapter). This demystifies the woman's problem, the therapist's "magical power," and the process of therapy itself.

I believe that this kind of demystification is essential if women are to achieve a sense of their own power in therapy. The demystification process must continue throughout the course of therapy in order to work actively against the posture of passive, powerless Patienthood. An argument might be made for the fact that much of the initial benefit that accrues from therapy comes from the Patient's fantasy of placing herself in the hands of an all-powerful figure who she is convinced holds the key to her rescue. In effect, this fantasy might be said to act as a kind of therapeutic placebo effect. The kind of therapy I am proposing cuts into this effect as soon as possible. For this reason, it may not seem attractive to people who cherish the rescue fantasy. But the erosion of this fantasy as early on as possible is a prerequisite for the genuine work of therapy. For no substantive personal change is possible without the client's increasing recognition of her own power to accomplish it. In this sense, therapy must be geared to helping the client see that she must be her own rescuer—that the power she longs for is not in someone else but in herself.

Another way in which I further the demystification process in the initial meeting is to help the client name her goal for therapy in concrete, specific terms. The question I ask here is, "How will you know when you are ready to end therapy?" Helping the client answer this question often takes up much of the initial session, since general or vague answers like "I want to be happy" must be refined in order for the client to have a more palpable grasp of what she wants and how to get there. In this way, we develop specific criteria of success against which we can both evaluate the therapy at the end.

In effect, this initial meeting encourages the client to trust herself as a person who is both knowledgeable and powerful, and to see the therapist as a person who is accountable for her end of the therapeutic relationship. It sets the stage for a demystified working relationship between two people.

I charge a nominal fee for this first meeting. Should we agree to work together, my fee is set on a sliding scale according to what the client can afford. It would be hypocritical to talk about therapy for women if it turns out to be a luxury that only the more well-to-do can afford. In this sense, the sliding-scale fee policy is an integral part of any therapy that seeks to serve women as a whole.

Just as I begin therapy with an initial meeting, I end it with a final evaluation of therapy: an assessment of how the client has changed and of how I have helped. In the last several weeks of therapy, my client and I share our thoughts and feelings about the work we have done together. The client evaluates herself in relation to the goal set for therapy in the initial session; and I give her my feedback. Often clients who have successfully reached their self-stated goals come to realize, through the process of therapy, that there is some other work they would like to do in the present or future. I do not believe that therapy necessarily has an absolute termination date. Since there was no disease, there is no final "cure."

These final evaluation sessions also include my clients' assessment of my work. I encourage clients to let me know what they have found helpful in the way that I've worked, as well as what has been less helpful. This feedback is then cycled back into my ideas about how to work in the future. The entire process furthers my own accountability in the therapy relationship.

From the outset, the kind of therapy I am proposing dispenses with the traditional taboo against "identification with the patient." For women working with women in therapy, this taboo can only be a blinder. It is clear that women who share a common social condition are bound to empathize or identify with one another in certain ways. The task of feminist therapy is not to root out this identification but to *use* it to the advantage of the client.

At the same time, it is important to acknowledge that therapy cannot be a totally equal relationship. The concept of equality does not apply to a situation in which one person is paying the second for help and in which the focus of the relationship is always on the first person. Also, Freud was correct in claiming that people exhibit transference in therapy. The very act of becoming a subject of any kind of therapy seems to elicit and exaggerate psychic carryovers from past authority figures. These carryovers are transferred onto a therapist fantasized as all-powerful. The fact that only the client's transference, and not the therapist's, is examined in therapy makes for an inherently unequal power relationship.

The solution is not to ignore transference or pretend it doesn't exist. (This is the mistake of the totally here-and-now orientation of many growth therapists.) Psychic carryovers from the past do affect the way all of us experience ourselves and others in the world. It is a psychological facet of human beings in general, not merely therapy patients, to perceive reality in a way that is colored by the past. The repetitive mapping of past scenarios onto the present distorts and inhibits the way all of us live. Often these transferences are debilitating; we end up sabotaging ourselves in unconscious ways. Much of the work of therapy lies in helping the client become more consciously aware of these unsatisfying or crippling patterns so that she can free herself from their influence. Finally, it is especially important to work with clients' transference fantasies of the therapist as all-powerful rescuer. (These fantasies invariably result in feelings of frustration, anger, and helplessness.)

The task of this new model of therapy is to work with the client's transference while at the same time encouraging a more equalized, authentic therapy relationship. The often antagonistic quality of the traditional Expert-Patient relationship is due to the failure of the therapist to recognize or validate the patient's genuine feelings, apart from transference. This has the effect of making the patient feel that she is nothing but a child of the past and that the therapist is not a person at all.

But transference, as important as it is, is not the only thing happening in the therapy relationship. It is my firm conviction that no therapy can be really successful without a basic, real relationship of mutual respect, caring, and trust between therapist and client. To cultivate such a relationship, it is necessary to validate the client not only as transference child but as adult person.

A good illustration of how to do this lies in the important issue of how to work with a client's anger at the therapist. As we have seen, it is common for traditional therapists routinely to interpret any anger on the part of the client toward the therapist as transference or resistance. But in my own practice, I have seen that there is no incompatibility between working with a client's unconscious transference toward me and also working with her "real" feelings toward me as a person. Anger is a key emotion for women. Most of us have learned in the course of our apprenticeship as women in this society to deny it and turn it inward against ourselves. Consequently, in most cases I regard a client's increasingly direct expression of anger at me as a sign of increasing strength. Usually, some of this anger is due to the client's transference. But sometimes a client's anger at me may *also* be directly related to attitudes or behaviors of mine that she finds legitimately vexing. Therefore, when a client openly expresses anger toward me, I consider it my responsibility to examine myself to see if she has a legitimate gripe, and if so, to admit my mistakes. Unlike the traditional Expert, the female-style therapist is not Mr. Right. She uses herself as a model of someone who has the strength to acknowledge her limitations.

Women in emotional distress do not need distant, male-style Experts. But good therapy for women does require a great deal of therapeutic skill. In my own experience, the major skills of the therapist in this new style of therapy relationship are an ability to listen to, intuit, empathize with and understand another person's experience—and to communicate that understanding to her; an ability to use one's own feelings toward the client as a tool of help; and an ability to educate the client toward a greater understanding of the social roots of her personal pain. Most of these skills are culturally female. In this new model of therapy they are not ignored or devalued, but heightened and cultivated: they become key elements in the proper work of therapy. These female skills are used to complement the therapist's traditionally "male" skills of theoretical expertise, distance, and discipline.

The word "therapy" comes from a Greek root which means "to treat" or "to attend to." The patient of therapy is someone who buys the attention of the therapist. I believe that in a great many cases, people consult therapists because they have no one else in their lives who will fulfill this function—no one who will really listen or take them seriously. The simple act of listening to the patient in this way may be the single most important factor in what is therapeutic about therapy.

The therapeutic skill of listening is the basis for good therapy with both men and women. But in the case of women it is crucial. Traditionally, women have not been listened to very well. Our stories have not been heard or validated from our own point of view. Rather, we have been made to fit the prevalent male theories of who we are or should be. I have argued that it is important for any therapist to have a feminist theory of women. But in the process of therapy, the theory itself must sometimes take a back seat to the simple but complex act of listening without preconceived judgments or hardened categories.

To be a good listener, the therapist must know how to open herself to the subjective experience of the person in front of her; to take in the point of view of the other without censoring or categorizing or in other ways modifying it to suit one's own beliefs. Anyone who has ever listened raptly to an enthralling storyteller knows the sensation of getting lost in the story. The therapist cannot become so absorbed in her subject that she loses the thread; she must always keep an observing eye on the process of therapy in order to guide it most beneficially. But still, there must be an ability to let go into the other person— that is, to hear without one's own ego interfering in what one is hearing.

For example, in the mass of information that any therapist receives from her patient, she is most likely to respond to themes that are especially important to her for personal and professional reasons. It is as though these themes jump out in bold type from an otherwise uniform page of script. (Hence therapists particularly interested in "bad mothers" see all their female clients or clients' mothers this way, etc.) This is, to some extent, unavoidable, and in and of itself not necessarily a bad

thing. Nevertheless, it is important for therapists to know how
to put these favored themes aside in the interests of finding out
which issues the patient considers to be most important to her.
(These may or may not coincide with what the therapist thinks
to be most important.) The therapist who is a good listener must
know how to respond to the patient's issues in the patient's
own terms, as well as how to guide the patient toward deeper
levels of awareness of her own experience.

To take another example: I often work with women who
are preoccupied with faltering relationships with men. Much
of my work here is to help them understand the dynamics of
these relationships in terms of sexual politics. At the same time,
I have often observed that the particular emotional intensity of
certain male-female relationships is connected to women's
early relationships with their mothers. Many women have had
the experience of mothers who seemed so starved for emotional
affection themselves that they were not able to provide the
nurturance that their children needed (this is quite common in
families with very cold or distant fathers.) The female children
in these families often end up searching for nurturance in a
"solid" masculine figure, hoping to find what they didn't get
from their apparently "weak" mothers. But because men in our
society do not generally learn how to nurture, such women
invariably end up feeling frustrated, deprived, and angry—just
as their own mothers did! One can easily see that an understanding of the sexual politics of these male-female relationships supplements rather than conflicts with a more traditional
family-oriented interpretation of these clients' problems. In
helping such women, I have found making flat-out declarative
interpretations of the issues often ineffective. Rather, the task
is to work with the client in such a way as to engage with her
own understanding of the issues involved. For the most part,
this is a matter of listening and asking the right questions. I
might, for instance, ask, "What about your relationship with
this man feels *familiar* to you, as though you've experienced it
before in other relationships?" While I often have something

specific in mind when I ask such questions, part of the skill of listening is being able to take in the client's response for what it is.

To a large extent, understanding a client is a matter of trial and error: of listening, questioning, and listening some more. We may go down a road only to find it a dead end. We must then return to the main track and continue. Unlike traditional therapy, with its preconceived "phases," there are no hard and fast rules here. Where there is no Expert, but only a relationship, therapy cannot be a rule-governed process. In place of rules there is the human connection between women, a connection supported by the therapist's respect and compassion and heightened by the therapist's empathy and intuition.

The skill of listening is related to those of intuition and empathy (two words one hardly hears in traditional training circles). Intuition is perhaps the height of good listening. It is also related to empathy. I can tune in to a client's suffering with greater astuteness if I have known that suffering myself. In fact, the information that a therapist gleans through empathic intuition is probably her most crucial aid in helping the client move toward greater self-understanding.

Using intuition as a key to understanding is, of course, tricky. The therapist must learn the art of distinguishing what she has in common with her client from what she does not. It is important for therapists to avoid overidentifying with, and thereby distorting, the client. In this sense, the traditional skill of distance is essential to good therapy. In my own practice, I have found that the skill of distance includes staying on top of the interaction between myself and my client; not losing myself in her emotions or in her maneuvers to avoid them; discriminating between occasions when a client's feelings seem to be expressions of unconscious transference and when they are also conscious responses to me as a person; having the temerity to work with a client's defenses against her feelings, even at the risk of her anger; not confusing my feelings with hers.

To use empathy skillfully, the therapist must know the difference between herself and her client. But this kind of distance must be distinguished from the traditional posture of emotional withholding. Emotional stinginess and appropriate distance are not one and the same. Nor is it necessary to cling to the sacred line that divides Patient and Therapist. Rather, *what is crucial here is that the therapist know who she is.* The therapist who is not willing or able to face her own ghosts, to know her own strengths and weaknesses, and to understand what in the client's story triggers her own feelings, is a therapist severely hampered in her work.

In fact, the successful exploitation of the empathic connection between the therapist and client includes the therapist's *use of her own feelings in therapy for the benefit of the client.* Nowadays, some therapists get their patients to breathe deeply, to scream, to remember past lives, to talk to pillows, and to take off their clothes. But the one thing that therapists rarely, if ever, do (from the most orthodox Freudian to the most "far-out" growth therapist) is reveal themselves in therapy. All of therapy seems to be built around this extraordinarily strong taboo against the self-disclosure of the therapist. Of course, this is only the ideal model. I know one therapist who has all of his office work done by his patients—for free. Another enlists recruits for an organization she belongs to from the ranks of her patients. It would seem from these examples that some ways that therapists have of being "real people" with their patients are not particularly valuable. They may even be harmful or coercive.

But the self-disclosure of the therapist can be a powerful skill when used appropriately. The goal is for the therapist to use her own feelings and responses to the client in order to help the client learn about herself through these responses. It is a matter of the therapist using herself *in the interests of someone else.* This is a distinctly "female" skill in our society. It is an art that must be developed. There are no schools that currently teach it.

I take my model from women's relationships, not from schools of psychology. Think, for example, of two women engaged in what gets called "girl talk." Any two women who ever engaged in such talk know the great comfort and strength it can bring. A male onlooker to such conversations would be struck by the lack of linearity in the interactions. My friend talks to me about what is troubling her. Perhaps she is depressed over a recent fight with a lover or husband or with a woman friend. I listen to her. Simultaneously, I am reminded of similar fights I've had with loved ones in my life. I empathize. I talk about how these experiences were for me and whatever I've learned from them. At this point, my friend is listening. We then return to her problem. There is a sharing there, a give-and-take, a loss of ego boundaries. My friend feels stronger just to know that she is not alone.

Patients and therapists are not friends in this sense. The agreement is that the focus is on one, not two. But this doesn't mean that there is nothing to be learned from the ways that ordinary people help each other. The particular therapeutic skill to be learned from the above example is how to reveal oneself to another without taking the focus away from that person. In my own practice, using self-disclosure is not a matter of exploring my problems with my clients or using them to fulfill my own needs. It is a matter of sharing, where appropriate, the understanding of their problems that comes from my own experience; of expressing empathy where their own pain touches on mine; of letting them know what I learned from an experience of mine that was similar to their own; of expressing certain feelings I have toward them in order to give them feedback on how they affect others. Connecting with clients in these and other ways often helps them to see themselves in a new way.

By way of example: sometimes a client plays out what I call a "stubborn streak". She is consistently passive, refuses to let me know what she's feeling, or refuses to take up on any of my suggestions about how to help herself get through an apparent impasse in therapy. As we have seen, women who are trained in turning anger inward and not expressing it directly will often develop these passive-aggressive or indirectly hostile ways of being angry. Sometimes, I will let such a client know that I am beginning to feel helpless or angry. My intention here is not to guilt-trip the client but to let her know that her way of behaving has certain effects on people. The client who feels powerless is often very surprised to hear that she has any effect at all on anyone—much less on her therapist! She is usually somewhat gratified to find out that her anger, as indirect as it is, is not quite as impotent as she thought it was. As a result, she is often able to express her anger at me directly. In many cases, her anger has to do with feeling that I am not "saving" her fast enough. Because she feels that this is an illegitimate emotion, she cannot bring herself to say it directly. Thus revealing my own responses to her is often just what it takes to help such a client move past her anger and move on in therapy.

The emotional self-disclosure of the therapist can be a valuable and even indispensable part of the therapeutic process— but only if it takes place within the context of a mutually respectful, trustworthy relationship. Modeling the ability to recognize and articulate one's feelings encourages the patient to do the same. It helps establish an atmosphere conducive to spontaneous emotion—an atmosphere necessary for successful therapy.

Finally, any model of therapy that takes empathy seriously as a therapeutic skill must recognize that the needs and feelings of the client are often akin to the needs and feelings of the therapist. Consequently, this approach to therapy entails treating the emotional needs of clients in a very different way than the traditional model does. A female-style model of therapy must acknowledge that not only children but adults have legitimate needs for caring, reassurance, nurturance, and support. The skills involved in legitimizing and responding to these needs are intricate. I have had to learn, for instance, when it is in the client's best interests for me to make reassuring statements and when it is best to hold off in order to encourage her to develop ways of supporting herself. The male-style Expert would say that gratification of *any* patient needs encourages dependence. But the traditional way of defining "dependence" (feminine and therefore unhealthy) is part of the problem. In this new model of therapy, such categories are transformed, and the painful and crippling internalizations that they have produced begin to change. (See Carol's and Laura's stories in this chapter).

Therapy of this kind sets up rather different transference patterns in clients than traditional therapy does. The emotional withholding of the traditional therapist is bound to elicit the patient's feeling that she is being deprived of nurturance or intimacy. The traditional patient essentially learns to accept this deprivation of contact and to work with the transference feelings it evokes. But a therapy based on the gratification of the client's need for emotional relatedness tends to evoke whatever fears of intimacy get in the way. Thus, working with my client's responses to my feelings in therapy is one of the best tools I know of for dealing with the client's feelings about closeness in relationships.

For instance, sometimes when I share something of myself, the client feels both guilty and resentful. She imagines that my revealing my feelings to her means that she has to drop what she is feeling to take care of me. She assumes that if I have shared a feeling, I need help, as though feelings were necessarily overwhelming and crippling. She finds it hard to imagine that I do not, in fact, need her to come to my rescue, that one can be both vulnerable and strong. Moreover, she doesn't want to rescue me, she wants to be rescued by me! So she resents what she imagines as my switching these roles. Exploring these various feelings is often the most fruitful work that a client can do in therapy. She comes to discover, for instance, that the stock roles of Victim and Rescuer are roles she takes in to all of her relationships; that these roles are as detrimental to intimacy outside of therapy as in therapy. She faces her fear of seeing me as a person, her desire to cling to her fantasy of me as an all-purpose savior figure. She confronts how much these feelings hold her back in therapy, as in life.

Most of the time, whatever else clients may feel about knowing me as a person in therapy, they also feel great relief that their problems are not as "crazy" as they thought. They eventually come to see that my being a person in this way will not infringe on their therapy but will advance it. Certainly, my self-disclosure influences clients. But the influence is much more direct and apparent than the invisible power of the traditional therapist.

Finally, no therapy for women is complete unless it includes the therapeutic skill of helping a woman understand herself in relation to her society. It is vital that women in therapy develop a strong consciousness of the social roots of female emotional pain. Without such a consciousness, it is impossible for the female client to claim an authentic sense of her own power, both individually and along with others. A new approach to women and therapy, in short, has to offer women a means of both personal and political change. Ultimately, *the goal is to help a woman see how her own power as an individual is inextricably bound to the collective power of women as a group.*

To accomplish this goal, the feminist therapist must know how to work with the Patient Identity of women who come to therapy so that the problems that appear as purely personal can be seen as an aspect of a social condition that is deeply internalized. A clear knowledge of what is, properly speaking, "outside" a person and what is "inside," and of how the two realms interact, can be very powerful "medicine" for Woman as Victim-Patient. It can help cut through the profound feeling of powerlessness which is the bottom line of Victim-Patient consciousness. Thus what has always been considered an intellectual matter of ideology—and therefore shunned in traditional therapy—is an essential ingredient of therapy with women in our society.

Therapy must respect the client's intellect as much as it does her unconscious psyche or her feelings. It is important for therapists to engage in the process of *thinking* with both male and female clients; of helping them rethink their conditioned beliefs about themselves and their world. This becomes all the more important for women who are not aware of their oppression and who, therefore, internalize it all the more.

Certainly, there are times when the client's thinking gets

in the way of her feelings and the therapist must know how to help the client stop intellectualizing. Nevertheless, the process of intellectualizing *with* the client is also an important therapeutic skill. (See Andrea's and Elizabeth's stories in this chapter). For feelings do not exist independently of beliefs, whether these beliefs are conscious or unconscious. In the last chapter, for example, Linda's feeling of worthlessness was connected to a belief that women who possess a sense of self-worth in the way that men do are conceited. It was only after I pointed out the double standard in her line of thinking that she was able to see that her belief was irrational. (By irrational I mean that it was unjustified. Understood in its social context, however, such "irrationalities" are paradoxically rational adaptations to a culture that attributes different characteristics to men and women and devalues the latter.) In consciously reflecting on her deeply ingrained beliefs, Linda was able to disengage from their power over her. This intellectual process of freeing her thoughts, in turn, allowed Linda to give up her attachment to her feelings of worthlessness; for those feelings were no longer supported by the thoughts she had about them.

In the kind of therapy I espouse, the therapist acknowledges and uses her values in the therapeutic relationship. As we have seen, the therapist's beliefs are bound to have crucial effects on the patient, even in those therapies that claim to be neutral and geared strictly to the patient's feelings. We have seen how the values of the therapist affect the patient in chapters five and eight, which chronicle Polly's encounters with the traditional and humanist therapists. To help her understand what was happening to her, and what she felt and needed, each of these therapists made certain choices regarding what to pursue and what to ignore in her account of herself. We can see from the different choices they made that *every therapy is, in fact, both a personal relationship and a political activity.* For the impact that these two therapists had on Polly affected not only what she felt about her work situation, but also what she believed about it and how she chose to act on it. In the traditional session, Polly ended up seeing her problem with her boss

as a matter of her unconscious Oedipal feelings. In the humanist session, she ended up releasing and pacifying her anger at
the imaginary boss in the therapist's pillows. But in neither
therapy did Polly come to feel a sense of her own power with
regard to challenging her boss's sexual harrassment.*

The task of feminist therapy is to use feminist values to
help women cease to comply with their own subordination consciously or unconsciously. This means helping Woman as Victim
see herself through her own rather than through male eyes. It
means helping women see both the crippling effects of our
oppression and the strengths we possess that have not been
properly valued in male culture. It means helping us understand and value ourselves in our own terms.

To accomplish this task is by no means a matter of indoctrination or lecturing. The consciousness-raising aspect of therapy
is an art requiring a great deal of subtlety, skill and good timing,
for the goal is to help a woman feel freed up by her raised
consciousness, not weighed down by the burden of the per-
sonal-political pain she carries. Making declarative statements
such as "you feel this way because you are oppressed as a
woman" is not skillful, and is no more effective than many
declarative interpretations made by traditional therapists. But
it is often helpful to tell a client that what she feels is common
among women, that, for instance, virtually all of my other female clients feel similarly, or that I have felt the same way
myself. Using self-disclosure (for instance, telling a client about
my own experience of depression and my understanding of it)
can be most helpful here.

The educational component of feminist therapy is embedded in a highly charged psychic journey that each client makes
in her own way. The therapist is there to help guide her toward

* Even where the client's problem is less overtly political than sexual harassment,
the hidden or overt influence of the therapist's beliefs on the patient are still crucial.
We must bear in mind that the issue of sexual harassment did not become "political"
until the women's movement redefined it. Before this, it too was considered a strictly
personal affair—and a titillating one at that.

an awareness of her power as a woman, and to help her learn how to trust that power, rather than give it over to others in the feminine style. This model of therapy is designed to help the female client learn about her own power *through the therapy process itself*—that is, through maintaining her power in the therapy relationship. Gradually, the client comes to learn one of the hardest lessons of therapy: to love and trust herself, to know her own strength. In the end, the therapist is no longer seen or needed in the same way.

A few words about therapy techniques are in order. Since therapy deals with aspects of a person's identity that are both painful and difficult to understand, it is often not enough simply to sit back and wait for the client to talk, as the traditional therapist does. Clients often get "stuck"—unable to move past a certain knot or block in their consciousness—in a variety of ways. They cannot talk; or they talk, but don't feel that what they are talking about is really what is going on; or they can name what is going on, but not feel it directly. At such times, various therapeutic techniques are useful. I borrow some techniques from the growth therapies and gear them to helping the client find her own direction in the work.

One such technique is the use of deep relaxation to help clients work with their unconscious in a deeper mode than in normal awareness. (See Dorothy's story). Gestalt therapy techniques are also quite useful. Here the client gives voice to a particular feeling or aspect of herself as though that feeling or aspect were an "I" that was speaking. For example, it might be suggested that a client have a conversation between the part of her that feels angry and the part of her that feels her anger is unjustified or bad. This is also an effective way of working with the dream symbols of the client. In effect, gestalt techniques encourage the client to take responsibility for the part of herself from which she has become alienated. It productively counters the externalization process I discussed earlier. (See Susan's story).

I also sometimes use therapy time to educate clients in healthy nutrition, meditation, or yoga as ways of improving their overall mental and physical health, particularly in cases of depression, psychosomatic pain, and sexuality problems. This is part of a general effort to teach clients to put therapy in perspective as just one means of getting help.

Finally, I often give "homework" assignments as a means of encouraging clients to do some emotional work on their own outside of therapy, and thereby to rely less on me and more on themselves. This homework may take the form of writing something (for example, a general autobiography, or an autobiography of a specific issue such as "The Story of My Sexuality"). Or the homework may be to read some relevant material or simply to think about a theme raised in therapy.

All of these techniques are just that: tools by which the powerlessness of the Patient can be challenged. As techniques, they are not necessarily autonomously useful: they take place in the context of a working relationship.

The therapist's role in this new approach to women and therapy requires a transcendence of the old divisions between feeling and thinking, emotional release and theory, love and work, female and male. The therapist must know how to combine the feminine skills of empathy, intuition, and relatedness with the masculine skills of discipline, distance, and theory. These latter skills are reinterpreted and integrated into a more balanced view of therapy. Therapy without a theory of itself gets lost in the uncharted swamp of feelings. Therapy without an intuitive, empathic connection between therapist and client becomes a sterile exercise in domination and intellectualism. Good therapy requires both a head and a heart. When both therapist and client can think and feel together, therapy works. It can be a vibrant and precious human relationship. Of course, the outcome is never guaranteed, for therapy, like any other human relationship, is an adventure with an unknown end.

In the stories that follow, my attempt is to show how this new approach to women and therapy works in my own practice. I have tried to present a variety of stories that illustrate some typical and key themes in women's lives at this time. In this work, my first task, and the one that continues to be important throughout therapy, is to help the client transform her consciousness of herself from Patient to person. This is sometimes harder than it sounds. Given the conditions of Victim-Patient consciousness which I have described, there is often a tremendous resistance to this process. Often, women will not let the Patient in them die an easy death.

Carol's story is a case in point.

2. Carol's Story: Undoing the Patient Identity

Carol was the first diagnosed chronic schizophrenic I met while training as a psychologist. She was a young woman in her twenties with a soft, intelligent look on her face and a wariness mixed with warmth in her eyes. A woman of extraordinary bulk, she was of medium height and weighed about two hundred pounds.

Carol was an Italian Catholic girl born and raised in a working-class town. But she did not talk like a working-class Italian Catholic. She talked like someone who was intimately familiar with *I Never Promised You a Rose Garden*. Like Debby in the book, she presented herself as someone who secretly awaited the therapist who would slowly get to know her chaotic inner world of demons and faeries and, eventually, help her to give them up.

In my initial Intake Interview with Carol, she immediately told me that she saw herself sitting in the chair in the room but it all seemed unreal—offering me a perfect psychiatric definition of the symptoms called feelings of "depersonalization" and "unreality." She said that she had difficulty separating reality from fantasy, was often confused and disoriented, and had frequent dreams of being dead. In addition, she heard noises that others didn't seem to hear, had trouble controlling her thoughts, and was depressed. Almost everything Carol said had a rehearsed quality to it, as though she had said it all many times before. I had the distinct sense that she knew that her impressive psychiatric symptoms were likely to attract her interviewer's close attention.

In short, Carol had the practiced air of the professional Patient, someone who had spent years making herself into an Interesting Case. What intrigued me most about her was just this: not so much her symptoms themselves as the way in which she used them to arouse my interest.

Given what I had learned about the symptoms of schizophrenia, there should have been no doubt in my mind about Carol's diagnosis. Her family and social history also seemed to confirm it. By Carol's own description, her mother was the classic picture of what some psychiatrists were fond of calling the "schizophrenogenic mother": a woman who was harsh, demanding, unloving, and rejecting as well as overprotective and intrusive. Carol hated her mother and would have nothing to do with her. She thought of her as someone who demanded everything and gave nothing. Her mother's major message seemed to be: Stay here and go away.

Carol's father, on the other hand, was presented as the weak-willed dominated husband who didn't know how to assert his power or his love for Carol. For example, when Carol was sixteen, she was expelled from home by her mother for being too much of a "burden." Though her father seemed saddened by this, he did not protest. In fact, he was the one who actually drove her away from home in his car, protesting all the while that he worried about her future. Carol referred to her father as her mother's "puppet."

With no way out of the double binds she felt she was in, Carol had slashed her wrists. After this, she was hospitalized twice, for a total of about one year. In the hospital she was first diagnosed as schizophrenic, a diagnosis that was subsequently repeated by the therapist she saw as an outpatient for several years.

During this time, her therapist had prescribed a variety of antipsychotic drugs for her. In addition, because Carol complained that she couldn't sleep, he had prescribed Quaaludes (a well-known and well-used drug among addicted adolescents). Carol had made it quite clear in her initial Intake Interview that, as much as she wanted to find a replacement for this therapist (who had moved out of state), she wanted to find someone who would continue to feed her drug habit. In short, by the time Carol got to me, her identity as a Patient was deeply fixed, both psychologically and physiologically.

Carol's medical chart from this period made no mention of any details regarding the onset of her "illness," or of her life at the time. It appeared, from the records, that Carol was a classic case of the chronic "schizophrenic": someone whose illness did not show up in her earlier childhood years, but broke suddenly in adolescence. The prognosis in such cases was considered poor. Schizophrenia of this type was supposed to continue a slow, insidious process of deterioration of the patient's cognitive faculties.

Nevertheless, I didn't believe that Carol was schizophrenic. Not only did I have a philosophical predisposition to distrust the very concept of "schizophrenia," but it seemed to me that, even if one accepted the psychiatric terms of definition, Carol had been misdiagnosed. If a diagnosis was necessary, it seemed to me that her adolescent wrist-slashing was probably the self-destructive acting-out behavior typical of female teenagers who felt trapped. The usual diagnosis in such cases was "adolescent adjustment reaction."

Yet clearly, by the time Carol got to me, she had learned the ropes of how to be a schizophrenic. Her report of her symptoms in our intake session had the clean, professional air of similar reports I'd heard in case conferences and seminars at the hospital. But the symptoms that Carol reported to me did not seem to be embodied in her as she sat and talked with me. The discrepancy was striking. She came across as a fairly put together young woman who was doing her best to prove herself crazy. Perhaps this was a kind of craziness, but it was not what psychiatrists generally referred to as schizophrenia.

The challenge of working with Carol was apparent from the start. A diffuse vagueness permeated her descriptions of herself. Often, when I asked her to clarify something, she would evade the question. She would say something like "I feel that I live in two worlds all the time"—yet refuse to clarify what she meant. Or she would say that she'd written something about herself for me to read but had decided not to bring it in, tantalizing me with hidden revelations. It was clear that her general psychiatric symptoms were much easier for her to talk about than anything specifically going on in her current life. (She refused, for instance, to talk about her job as a welfare worker.) Though she reported many apparently intimate details of her psychic life, she was very difficult to get to know. She used her symptom reporting as a way of keeping herself distant from me—and other people in her life. This was the paradox of what I came to call Carol's Patient Routine: in revealing herself as a "case," she concealed herself as a person.

At one point early in our work, Carol said: "I play roles all the time. I only function because I have to." My response was that I didn't think anyone *had* to function, that she had the choice of letting it all go to pieces if she really wanted to, and that perhaps she was not giving herself credit for the ways in which she did manage to take care of herself.

Carol looked startled at first, then angry. She told me coldly that she didn't see things that way. When I asked her how she did see things, she evaded the question, instead giving me a rambling account of her latest symptoms while staring at a spot on the wall above me. My suggestion that Carol might have some hidden strengths she wasn't acknowledging was greeted with hostility. Traditional psychologists speak of resistance to unconscious material. What I saw in Carol was a massive resistance to being seen as anything other than a Patient. She found many ways (all of them fairly indirect) of letting me know that she objected to my seeing her as an active agent in her own life, rather than as a victim of her illness. (Her "psychotic" diversion when I suggested that she might credit herself for functioning was one such maneuver.)

It was not that the symptoms Carol reported were not real. Indeed, Carol suffered from a great deal of identity confusion. She *did* play roles all the time. (The Patient role was the one she most adamantly refused to acknowledge!) She suffered from inordinate feelings of anxiety and dread and had some strange compulsions, phobias, and perceptual distortions. She lived in fantasy a good deal of the time. All of this was true enough. But to pursue the content of these symptoms without exploring how Carol used them to keep herself from authentic relationships with people would have led nowhere. At the tender age of twenty-four, Carol was already so steeped in her identity as a schizophrenic that I feared she would indeed end up being a chronic patient all of her life—forever getting hospitalized, having so-called remissions, and getting hospitalized again. I had seen such cases in the hospital, and I hoped to help Carol avoid this fate.

My first opportunity to offer help came after only two months of therapy, in what I came to call the episode of Carol's test.

Carol came in one day and asked if I could see her twice a week. She said that she was feeling increasingly anxious and that her inner world was getting more and more out of control. I saw no reason not to say yes, but I knew that I would have to reject her request. My supervisors had already cautioned me not to allow myself to be "manipulated by Carol's neediness."

Professionally, I was obliged to say no to Carol's request while advising her to use our one session per week to explore her need to see me more often! Carol's last words to me in this particular session were "It's really hard to tell you just how bad I feel." I had a hunch this meant that she would have to find some way to let me know how angry she was that I had said no.

She did. Her way was to play the part of the Patient to the hilt: to "go crazy." After missing several sessions, she walked in one day looking bedraggled and wild. She had black and blue marks under both eyes. When I asked her what had happened, she evaded my question. Instead, she told me that the room was floating and that everything was unreal. She was distraught, anxious, and frightened. Her message was "See me now—I'm crazy! Now you *have* to see me twice a week!"

With some urging, she sat down. After talking with me for a while, she placed her hand next to mine on the desk. I did then what I was expressly trained *not* to do: I touched Carol. I asked her if she wanted me to hold her hand, and when she said yes, I did so. Then I looked at her and said, "Is this the only way you know how to get your needs met? There must be some other way. I know you wanted me to see you more often, but I've been advised not to do that. Still, there must be some other things you can ask for and get in our sessions together, and other ways to ask besides acting crazy."

Carol looked visibly relieved. I believe that this was the genuine start of our therapeutic relationship. We spent several sessions after this one exploring her need to play the role of crazy Patient, both as an attempt to get people to care for and protect her, and as a way of keeping herself from getting too close to people. We talked about the self-destructive aspects of this role, and how it masked her deep fear that no one would ever love her or be there for her if she did not behave in this way. The major issue of Carol's therapy for the next four years was named: her ambivalent wish for and fear of nurturance; how much she needed to be loved and yet how much she feared getting close enough to people to get what she needed. What emerged was that, for Carol, being nurtured was bound up with being controlled—for it had been this way in her relationship with her mother. Our work was set out for us.

What could have turned into a major "psychotic episode" and another psychiatric hospitalization thus turned into a rich opportunity for Carol to be honest with herself and with me— in the process beginning to shed a skin she no longer needed in the same way. Of course, this was not an overnight matter. But it was a turning point. From this point on, Carol was able to handle being in therapy without taking any medications, including Quaaludes. She had taken a crucial step in the direction of undoing her Patient identity.

Carol's request to see me twice a week was interpreted by my supervisor as evidence of her increasing transference to me. It was thought that, in asking for more from me, Carol was manifesting an unconscious desire for maternal nurturance; she wanted me to supply what her mother had failed to give her. As her therapist, I was supposed to explore her dependency needs and their roots in her transference to me as mother-surrogate, while refusing to "gratify" this transference. (Another way of putting this is that I was supposed to paternalize her. In fact, this entire process was dubbed in therapy circles "setting limits with the patient"—as one would with a child.)

In physically touching Carol I had, in effect, defied the traditional role of the therapist. I had responded to the closeness she craved, rather than denying it. I had gratified her transference. We may recall that the psychiatric taboo against doing this rested on the idea that a certain tension was necessary between a patient's unconscious needs and their gratification, in order for therapy to work; that unconscious material would not surface unless this tension was maintained. But in our example, the opposite was true. It was my breaking out of the traditional role that had furthered our work. Far from preventing the emergence of Carol's unconscious feelings about nurturance, the physical and emotional connection between us helped her to open herself both to me and to her own unconscious feelings. Once she had some reassurance that I cared about her, Carol could gather the courage it took to talk about the part of her she considered "evil": her dependency on others. I am convinced that the traditional posture of withholding would only have delayed this exploration: for why would anyone (patient or otherwise) who is afraid to need allow herself to open up to someone who appears so distant and invulnerable?

It is important to clarify that I am *not* saying that it is always wise to grant any request that a patient makes of a therapist. The folly of this approach is best illustrated by the request of one young man who asked me to help him "avert an indeterminate sentence to mortality." His goal for therapy was to get over his "block against suicide." I know of no therapist in his right mind who would honor such a request (though I do know many who would not think twice about hospitalizing such a man against his own wishes). The question at hand is not "Should therapists always grant their patients' requests?" but "How should therapists respond to their patients' needs for nurturance?"

The traditional answer to this question is that the therapist should not respond—he should interpret. The patient's dependency needs are seen as, by definition, immature. They are thought to be fixations or regressions to infantile needs. (The very word "neediness" rings with this judgment that to need in the way that Carol did is basically unhealthy.)

Yet it seems reasonable to suppose that in Carol's request for more therapy, whatever infantile transference feelings may have been involved coexisted with a more mature or adult sense of what she needed in order to take care of herself. In denying the reality of this latter kind of need, the traditional approach actually ended up by infantilizing her. Despite the intentions of traditional therapists to minimize their patients' dependency needs, such needs are actually *prolonged* through denial. For there is nothing more likely to provoke and perpetuate a patient's infantile dependency needs than infantilizing the patient!

Strangely enough, the psychiatric system's entire approach to Carol's "neediness" bore a striking resemblance to the approach of Carol's so-called schizophrenogenic mother. As a child, when Carol cried and needed to be held, her mother would instead scold her, saying, "You mustn't behave this way! Be good!" Carol's mother had not known how to tolerate the natural needs of her child. As a result, she blamed the child's needs—treating them as though they were bad, wrong, or even sinful. Carol had repeatedly learned that to need is bad. But this did not make her needs disappear. She learned how to shut them off, and to get some of the nurturance she longed for from fantasy figures whom she made up in her child's play. This world of her own then became something she possessed quite separate from her mother: a world into which she would not let her mother enter.

This pattern laid the groundwork for Carol's eventual use of her Patient Routine in therapy. Psychiatry, like Carol's mother, saw her needs as "bad": to be controlled and managed, rather than met. The therapist in this scenario became another withholding mother, unable to tolerate the patient's needs and blaming the needer instead. The traditional psychiatric view reflects a masculine contempt for and fear of dependency which, paradoxically, ends up heightening the dependency of patients on their therapists.*

It is true that Carol knew how to manipulate others in an attempt to get her needs met. She did so because she had learned that to ask for what she needed was dangerous or guaranteed failure; because she had internalized the message that to need is bad; and because she was frightened that to get her needs met implied being controlled and manipulated herself. Carol's request for an additional session had been interpreted as her "manipulation"; on the contrary, it was a direct appeal for what she felt she needed. Rather, the Crazy Patient Routine she played with me afterwards was her manipulation—an attempt to test me to see if I could be manipulated into giving her what I had denied her. As a strategy of manipulation, going crazy was well matched with the psychiatric system, which inherently rewarded crazy behavior. After Carol's "decompensation," my supervisors recommended that I see her twice a week until she felt better!

The results of the traditional approach to Carol's dependency needs are thus well illustrated by the episode of Carol's Test. In not responding to her direct appeal for additional therapy, I only succeeded in encouraging her to behave in a self-destructive way. Then, in granting her initial request only after she had acted out, I had, in effect, reinforced both her view of her needs as bad, and her conviction that she had to act crazy in order to get them met! Therapy of this kind ended up reinforcing the very pathology it was attempting to cure.

* At work here is a male approach to what it means for one person to need another. Culturally speaking, it is not manly to need. Men are not supposed to need; they are supposed to take care of others who do. Needing belongs to the realm of women and children. Because the need for emotional nurturance is in this way culturally "tainted" with the feminine, it is considered a deviation from the (male) norm. As a result, feminine "dependence" (which affirms the need of human beings for connectedness with others) is considered less mature or healthy than the masculine norm of "independence" (which stresses the need for separation of one person from another). We shall have further occasion to look at the issues of dependence and independence in women's lives in section four of this chapter.

Carol did not need a therapeutic system that stressed her pathology, rewarded her for acting schizophrenic, and regarded her needs as part of her illness. She needed a therapeutic system that stressed her strengths, rewarded her for authentic and close interactions with people, and honored her dependency needs as legitimate. She did not need a therapist's cold manipulations. She needed a therapist who was not afraid of intimacy, as she was.

Only after Carol and I started to work together outside the traditional system could I offer her such a therapy. After my training, I saw Carol privately for three years. During that time, I engaged in a gradual and arduous process of "remothering" her: a process of treating her dependency needs as valid rather than sick, and of helping her get what she needed without harming herself.

The new rules of this therapeutic relationship were overtly stated and mutually agreed upon. The first of these was that it was permissible (and in fact, encouraged) for Carol to ask for what she wanted or needed from me—including physical and verbal support—as long as she was also willing to explore her feelings about asking, taking, getting, and not getting. In traditional terms, I was allowing Carol to regress as far back into her infantile wishes as she pleased, while simultaneously stressing her adult capacities to understand her needs and act responsibly to get them met. (This included helping Carol distinguish between needs that belonged to the child part of her, and those that felt more adult.)

Because Carol was so firmly convinced that her needs were bad, a great deal of this work involved helping her get to the point of asking for what she wanted. For instance, I encouraged her to use the option of telephoning me at home if she wanted to. This is in contrast to the traditional rule that all therapeutic work should take place within the confines of the fifty-minute hour. Most therapists do not welcome calls at home unless it is an emergency. But my attempt was to help Carol recognize and act upon her needs before they became urgent enough to be called emergencies. In this sense, I considered it a sign of progress, not regression, when she could call me to tell me that she was feeling scared or depressed and needed to speak to me. Like most of the women I see in therapy, it took Carol a long time to learn to ask.

In effect, I was engaged in reeducating Carol in a new approach to her needs for nurturance and dependency: an approach that regarded them as potential strengths, rather than inherent weaknesses. Through this process, Carol began to come out as a needer! Her old lesson, "It's bad to need," began to erode as she found a new respect for herself, including her "neediness." It was only after this process was well under way that the final stages of our work could begin: the phase of Carol's weaning herself from her dependence on me as a mother-like figure. Once Carol became more adept at asking for what she wanted and taking it, the rules of therapy were somewhat modified: it was still acceptable for Carol to ask, but this time, we put more emphasis on how she felt to be denied her wishes. The inner sense of emptiness that Carol tried to fill by depending on others was examined more closely. Carol came to realize that she was less needy than she thought, that she was more capable of meeting her own needs. Indeed, there was a process of limit setting going on here—but the parameters of the limits were much greater than imagined in traditional therapy.

Throughout my work with Carol, my goal was both to re-mother her and to treat her as an equal in a way that her real mother had not. This entailed more than encouraging Carol to bare her own needs and feelings. It included using myself as a model of someone who could be both strong and vulnerable. Thus the rule that Carol divulge her feelings and open herself to needing was paralleled by the rule that I was someone who would respond to her behavior honestly and directly.

One of the most obvious examples of this was how I used my feelings of anger at Carol when I felt manipulated by her. The fear of the patient's manipulation was, we recall, behind the traditional posture of withholding. Rather than retreat into this stance, I announced to Carol that I would let her know directly when she angered me, and why. At first, this was difficult for her to handle. But eventually, she came to appreciate that my anger was something that she could tolerate—and that, once expressed, it was not something I hung onto. This modeled both a way of staying close while feeling angry, and a way of letting go of anger—and helped Carol to do the same.

In the years that we worked together, Carol came to learn that it was possible to be nurtured without being controlled—an experience she had not had with her own mother, or within the psychiatric system. She came to feel that it was possible to be both dependent and independent, vulnerable and strong, open and honest about herself and yet get what she needed. She learned that she did not have to be a "Case" to be an interesting, involving person—someone worthy of attention and love. This was the "corrective emotional experience" that traditional theory recommends and considers the heart of therapeutic work. But it could not have been accomplished with me in the role of omniscient, omnipotent Expert and Carol in the role of Interesting Crazy Patient. To reach the goal of therapy, both of us had to surrender these roles.

After four years Carol graduated from therapy. The two-hundred-pound woman, considered an incurable schizophrenic by psychiatric experts, was transformed, both physically and emotionally. During this time, in addition to working as a welfare worker, she had put herself through college; been accepted by several graduate schools (she once thought that she was incapable of doing academic work because of an organic brain disorder!); overcome her dependence on drugs; and reclaimed a sense of herself as a competent and beautiful person —which she most certainly was. In the process, she had lost most of her fat. She looked as well as felt like a new person.

This is not to say that Carol's was a total Success Story. Though we both agreed that it was time for Carol to terminate, Carol left therapy protesting that I never really understood the depths of her "craziness." Perhaps I hadn't. I had never seen Carol as schizophrenic, and it's quite possible that I had missed parts of her that did not conform to the way I perceived her. Every perspective has its limitations. Carol never fully gave up her Crazy Patient Identity. But she gave up much of the Patient's powerlessness, and came into her own as a woman.

3. From Headshrinking to Consciousness-Raising: Turning Women's "Weaknesses" into Strengths

Most, if not all, of the people I see in therapy suffer from seeing themselves as Patients. Everyone has her unique Patient Routine. This is true even for the most educated and highly politicized feminist women. Outside of therapy they may be deeply involved in political struggles, but once in the therapy room, the most sophisticated analysis of women's oppression often recedes in favor of understanding one's problems in narrowly psychological terms—as products of personal emotional inadequacies unrelated to the social world.*

I have said that female symptoms arise as a response to an untenable psychopolitical situation. This is true even where it is not immediately or directly apparent in the woman's own life. All one need do is look a bit further down the genealogical line—to the woman's mother or grandmother or to other important female figures, and the situation that breeds the symptoms becomes apparent. Carol's "schizophrenia," for instance, was a way of coping with her mother's inability to nurture her as a child. In her own fantasy world, she could get some of what she needed; and in this way she could also attempt to separate herself from a "symbiotic" tie to her mother. Her mother's inability to nurture Carol, in turn, was related to the fact that her mother was a Catholic woman who was culturally expected to bear and raise children, though she was clearly not emotionally prepared to do so. In therapy, it was important for Carol to realize that her mother did not intend to hurt her but was trapped in her own socially induced inadequacies. In order for Carol to forgive her mother and thereby let go of the hatred that

---

* These Patient Routines are often very sophisticated. Many of my clients are forever diagnosing themselves, referring to their feelings and behavior with epithets like "masochistic," "hysterical," "borderline," etc. These words always seem to carry the same weight as the more informal diagnosis of "fucked up." They are ways the Patient has of blaming herself and being stuck in the tunnel vision of Patienthood.

poisoned her own life, Carol needed to know that her mother was simply incapable of—or perhaps never wanted—the role that motherhood demanded of her. The social background behind Carol's so-called schizophrenogenic mother was thus an important part of the picture of how Carol came to be who she was as a person, and an understanding of this background became a necessary part of Carol's consciousness-raising in therapy. To give up her "illness," she had to learn that the symptoms she had once adopted as a way of protecting herself from her mother's neglect and double binds were no longer needed.

I often tell the people I work with that their symptoms will begin to disappear when they stop seeing them as symptoms. They will be cured when they realize that there is no disease. They will stop suffering when they let go of this idea of their symptoms and realize that these are merely aspects of themselves that arose for very good reasons (usually as a way of protecting themselves from harm) but which they no longer need. *Within every symptom there is a seed of strength which lies dormant.* This seed can grow and flourish, given the proper conditions. It is the task of any feminist therapy to provide these conditions. To accomplish this task, therapy with women necessarily entails a process of consciousness-raising. Women often leave traditional therapy feeling worse than when they started, because they have learned to accept the negative, male, psychiatric view of parts of themselves they already hated. (This was obvious in the case of Carol's feelings about her dependency needs.) Any therapy geared to women must look to the seed of strength behind every symptom and help women transform what has always been regarded as feminine "weakness" into a source of energy to help us in our development as people. We shall see how this consciousness-raising works in the following stories.

DOROTHY'S STORY: CRAZINESS AS FEMALE WISDOM ■ Dorothy came to therapy with a commonly expressed concern of Woman as Patient: she was afraid that she was going crazy. Since childhood, Dorothy had experienced vivid visions. Sometimes these visions came to her unbidden, delighting her with fascinating, colorful images or frightening her with fearful ones. Other times, all Dorothy had to do was close her eyes to automatically conjure up a host of images. Dorothy regarded some of these visions as products of her own unconscious imagination and others as clairvoyant in nature. For the most part, she treasured her "psychic" capabilities and saw her visions as a means of helping herself develop spiritually. But just prior to therapy, she had begun to think that perhaps her visions were a sign of her incipient madness. She had been depressed for months and had experienced certain visual distortions that reminded her of tripping on LSD. Dorothy did not know how to interpret these experiences. She began to wonder how healthy her visions were. She knew that she had derived much satisfaction from them as a child and that they were still valuable to her. But she also knew that she could use these visions in escapist ways: turning to them when she didn't want to face something in herself. More and more, Dorothy came to distrust her own perceptions. This self-doubt and confusion made her feel that she was "going crazy."

In searching for a therapist, Dorothy had been careful to find someone who would not regard her visions or her powers of extrasensory perception as *a priori* evidence of psychosis. Her caution was certainly justified, for I am quite sure that some of the visions Dorothy described to me would be psychiatrically diagnosed as visual hallucinations which should be chemically controlled. Clearly, much of Dorothy's suffering (her feeling that she was going crazy) was related to a confusion regarding how to understand or make sense of her visionary experiences.

In her own family, there was a marked difference of opinion on what these experiences meant. Dorothy's father, a respected scientist, regarded them as so much bunk. Her mother, on the other hand, had visions herself and considered them spiritual manifestations. But in her family, as in most, her father's opinion prevailed; for his word was considered more knowledgeable and inherently valuable than her mother's. Her father had always regarded her mother as a woman who was hysterical and out of control. Indeed, her mother had been severely depressed while Dorothy was growing up and had tried to kill herself when Dorothy was a teenager. In short, in Dorothy's family, her father was the Expert and her mother was the "identified patient." Dorothy, as someone who was "like her mother," had inherited her mother's "craziness."

In finding a therapist who would respect her visions as valid (as her mother did) rather than denigrate them as pathological or merely silly (as her father did), Dorothy was, in effect, taking the more woman-identified side of her ambivalent appraisal of these experiences. She chose, in effect, to honor her visions and work with them, rather than to deny their value.

Fortunately, this choice worked to Dorothy's benefit in therapy. Once she was assured that I did not regard her experiences as pathological, her preoccupation with whether or not she was going crazy literally evaporated. Far from evaluating her visions as "psychotic," I saw them as gifts from her unconscious which were rich with symbolic meaning and represented an extraordinary source of power. Dorothy's facility for tapping her unconscious images was a valuable female skill. We entered on a course of therapy that sought to use this skill to her advantage, rather than to make it disappear.

We agreed that we would use a deep relaxation technique to help Dorothy fully move into her visions and use them as a source of understanding what she was feeling and how to move on in her life. Each week, Dorothy would enter into a deep trance state and allow her mind to come up with its storehouse of images. For the most part, we worked with Dorothy's images while she remained in this trance state; but at the end of every hour, we set aside some time to talk about the session's work while Dorothy was once again in her "normal" consciousness.

The speed of this kind of work was extraordinary, for Dorothy had conscious access to her unconscious in a way that most people do not. Dorothy's depression lifted in several weeks, after she saw its relation to her conflicts about her vocation as a pianist (a profession her father devalued and her mother had given up in order to marry). She quickly understood how much of her preoccupation with craziness was a way of staying connected to her mother. And she realized that much of her lack of self-esteem came from seeing both herself and her mother the way that her father did. Outside therapy, her behavior toward her parents was changing. She found new ways to be with her parents that did not entail the self-contempt of seeing herself as crazy.

Dorothy's therapy was short-term. After only twenty-one weeks of this kind of work, Dorothy concluded that she was finished. She left feeling that virtually all of the major areas of her life—her work, her relationships with her parents and her lover—had vastly improved. Through therapy, she had transformed her preoccupation with craziness into a sense of confidence in her extraordinary capacity for intuitive forms of knowledge. She came to value and use this feminine strength in a new way.

BONNIE'S STORY: FAT AS THE GREAT REFUSAL ■ Have you ever met a woman who thought being fat contained a kernel of great strength? Not likely. As we know from the huge profits made by industries that thrive on women's terror of being fat (diet foods, diet pills, and diet books) women tend to see their excess inches as ugliness born of weakness. (This is true even when an impartial observer cannot detect the excess inches.) Bonnie was one such woman. She exemplified one of the most typical women of our time: the woman obsessed with being fat. After fifteen years of compulsive eating and compulsive dieting, she was still fat.

Bonnie's Patient Routine included a sophisticated psychological analysis of her fat. She saw it as part of her "control issues": her need to feel in control of everyone and everything around her, and her fear of being controlled by others. Being fat, she thought, was a manifestation of her unconscious wish to have a layer of protection against others. Her control issues, in turn, were thought to be caused by her relationship with an extremely "over-intrusive" mother. Bonnie saw her fear of being controlled by others as a figment of her unconscious imagination: a feeling she transferred to others from her relationship with her mother.

As a result of this analysis, Bonnie concluded that she was severely neurotic. This conclusion, of course, made working on her "fat issue" very difficult, for there was always the belief that whatever Bonnie felt about being fat was a symptom of her neurosis. Thus mired in her identity as a Patient, the chances of her shedding her fat were quite slim. Her identity as Fat Woman and her identity as Patient were inextricably intertwined.

Again, it was not that Bonnie was wrong in her analysis. It was just that her analysis was incomplete and suffered from a male cultural bias: against fat "neurotic" women. Like all Patients, Bonnie was very good at using this analysis against herself. What Bonnie failed to see was that some people *were* trying to control her! What she did not take into account in analyzing the genesis of her control issues or her fat was that, in patriarchal society, an entire group of (male) people in fact controlled, or attempted to control, the lives of women in very definite ways. The cultural dictate that women must form their bodies to suit men was one of these forms of control. Especially in this era, staying slim was one of the more obvious necessities for women who wanted to be considered beautiful, desirable, and feminine. Given this context, Bonnie's fat was the outward and indirect manifestation of a suppressed wish to defy the cultural convention by which women are groomed to be beautiful objects for men. Her fat was the Great Refusal against the socially ordained role of Woman as Body. Like other female symptoms we have seen, Bonnie's fat contained the seeds of an unconscious rebellion against the gender identity prescribed for her in patriarchal society.

Bonnie's "paranoia" about being controlled could be used to help her develop a heightened awareness of the power that men as a group have over women in patriarchal society. Bonnie was indeed aware that her fat kept her from seeing herself as a sexual being with men, that it neutered her, both in her own eyes, and in the eyes of men she knew. She was aware that, in being fat, she kept a lid on her sexuality. She knew that sexual autonomy frightened her. She was one of the many women who fake orgasm because they don't want to disappoint the man. With some work, she was able to see that her fear of letting go in sex and her faking were also related to her anger at and terror of being controlled by men.

But no matter how deeply we got into these sexual-political issues, Bonnie always, in the end, came back to her relationship with her mother as the source of her "control issues." It was as though for Bonnie there was only one person who ever controlled anybody: her mother. She could see that her anger at a distant and nonexpressive father might have some bearing on her fear of getting close to men. But as soon as we got into this anger and her anger at men in general, Bonnie's mind would go on strike. The consciousness-raising process of seeing the inherent seed of power and resistance in her being fat stopped right here. After many hours of trying to get past this impasse in therapy, Bonnie at last admitted that she really did not wish to explore her anger at men. "I'm scared," she said, "that if I get into my anger, I will never be able to have a relationship with a man." Beyond this, Bonnie was also convinced that her anger would turn her into a lesbian—a prospect that terrified her.

This refusal to look further into herself was, of course, a testament to just how strong her anger at men really was. The energy behind her anger was the same energy that kept her fat. But as a veteran Patient to the end, Bonnie preferred to see herself as someone with "control issues" than as a woman with the deeply internalized social problems of Woman as Body. Of course these two ways of seeing Bonnie were not incompatible. Both were true. But the first way was less frightening and entailed only her anger at her mother—an anger with which she was quite familiar and comfortable—whereas the second way entailed her anger at an entire male universe. Indeed, someone with control issues would find it hard to tackle this latter feeling. Bonnie feared that, if unleashed, her rage would be out of control.

Bonnie's story illustrates the limits of consciousness-raising in therapy. To say that there is a seed of enormous strength in every woman's symptom is not to say that every woman desires to tap this potentially terrifying power. (We shall see how to work with the rage from which Bonnie turned away in section five of this chapter, "Every woman's Story: Internalized Anger.")

PAM'S STORY: FEARING MEN AND LOVING WOMEN ■ Pam came to therapy with another familiar female goal: she wanted to raise her self-esteem. She had been a lesbian for several years and was, for the most part, comfortable with her sexual identity. As an attractive woman, she was sometimes approached by men who wanted to date her. In the course of therapy, she realized that she was afraid of the sexual advances of these men. She began to think that perhaps she had chosen to be with women because she was afraid of men, and to fear that her identity as a lesbian was somehow built on an "unhealthy" foundation.

Questions of sexual identity at this point in history are more open—and therefore more confusing—than ever before. I do not believe it is the business of any therapist to prescribe the "correct" sexual orientation for anyone. (Indeed, the American Psychiatric Association finally learned this lesson and rescinded its professional hex on homosexuality several years ago.) In therapy, my aim was to help Pam explore her sexuality and identity as a lesbian without assuming that the choice of heterosexuality was inherently healthier than that of homosexuality or bisexuality.

In this process, Pam revealed that she was clear about one thing: she did not want men as lovers. She regarded her identity as a lesbian as fixed. But she was attracted to some men as people. She shared some passions with men that she knew, including an avid interest in sports, car mechanics, racing cars, and other culturally male pursuits. She wished to befriend some of these men, but feared that if she made it clear that she did not want to relate to them sexually, they would not want to relate to her at all. She was unsure about how close she wanted to get to these men, or whether she should come out to them.

In exploring these issues, I learned that when Pam was a lonely teenager, she had been befriended by an older, married man who said that he thought of her as a daughter. Apparently this did not stop him from attempting to have sex with her and becoming cold and distant when she turned him down. (Shortly after Pam said no to this man, he had sex with her best friend.) More recently, Pam had become friendly with a man with whom she shared her work as an electrician. When she told him she was a lesbian, he turned away in disgust.

It was clear that it was not in relating to men as equals (for example, in sharing her work or her hobbies) that Pam felt ill at ease with men. But when these men approached her sexually, she became confused and frightened. These feelings then became evidence by which Pam converted her lesbianism into an illness.

Without entering into a discussion of why and how people come to choose their sexual orientation as homosexual or heterosexual, I want to make the point that there are no one-to-one correlations between cause and effect in the complex matter of sexual preference. Moreover, regardless of Pam's reasons for choosing to love women, her fear of male sexuality in no way invalidated her lesbianism. Pam's choice of homosexuality was no more exclusively caused by her fear of men than any woman's choice of heterosexuality is exclusively caused by her love of men. Women who choose to be heterosexual do so, at least in part, because they have internalized the culture's heterosexual standard for sexuality, as well as its homophobia.

Moreover, Pam needed to understand that her fear of men who approached her sexually was not altogether "unhealthy" or irrational. Certainly, the caution she felt was based on her experiences with men who would not or could not relate to her as an equal and who could not tolerate her lesbianism. Such men are hardly the exception in our culture. Given a culture of misogyny and the sexual politics of patriarchal society, it is not unreasonable to expect that all women—homosexual or hetero-sexual—have a nice, healthy dose of caution about trusting male power and male sexuality. In this sense, the fear that Pam thought was a weakness had the seeds of an essential strength: the instinct toward self-protection that lesbians in a homophobic society (and all women in a woman-hating society) must have in order to survive.

This does not mean that it is wise for women to be scared of men. It is important for women to conquer the fears that only make us more likely victims of male abuse. But neither is it wise for any woman, including Pam, automatically to open herself to men without discrimination. Pam needed to look at her fear of men without seeing that fear as the sole motivation for her lesbianism and without using it to devalue the obviously authentic love she felt toward women.

For Pam to do this required a process of consciousness-raising in therapy. In exploring her fear of male sexual advances and of intimacy with men without using this as a weapon against herself, Pam came to see that her love of women was a strength, not a necessary evil born of weakness. And she came to understand the power that lay within her "fear" of being treated like Woman as Body by men with whom she wished to relate as an equal.

ANDREA'S STORY: AFTERMATH OF A GANG RAPE ■ The potentially disastrous consequences of not possessing a healthy fear of men was painfully illustrated by Andrea's story. Andrea was an intelligent and creative woman, fiercely devoted to her independence. She was single and supported herself as a carpenter and artist. She prided herself on her fearlessness, physical strength, and lack of physical intimidation. One evening, her car broke down and had to be towed. She visited with a friend nearby until around midnight. Then, rather than take the subway, she decided that she would try to hitch a ride. She was picked up by two men who took her for a long ride, brought her to a house, threw her on a bed, and called several of their friends. For the next several hours, Andrea was raped at knife point by seven different men. In between rapes, the man with the knife would urge her to tell him how much she enjoyed it. Afterward, she was blindfolded, taken for another ride, and dropped off on the street in an unknown neighborhood.

No woman recovers from an experience like this very easily. The climb back is hazardous and full of pain. For the first few days, Andrea was numb—she could feel nothing at all. Like many rape victims, she told no one what had happened to her. Prior to the rape, Andrea had always kept a firm lid on her feelings. But her instinct for survival now told her that she would have to get to the bottom of what she felt. With just a little encouragement from me, her feelings came gushing out in great torrents; terror, rage, shame, helplessness, and vulnerability overwhelmed her. She saw a rapist in every car. She distrusted men and wanted nothing to do with them—including the male friends she had known before the rape. She was ashamed of her body, which felt numb and dead. She wanted to kill or maim or castrate the men who had raped her.

Prior to the rape, Andrea had thought of herself as a "free spirit." Now, her innocence was permanently shattered. On the streets she used to love she felt like a "prisoner." The streets were no longer safe; nothing was safe. There was nowhere to hide—not even in her own home. She felt like a "caged animal." Her former fearlessness was replaced by an abiding terror. She felt utterly powerless. The entire world seemed to seethe with male menace.

How could therapy help Andrea make sense of and get past these feelings? The conventional expertise on rape would have it that Andrea's feelings of terror, rage, and powerlessness are the inevitable, if somewhat irrational, consequences of the victim's individual trauma. The goal of any therapy that subscribed to this view would be to help the rape victim express and resolve her feelings. Presumably, such resolution means that the rape victim eventually learns to put her ordeal behind her in order to "get back to normal." She works through her feelings in order to resume "normal" relations with men.

The limitations of any therapy that treasures the myth that "It's all in your head" are nowhere more obvious than in the case of a woman who has been raped. The feeling bias of such therapy—that is, the belief that once a person has discharged her feelings, she is free—is bound to leave the victim of rape exactly where Andrea started off: with a false sense of her own power and freedom. What the conventional view of rape as an individual trauma ignores is the fact that getting back to normal for any woman means getting back to the reality of rape as a normal fact of female life. In fact, the normal relations between men and women in patriarchal society include rape as a pervasive social phenomenon for women.*

The conventional therapeutic view of rape as an individual trauma misses the point: that rape is the basic male weapon in the patriarchal war on women—a war that affects all women, not just a handful of unlucky ones who suffer the "accident." Any therapy that views rape in this way is thus likely to miss the boat in understanding and helping Andrea with the overwhelming rage and powerlessness she felt.

Like many women who have been raped, Andrea was not, in fact, eager to resume normal relations with men as soon as possible. But she was driven by an urgency to make sense of what had happened to her and why. To help her do so, therapy had to offer Andrea more than an opportunity to ventilate her feelings; it had to help her reconstruct her sense of herself as a woman in a man's world. Andrea now knew, in a visceral way, that rape was not only an act of violence against a woman's body: it was a violation of her very identity as a person. The men who raped Andrea not only demanded free access to her body, they demanded an acknowledgment that Andrea "en-

---

* On the average, one woman gets raped every three minutes in the United States.[1] Most rapes are committed not by strangers but by friends and acquaintances. (This does not include the incidence of women raped by their husbands, which, in most states, occurs with legal impunity.) Women old and young, black and white, beautiful and plain, are all victims or potential victims. Women are approximately eight times as likely to get raped as they are to get killed in a car accident. Women lucky enough to avoid rape know that their time may yet come.

joyed" her humiliation. They wanted her to admit that she was a willing subject of degradation. What they wanted, on threat of her life, was for her to "beg for it"; to surrender herself as a subject; to become a total victim. Stealing Andrea's body was not enough: the rapists wanted to steal her being.

In order to survive this terrifying ordeal, Andrea had no recourse but to retreat as a person. During the hours that she was raped, she began to see her own body as an object rather than to experience it as a subject. In one sense, she adopted the rapists' view of her. But in another, she was refusing to submit to them in the only way available to her. She gave them her body, because she had to, but she did not surrender her mind. Instead, she took her mind away. Her situation was so dehumanizing that, paradoxically, in order to survive as a person she had to depersonalize herself. (This way of defending herself was actually a way of coping common among survivors of situations of inordinate dehumanization—for example, survivors of the concentration camps.)

Once this process has taken place, the road back to life is difficult. Any genuine sense of Andrea's autonomy, personal integrity, power and humanity as a woman had to be based on a different foundation than before.

Before the rape Andrea had intellectually understood that women in our society were at a disadvantage. But she had thought of herself as somehow above these limitations that most women have to face. She was, in fact, what many people nowadays would refer to as a "liberated woman." She had succeeded in transcending the stereotyped roles prescribed for women in our society. She had many "male" skills, including carpentry and physical prowess. (She was proud, for instance, of being able to lift heavy objects as well as or better than most men.) She had taken both pride and pleasure in her body and in her autonomy. She thought, in short, that she was free in a way that other women were not.

Andrea's pre-rape sense of her own freedom was what many therapists would consider the final goal of therapy. (This includes some therapists who identify themselves as feminist.)

The inadequacy of a strictly psychological definition of what freedom or liberation means for women is blatantly obvious in the case of Andrea—or any woman who has been raped. For it was precisely Andrea's pre-rape conception of her own freedom that had most betrayed her. It was itself an irrational refusal to acknowledge the real oppression of women, a denial of the danger that women risk, for instance, when they get into a car with two strange men at midnight. Given the patriarchal norms, Andrea's hitching at this hour had the cultural value of a come-on to men, an invitation to be violated. The popular wisdom holds that (to put it in the colloquial) "she was asking for it." It was the internalization of this patriarchal norm of "justice" for women that made Andrea feel, after the rape, that she was responsible for provoking it, and that she in some way deserved it; In short, that she "got what she asked for." This sense of shame is another aspect of the psychic harm that rape inflicts on women. One of the trickiest tasks of therapy was helping Andrea to see that, given the reality of female oppression, her innocent trust of men was misguided; but that this did *not* mean that she either provoked the rape or deserved it.

After the rape, it was the sudden loss of Andrea's sense of freedom, more than anything else, that she mourned. She feared that she would never again be able to enjoy the ease of walking down a city street; that she would never be able to take pleasure in the integrity of her own body; that she would never again feel that she was as capable as any man and could do what any man could do. Suddenly, she had seen what men could do to women in a new way: men were Rapists, women were Victims.

After the rape, Andrea no longer felt exempt from the general lot of victimized women in the world. Her old sense of being special vanished. The wall that had separated her from the majority of women began to crumble. To the men who had raped her, she had not been Andrea the female carpenter and fearless, free woman. She had been just another female: just another target, just another victim, just another cunt.

Andrea's pre-rape sense of freedom had been the false consciousness by which she denied how "caged in" women in our society actually are. Her post-rape consciousness of her vulnerability as a victim, unfortunately, was in some ways more appropriate to the reality of female oppression. After the rape, Andrea could no longer afford her previous sense of freedom: it no longer made sense. In the process of getting raped, she had lost both her previous sense of power as an individual, and her previous identity as an exceptional woman.

Therapy had to help Andrea turn her losses into gains: to offer her a new basis for a sense of identity and power as a woman.

One of the best ways to do this was to work with Andrea's newly found sense of outrage. This burning outrage was like nothing else she had ever experienced. She simply could not understand how any person was capable of doing what these men had done to her. Like all victims, she could not help asking, "Why me?" But beyond this, she wanted to know: "Why any woman? Why do men rape? How will I ever feel strong and free again?" Andrea's fierce outrage was like a bomb exploding in her head. It, more than anything else, motivated her to piece her world back together again. Her consciousness was open in a way that it had not been before. In this lowest point of Andrea's life, therapy could help her make use of this openness, for it was her greatest strength in the task of surviving and recovering with a renewed sense of her power in the world.

Andrea's consciousness of herself after the rape contained the seeds of a very powerful new awareness: that her fate as a woman was inextricably bound to the fate of women as a whole; that she could not be the exceptional free spirit as long as women as a group remained oppressed. This new awareness was the bridge to a new basis for her sense of power as a woman. With her consciousness raised, Andrea came to understand that her post-rape emotions of terror, rage, and powerlessness were supreme exaggerations of the "normal" way that women feel in our society, whether consciously or unconsciously. She saw that her old brand of freedom before the rape was, in part, a denial of these feelings and an escape into a pseudo-haven which did not really exist. At the same time, she saw that none of this meant that she had to feel terrorized or helpless all of her life—that in unity there was strength; that there was a different way to feel powerful in concert with the women with whom she now closely identified.

One year after Andrea was raped, she took part in a "Take Back the Night" march and rally in her city. Thousands of women walked together in that city and others across the country. When she marched that night, down the very streets that had once seemed so dangerous to her, Andrea found a new and exhilarating sense of freedom which she had not known before. It was a symbolic moment, a flowering of the new awareness of her identity and power as a woman which she had gained through examining her rape experience in therapy.

NORA'S STORY: RESISTANCES TO CONSCIOUSNESS ■ Andrea's story vividly illustrates the way in which any therapy geared to the needs of women must address itself to matters of consciousness-raising: that is, to helping women integrate—in a radically new way—feelings and beliefs about what it means to be a woman in our society.

This process can be more or less successful; it was, as we have seen, more successful in the work with Andrea's rape experience than it was in the work with Bonnie's monomania about being fat. The success of consciousness-raising in therapy depends, to a large extent, on the degree of resistance to consciousness in the patient. In traditional terms, resistance is defined as an unconscious phenomenon that pertains strictly to *feelings*: the patient resists the surfacing to consciousness of long-repressed feelings that are a threat to the patient's ego or superego. But in working with people in therapy, I have seen, again and again, how resistance applies to the patient's *beliefs* as well as feelings. Women often have a powerful resistance to seeing their oppression clearly; for the Victim is easily overcome by the magnitude of the subordination of women in our society without feeling a commensurate ability to fight that subordination. Because it all seems too big to tackle, the Victim makes a hasty retreat, refusing to confront that which has already vanquished her. In such ways, women unwittingly comply with our oppression. This was the case in Nora's therapy.

Nora came to therapy after a serious suicide attempt and a brief psychiatric hospitalization. Like Linda in the preceding chapter, her hospitalization had not succeeded in helping her overcome her depression. She had tried to kill herself as a way out of a deteriorating marital relationship. Six months earlier, her husband had found out that she was having an affair and had threatened to leave her. Rather than endure the prospect of being abandoned, Nora had taken an overdose of sleeping pills. Her suicide attempt was also a way of trying to manipulate her husband into staying with her.

After several months of therapy with me, Nora realized that her relationship with her husband was not, in fact, meeting her needs, and that divorce was a better option than suicide. But like many women, whenever she thought about exercising the power to end her marriage, she was overcome by a kind of paralysis. She felt like a "puppet on a string trying to get up and walk." Like Linda, she was an inveterate man-junkie: she simply could not imagine living without a man. Even if the man was not what she wanted, something was better than nothing. And "nothing" was the way she thought of life without a masculine benefactor.

In one of our sessions, Nora admitted with a mischievous grin that she was bisexual: the affair that had enraged her husband had been with a woman. But this did not mean that Nora saw relationships with women as an alternative to relationships with men. On the contrary, her sexual liaisons with women only confirmed her deeply held belief that only men had real, lasting value.

We spent many sessions exploring how men came to be vested with such value. Asked to free-associate to the word "feminine," Nora came up with: frilly, sexy, dependent, pathetic, weak, negative. Her free association to the word "masculine" was: mechanical, independent (especially economically), into sports, strong, positive. Having come up with these associations, Nora expressed dismay and confusion at knowing that she was more feminine than masculine. She hated herself for (in her own words) "using my face to manipulate men." (Nora was strikingly attractive.) Yet she also took pride in her ability to do so. The more we talked, the more Nora realized that much of her attraction to men was based on their power. She saw men as persons capable of providing her with money and status, and of making her feel okay about herself. She thought of men as teachers. She also enjoyed turning men on sexually, explaining that "sex is the only thing I'm good at."

Her attraction to women, on the other hand, was what Nora described as "just physical." She saw women as bodies that had an innate sexual interest. But they had no power to make her feel good about herself. They had no inherent value: they were negative, not positive. Nora had internalized the male view of Woman as Body. Her bisexuality seemed to offer little opportunity for increasing her own sense of power and value as a woman.

In the course of therapy, Nora did achieve a new awareness of herself as a woman. She realized how much she devalued herself and women in general. She developed a fuller understanding of her identity as a "bad girl." Her bisexuality, her marriage to a man her father disapproved of, and prior to this, her unwed pregnancy and abortion, and her adolescent involvement as a juvenile delinquent were all part of this bad-girl role of which she felt both proud and ashamed. She reached an understanding of the self-destructive aspects of this role and, in the process, regained her will to live. After nine months of therapy, she announced her desire to terminate. She had separated from her husband and no longer felt depressed or suicidal. In this sense, she had accomplished her goal.

Though she recognized that she could benefit from further work on her relationships with men and women, she did not want to do this work. It was only at this point in the therapy that Nora admitted that she was, as she put it, "down on women's lib." When I asked her if my open identification as a feminist (which I announce quite clearly at the onset of therapy and which is obvious throughout my work) in some way made her feel pressured to be similarly involved, Nora denied this. She explained that she saw my identity as a feminist separate from my skill as a therapist; that she had benefited from the latter and tolerated the former. In this way she split what were, in fact, inseparable aspects of my therapeutic work. She resisted seeing the connection between the value of feminism and the value of therapy in her progress from suicidal depression.

From my point of view, Nora's desire to terminate therapy expressed not only her achievement of her stated goals for therapy, but also her desire to maintain her bad-girl identity. Most people fear that therapy will rob them of something that makes them unique. For Nora, that uniqueness resided in her bad-girl quality. She did not fully understand how her bad-girl identity contained the seeds of a potential freedom from the conventional feminine role, which she ultimately accepted. Through therapy, she had learned to appreciate herself and her power enough to overcome her depression and her desire to die. This was no small accomplishment. But she had only partially transformed her image of women (and of herself) as essentially pathetic, crazy, sexual objects that were imbued with value only through their association with men. The consciousness-raising process had gone only so far.

ELIZABETH'S STORY: CONFLICTS IN CLASS- AND SEX-CONSCIOUS-NESS ■ The effectiveness of using consciousness-raising as a therapy tool is most immediate in short-term therapy. In such work, there is an agreement to focus on one specific issue for a time-limited period. (Ordinarily, I work with people for twelve weeks and then renegotiate if they want to work further.) I have done short-term therapy work with women who have wanted to focus on virtually all of the female symptoms familiar to us by now, including depression; body image and sexuality; psychosomatic ailments such as migraine headaches, colitis, etc.; relationships with men; divorce or separation from a spouse. In addition, I do a great deal of this work with couples—both heterosexual and lesbian—who wish to work on their relationship. With virtually no exceptions, all of these short-term clients experienced significant improvement in the areas on which they focused.

One of the advantages of this kind of work is the fact that the short-term therapy relationship is bound to be less characterized by the patient's transference to the therapist than is long-term therapy. Since the relationship is short-lived and the specific focus is on current problems, there is less chance for the client to develop the unconscious (or conscious) attitude of a child toward a therapist who is experienced as a parent or parental surrogate. The "larger than life" quality of the therapist recedes in favor of a more equal tone to the therapeutic relationship. Furthermore, the time limit tends to enhance the patient's motivation. Often, patients will notice significant changes in only a few weeks; this, in turn, leads to a renewed sense of power which furthers the work. All of these factors in short-term work combine to help undo the Patient Identity more effectively than in long-term individual therapy. Finally, though the client doesn't necessarily leave therapy feeling transformed, a substantial change in one specific area of a person's life often has a domino effect: it leads to further changes in the person's life outside of and after therapy.

Elizabeth came to therapy seeking relief from acute anxiety about her work. She was an airline flight attendant promoted to the rank of supervisor, whose success precipitated a terrible crisis in her life. As a flight attendant, she had enjoyed her work but disliked its low status. After her promotion, she felt good about the increase in her status and her salary, but found herself in a state of almost constant anxiety about the work. She found it excruciating to evaluate her underlings' performance, dreading that she would hurt them by her evaluation, alternately feeling guilty and responsible for their fate or feeling resentful about people who tried to take advantage of her as a "soft touch." Her anxiety mounted daily, till it got to the point that she found herself tempted to drive right past the airport and never go to work again. Typically, she began to fear that she might be "going crazy." It was at this point that she sought therapy.

Elizabeth was not going crazy. But her fear that she was, was based on some profound role conflicts in her work. Elizabeth had been raised by a working-class mother who was in and out of mental hospitals, alternately taking care of and abandoning Elizabeth. Her father had left when she was a baby. From an early age, she had learned to take care of herself, both emotionally and financially. She had taken a variety of jobs, all "woman's work": waitress, maid, flight attendant. Now, for the first time in her life, she had a "man's job." She was responsible not for serving people, but for judging them. Her inbred sense of feminine responsibility for nurture in relationships was at odds with her new masculine task of exerting authority over others.

Elizabeth's greatest fear was that she would hurt people through her evaluations. Like most women, she felt that to hurt someone else, even inadvertently or unintentionally, was a heinous crime; she preferred to hurt herself. As we talked about this in therapy, it became apparent that the hurt she inflicted on others was more often imagined than real. It was the act of evaluation itself, her *power* to affect others' lives (whether or not that power resulted in penalties for the worker) that made Elizabeth feel guilty. At the same time, she carried a great deal of unconscious resentment at those whom she felt she was failing to protect. Elizabeth's dread of her own power belonged to a distinctly feminine sense of identity. (It is quite common in women's therapy, rare in men's.)

This central conflict between Elizabeth's feminine identity and her masculine-style job was complicated by the conflicts between her present managerial position and her working-class past. All her life, Elizabeth had been the one to be evaluated, not the one evaluating; she had been the worker, not the manager. When she evaluated those beneath her in the work hierarchy, the "worker" in her experienced an undercurrent of profound resentment at her own bosses, whom she felt were making her harm others. She identified with the people she evaluated and thus felt guilty about what she was doing. On the other hand, the "manager" in Elizabeth was proud to be "above" those "on the line." She enjoyed a kind of superiority that she'd never known before. Here again there was a guilt in feeling superior. The flip side of most guilt is resentment: and indeed, underneath it all, Elizabeth harbored massive resentment at those both below and above her in the hierarchy.

Like most women, she experienced a feminine compulsion to please all the people all of the time. But in her situation, this was impossible. She felt that she was failing either those whom she supervised or those who supervised her. Thus, in her most successful moment in the airline industry, she felt like a failure.

Not surprisingly, the only solution to her current distress that Elizabeth could imagine was returning to her former job as a flight attendant. But while she knew that being a flight attendant would get rid of her anxiety, she also felt that returning to this former position would be an admission of even greater failure. As a result, she felt stymied: there was no way she could come out feeling she'd made the right decision. So instead of acting, she became paralyzed. This, in turn, fueled her feeling that she was going crazy.

Elizabeth's therapy centered on the conflicts in sexual and class identity which were at the core of her current problem. My task was to help her realize not only *what* she felt, but *how to think about what she felt.* For instance, in talking about her early life as a child, Elizabeth experienced a strong sense of shame which she thought was connected to her memory of her mother as an "inadequate," psychiatrically institutionalized alcoholic. With some help, she came to see how much of this shame was also related to her working-class roots in general: to the life that she had left behind in becoming an airline manager. At the same time, she felt a fierce kind of loyalty to those people.[2] She began to realize how much of her current distress was related to her unconscious feeling that she was betraying her class. Similarly, she came to a new awareness of the conflicts between her feminine passion to nurture others and the masculine authority her job demanded. It became apparent to her why the only solution she could imagine to her current dilemma was to return to the conflict-free feminine role of air-line hostess.

The consciousness-raising aspects of Elizabeth's therapy coexisted with a more conventional analytic approach to her problems. For instance, we explored how much her current anxiety at work was related to the fact that, in becoming a manager of others, she felt she was relinquishing the family role she had as a young child: that of caretaker of others (including her mother). Like Dorothy, Elizabeth saw that her fear of going crazy—and her desire to become a therapy patient—were also ways of connecting to her dead mother (whose family role had been that of "crazy patient"). And so on. These family underpinnings of Elizabeth's pain existed alongside her sex and class conflicts.

In the course of Elizabeth's sixteen weeks of therapy, she became aware of how all of the sources of her pain worked together. She also used our sessions to release a great deal of stored-up anger and resentment: both the long-repressed anger at her mother, and her more recent anger at her supervisees and supervisors. Certainly, there was room to go deeper into all the themes we had touched upon. But once her conflicts became clear, her panicky fear of going crazy vanished: she could see the source of her confusion. Naming and clarifying her conflicts and experiencing her feelings of guilt, anger, and resentment helped her to rethink what she wanted to do in a clearer way. She no longer felt pressure either to quit her new job or to stay in it indefinitely. By the end of therapy, she had not, in fact, decided whether to remain a manager, though she thought she probably would. But the problem of anxiety was gone. She no longer felt trapped and crazy.

4. Dependence/Independence: Dilemmas of the "New Woman"

LAURA'S STORY: NEEDING TOO MUCH, OR THE SAD SONG OF WHY I CAN'T MAKE IT WITH A MAN ■ We have seen in the stories of Linda, Diane, Carol, and Nora the centrality of the issue of dependence for women. Both Linda's and Nora's depressions were related to their dependence on men to give their lives value and purpose. Diane's fear of being alone was part of a dependence on others which crippled her capacity to feel whole. Much of Carol's therapy centered around her dependence on others, and her view of it as evil.

The question of how women in our society can achieve independence has become one of the hottest questions of our time. According to TV talk shows and serials, to advertisements and magazine feature stories, this is the era of the New Woman. The New Woman, we are told, has put her old patterns of dependence and subservience behind her and has embraced a new, "liberated" life-style. If she is single, she enjoys her new-found sense of freedom from domestic dependence. If she is married, her husband is the New Man: someone who shares the housework and child rearing and is an equal partner in life. The New Woman manages to juggle family and career without falling on her face. Like Jill Clayburgh in *An Unmarried Woman*, she is soft, vulnerable, and sexy (like the Old Woman) but she is also competent, assertive, and tough (like the Old Man). The New Woman is physically alluring and mentally able. She is not working-class. She has a satisfying, high-powered career from which she derives a great deal of self-esteem. Nor is she a lesbian. She likes men, but she doesn't cling to them, the way that the Old Woman did. Like a man, she values her independence above all else.

Indeed, many women today are grappling with the themes of dependence/independence in their lives, trying to come up with genuinely new ways to define these terms and live them out. But the New Woman image is more likely to harm than help us. It is yet another male fantasy of what women should be in the era of feminism. Living up to the new myth of Super-woman has created a whole new set of problems for women who feel that they should, but do not, measure up—and who feel that measuring up is simply an individual matter of liberation from old patterns of female psychological dependence ("It's all in your head").

We have already seen how the socioeconomic structure of our society still militates against the needs of women who wish to achieve their independence through paid work, or through combining work and family. The New Woman is a rare exception to the institutionalized socioeconomic disadvantage that women as a whole still face. The New Woman image also tends to feed into men's fantasies of having their cake and eating it too. That is, the New Woman, as an ideal, has all of the charms of the Old Woman's feminine capacity to nurture men without any of the old claims that women once expected in return for their domestic services (financial security, fidelity in marriage, etc.). In practice this easily results in a new kind of male oppression in personal relationships: the New Man who expects his New Woman to be there for him when he wants her, and to be "independent" when it suits him.

Women trying to achieve relationships with men in which both partners are equally dedicated to the woman's independence are still, for the most part, up against a very difficult struggle. In fact, some of the most independent women I know tend to have a hard time even finding men who are not put off by female independence. Even those men who intellectually support it often tend to find independence in women a profound sexual turn-off. In many cases, men who profess to want their women to be "liberated" and who disapprove of old-fashioned female dependence nevertheless still want women to treat them with that old-fashioned reverence. (There is nothing more threatening to these men than a woman who treats men as simple sex objects who are useful for their bodies but not particularly important or valuable otherwise—women who turn the tables on men sexually tend to be *Playboy* fantasies which, in reality, frighten men off.) In short, the New Woman has a great deal more than her own psyche to contend with in her attempts to achieve independence, both socioeconomically and in personal relationships with men.

Several years ago, I gave a talk at a local mental health center in a white, upper-middle-class neighborhood—the kind of neighborhood in which New Women are supposed to abound. By way of preparation for this talk, I consulted the Intake Counselor at the center (the person responsible for interviewing patients when they first came in) to find out what kinds of "presenting problems" these women were bringing to therapy nowadays. I learned that approximately 70 percent of the people using the center were women ranging in age from twenty-one to forty-five. The chief complaints of these women, in order of frequency, were : (1) "I'm depressed"; (2) "I have no sense of where my life is going"; (3) "I've just lost a husband [or lover] and I'm depressed"; (4) "I want to work on my dependency on men"; (5) "I want to work on how I set myself up to be hurt in relationships with men"; (6) "I want to work on having a good relationship with a man (I get depressed without one)"; and (7) "I'm having problems with my career."

The most striking fact about the New Woman in therapy, judging from this list (and from my own practice), is that, like the Old Woman, depression is still her number-one problem. The second most striking fact is the great preponderance of female complaints having to do with relationships with men: having them, finding them, losing them, needing them, and setting oneself up for bad ones. It is remarkable that the concern with career-related issues appears last on this list of grievances. (Moreover, three of the requests—4, 5, and 6—indicate that women still believe that their problems in their relationships with men are a result of their own psychological defects.)

The third most striking fact is the appearance of "I want to work on my dependency on men." From my own experience in working with women in therapy (as we will see from Laura's story), this request is gaining prominence in the list of reasons why women want therapy. There may very well be a connection between these three facts (the New Woman's depression, her preoccupation with relationships with men, and her concern with being overly dependent): the New Woman still tends to believe that she is primarily responsible for making relationships succeed. Consequently, she is more likely than a man to conclude that problems in relationships are essentially *her* problem. If these relationships are not working, it is all too easy for the New Woman to see her dependence (or other patterns) as the cause. The New Woman Patient thus often finds a way to use feminist ideology as yet another way to bludgeon herself with self-blame.

Many women today are finding it increasingly confusing to figure out how to be independent and yet get what we want in intimate relationships with men, or how to succeed in careers without adopting the traditional masculine style of competitive independence which we both shy from and dislike; or how to sort out our priorities in the realms of career and family; or how to keep our own sense of femininity in a high-powered workplace in which we are expected to work like a man but still be "womanly." We must remember that the social context for working out these various new dilemmas is still a culture that views any form of dependence as immature and conceives of independence in strictly masculine terms.

In facing these dilemmas, women often fall into the trap of thinking that we have to give up our former feminine subservience and replace it with a male style of autonomy that rejects all forms of dependence as unhealthy. We shall see some of the problems that result in the following story of Laura.

Laura was a thirty-three-year-old single woman, a hard-working and competent social worker, and an avid feminist. She shared an apartment with two other women and the daughter of one of them. She lived what the media would call an "alternative life-style". Her life was busy and full, yet she came to therapy, like so many women, because she was depressed about her relationships with men. She had recently broken up with a man whom she thought of as her "last hope" for a stable relationship.

During the course of our initial meeting, Laura said, "It's hard for me to admit, but the reason I'm depressed is that I'm thirty-three years old, single, and have no children. I want to be married. But I doubt that I ever will be." When I asked her why, Laura's answer was an extensive analysis of her predicament: "I set myself up for failure in relationships because I need too much. Men pick up on how needy I am and get turned off. I keep losing men this way. If I didn't need so much, I'd probably be able to find a man. This is the pattern I want to change."

Like many women, Laura had the identity of a "reject": an object men would always leave on the shelf. She attributed this to her "neediness." Like her lovers, she regarded her needs as childish, unruly, and extreme: to be eradicated rather than met. When I asked Laura what she meant by her "neediness," she answered that she felt her entire identity was built around her relationships with men. In response, I pointed out that however dependent she felt, it was clear to me that her identity was not, in fact, entirely geared to men: that she had a strong commitment to her work and to feminist politics, as well as very real and important relationships with women in her life. This simple observation seemed to startle her. It was as though this thought had never really registered with her. Certainly, she knew that her work, her politics, and her relationships with women were important. But somehow this never affected her view of her own dependency.

The more we explored her dependency, the more apparent it became that quite a variety of needs were included under this general category. One thing Laura meant by her dependency was her need to have a man in order to feel that she was not a reject or a loser: that she was worth loving. She needed a man to prove to herself—and her mother—that she was okay. She had fantasies about taking a man home for her mother's approval: a "good catch." She described her mother as cold and mechanical, someone who didn't seem to get much from marriage except financial security and status, yet who was always praising the institution. She thought of both of her parents as sexless and incapable of real intimacy, cold and proper as parents, not very loving to each other or to their children. Her mother had always advised Laura to "hold off" for the right man, yet, at the same time, not to be too "picky."

Laura was living out her mother's double message in her relationships with men. She put men in essentially two categories: the "good catch" and the "bad catch." The good catch was a provider type; the bad catch a sexy type. The good catch provided a woman with status, security and companionship, but was sexless (like her father). The bad catch provided sex but was unreliable for anything else (the anti-type of her father). But what all her men had in common was that they were emotionally distant, and that they found Laura "too needy" (like her father). With none of these men did Laura feel she could get the closeness or warmth that she needed. In the end, she would angrily dump both of these types of men, blaming them for not being "right," and blaming herself for not being able to make it with a man.

In short, Laura felt that it was impossible to get what she needed with any man. Ultimately, no man was worth marrying. Once, when I pointed out that, in a sense, she was choosing to remain single, Laura denied that this was a choice. She did not experience her own power to choose. She experienced herself as someone not chosen: the rejected, not the rejector. Laura's sense of her dependency centered around this way of experiencing herself as a Victim.

But there was another meaning to Laura's dependence which it took some work to uncover. Essentially, Laura saw all of her needs for warmth, companionship, sex, intimacy, and nurturance under the general heading "neediness." It was as though all of these needs proved her inherent lack of control and independence. By lumping both her need for a man to give her a sense of self-worth, and her need for sexual/emotional intimacy with a man in the same general category of neediness, Laura ended up by invalidating both kinds of dependence. Hence she never saw the part that her men played in her relationships. She never saw the problem that they had with giving emotional warmth or nurturance, with knowing how to depend on someone, or to open themselves to a certain kind of vulnerability in intimate relationships. She saw only her own "ugly" dependence and her own "ugly" anger—neither of which she felt was justified.

For Laura to overcome her first type of dependence (the impossible feminine demand that a man can make her feel good about herself) she had to reclaim her right to the second type of dependence: her authentic need for intimate connection. Strangely, Laura felt that her need for intimacy with women was legitimate, whereas the same need with men was not. In our therapy work, we traced Laura's view of her neediness to its sources, both in her family and in her experience with men. Her father was a respected lawyer, her mother a modern woman active in various social organizations. They were wealthy people who, ostensibly, gave Laura "everything." Yet, as a child, Laura was often sad. She felt an unnamed longing for something from her parents that she never got: warmth. Consequently, she was sent to a psychiatrist at the age of six. This confirmed her parents' message that, since she was getting everything, her needs were clearly excessive and her sadness pathological. She got no more warmth from her psychiatrist than she got from her parents. But she learned to bury her need for it and to see it as bad.

This parental message about her needs was confirmed and reinforced in virtually all of her later relationships with men. Laura was caught in the cultural double bind by which women are conditioned to feel and see themselves as dependent on men and then flogged for this very attribute in their relations with them.

In one of our sessions, we used the gestalt technique of giving a "voice" to Laura's various feelings. Her "top-dog" voice—the tyrannical voice that ruled her consciousness—told Laura: "You are too needy. Your needs are ugly and bad. You are too angry." Her "under-dog" voice—the voice of her internalized Victim—responded with "I can't help it. I'm trying to be better." What Laura learned in this session was that she believed her "top-dog" voice represented a reasonable assessment of her as a person! Her conscious ego identified with this ruthless voice of parental and masculine authority. It took some time for her to locate a third voice inside her which said, "You have a right to your needs for warmth. Your neediness is not bad. It's there for a good reason." My role was to be this voice when Laura could not muster it; to help her hear it so that she could eventually overcome her resistance to internalizing it.

By the sixth of our twelve sessions, it dawned on Laura that her problem was not so much that she was too dependent but that *she didn't allow herself to feel dependent on men* at all!

Rather than really experiencing her needs for intimacy, she converted her valid longings and frustrations into a posture of constant complaint about her neediness. She turned her needs into self-hate. She began to realize that, in short-circuiting this process through validating her own needs, she would no longer need men in the same way. For it became clear to her that the more she saw her needs as bad, the more she needed men to prove to her that she wasn't bad for needing—to make her feel good! Certainly, her dependence on men to provide her with a sense of self-worth was not working for her: it was an impossible demand which left her feeling perennially angry at men and inadequate as a woman. On the other hand, she began to see that her needs for warmth and vulnerability from men were difficult for many men to meet because of their own culturally induced fears of dependence.*

Therapy also helped Laura identify her various angers: the anger of the child inside her at her parents' coldness; the Victim's anger in her that came from an unrealistic fantasy of finding the perfect "catch" to redeem her; and the adult and legitimate anger at men for their oppressive invalidation of her needs. In the process, Laura came to expect both less and more from men: less of the Total Rescue Mission she had dreamed of, more of the warmth she deserved.

Laura's story reveals some of the complexities of the issues of dependence and independence for women today. She came to therapy having internalized a clearly masculine view of her feminine dependence: of feminine needs as weakness. Many women come to therapy wanting their therapist to collude with

* The process by which women convert their legitimate needs for warmth and closeness from men into self-criticism has an important psychic function. It is a doomed effort to control reality that grows out of the myth that "it's all in your head." It expresses a woman's belief that her problems in relationships with men are totally within her own control: all she has to do is get her head together. This way of thinking (consciously or unconsciously) is often more comforting (despite the pain it causes) than thinking that there are few men available nowadays for independent feminist women. The men who can emotionally match such women (who are not afraid of these women's independence, and who are not afraid of their own dependence on women) are not in great supply.

them in the attempt to do away with their needs. And many traditional therapists have been all too willing to do this because they share a male cultural bias against the needs of women, a view of women's needs for nurturance as excessive when compared to the more independent qualities of men. (Or, worse still, because they have shared society's traditional expectation that women should be geared to the needs of others while suppressing their own.) In my work with Laura, my attempt was clearly to help Laura see the legitimacy of her needs, rather than to help her wipe them out.

This was not only a matter of validating her genuine needs for intimacy and nurturance in her relationships with men. It was also a matter of helping her see that even in what she took to be her greatest weakness there was a strength. For instance, her fear that she would not marry was actually the conscious side of an unconscious wish not to marry. Her "I can't make it with a man" and "I can't make it without one" was also a way of refusing to find a "good catch" and to settle down into comfortable financial dependence, as her mother had. The seed of strength in Laura's "dependent" terror of not being married was a powerful desire to be independent in a way that her own mother had not been.

Laura's mother had given up a career in order to get married and have children. Yet there was a cold emptiness to her role as wife and mother, an emptiness that characterized the lives of many women of the Feminine Mystique. Her mother's lack of warmth for her role, in turn, had helped create a certain neediness in her child. But Laura enjoyed a degree of financial, sexual, and emotional independence that her mother had never known. She was responsible for herself in a way that her mother had not been. She had been raised to value her feminine dependence on men, but she had come of age in the explosion of contemporary feminism. One result was Laura's conflicted feelings about her independence: about being thirty-three years old, single, and childless. Laura's painful emphasis on her dependence on men paradoxically reflected an unconscious attempt to hold on to a traditional sense of her own femininity which was threatened by her more independent life-style.

There is something genuinely historically new about Laura's story. She had come to therapy with an ambivalent request: she wanted therapy both to help her find a husband and to help her eradicate her need for one. (In our initial session, when I asked Laura how she would know when she reached her self-proclaimed therapy goal of becoming more independent, she half-jokingly replied: "When I find myself a man.") I doubt very much whether, before the 1970s, there were any women who came to therapy to overcome their need for husbands. After all, female dependence had been defined by Freud as an essential attribute of femininity. Decades ago, women did not worry about it as a sign of pathology. If anything, they came to therapy because they felt insufficiently feminine to catch a man. They came hoping to discover and cure the psychological defect that kept them from marrying.

By contrast, in the era of feminism, female dependence has come to be seen as "unliberated," yet another reason for women to become patients of therapy. But whether it's the old refrain "I need a man to love," or the new refrain "I shouldn't need a man in order to be fulfilled," what hasn't changed is the profound feminine conviction of Woman as Patient that "there's something wrong with me."*

Dependence, a once accepted attribute of femininity, is no longer wanted—by women or by men. Books like *The Cinderella Complex* by Colette Dowling find a wide readership of men and women who feel that if women want the privileges of liberation, they should cleanse their minds of unsightly feminine dependence. The basic message here is, No more waiting

* Several years ago I participated in a panel discussion with a psychiatrist from Missoula, Montana. In his talk, he named the search for a husband as the number-one reason his female patients came to therapy. There may be some regional differences involved in how much women today are actually internalizing the ideology of the New Woman. Nevertheless, the fact that this psychiatrist's patients came to therapy, rather than to a computer dating service, to solve their problems of being without a man, is evidence of the continued existence of Woman as Patient.

for Prince Charming, girls; get out there and fight like a man! What gets lost in this message is the inherent value in women's capacity to depend on others, to make themselves vulnerable, to know that they sometimes need help, that they are not islands unto themselves. These qualities are quite human, and belong to men as well as women. The difference is that men have traditionally denied these needs in order to be masculine. And women have traditionally heightened them in order to be feminine.

But dependence is no more inherently healthy than independence. People who fear dependence are just as crippled in forming intimate relationships as people who fear independence. The words "dependence" and "independence" themselves betray the masculine bias against female attributes. Both men and women are dependent and independent, in different ways. Female-style dependence, in its extreme, is a form of subservience in which one's sense of identity is contingent upon the presence of another compared to whom one feels inferior, and through whom one tries to get the self-worth that is felt to be missing. (We have seen the crippling effects of this kind of dependence in the stories of Linda, Nora, and now Laura.)

But male-style independence, in its extreme, is a kind of autism, a denial of the ways in which men depend on women for emotional nurturance, as well as a refusal to acknowledge the very real ties that bind all of us to one another. (Men who are independent in this way end up feeling hollow inside too, but in a different way from women.)

From the culturally male perspective, women's dependence has been seen as feminine weakness, whereas male independence has been overvalued. Furthermore, male dependence on women has gone unnoticed. This is largely because the culture has provided for the satisfaction of male dependence in a way that it hasn't for female dependence. Men have had "wives"—women who fulfill their sexual, emotional, and domestic needs (and who do so for free because they see these tasks as a function of femininity). The rock of a man, who appears to all of his colleagues (and to his own wife) as the epitome of independence, goes home, where his wife cooks his meals, massages his ego, raises his children, and cleans his house. This man builds the rock of his character on the invisible foundation of his dependence on his wife.

Many women believe that they are dependent on men because they want to be taken care of. But this is part of an elaborate game of patriarchal doublethink. Emotionally, it has been women who have taken care of men. But men have traditionally denied or disguised this need while getting it met: for it has been the woman's job to take care of men's needs for nurturance. Women have felt more needy than men for nurturance precisely because, by and large, they have not gotten this need met by men. Nurturing is not an attribute of masculinity. Men have just not learned to nurture as women do. As a result, nurturance is something most men have gotten (and still get) from women but have not known how to give. The male dependence involved in this traditional relationship is overlooked because it has always been taken for granted that women will do the work of nurturance.

Women have not had wives. We have had husbands who are supposed to provide us with financial protection—that is, a built-in marital guarantee of female financial dependence. In many cases, women have not had even this much. We have had to carry a good part of the financial burden, as well as to do all of the emotional and physical work of maintaining the family. Certainly, women today are trying to break away from this kind of dependence on men.

But this process is only hampered, not furthered, by the ideas of books like *The Cinderella Complex*. It is not helpful to blame women for the kind of dependence that cripples us while ignoring the fact that society still continues to accommodate male independence and thwart women's. This is merely another blame-the-victim trap.

Women who fail to recognize their strength in being able to depend on others or who fail to recognize the ways that men depend on women, end up thinking of women as "dependent" and men as "independent." Such women often feel they've failed when they don't adopt a male style of autonomy—both in relationships and at work. But in many cases, this "failure" is due to the fact that women do not really *want* to become autonomous in the way that men have been. They do not wish to become competitively embattled against others, or to see their own individuality as contingent upon the renunciation of their needs for intimacy or family.

For example, Abby was a career woman who suffered from a lack of self-confidence in trying to establish herself as an architect—a field heavily dominated by men. She had recently finished a large architectural project. Though she had been responsible for overseeing this project, many people had worked on it, including several women "draftsmen." In one particular session, in an effort to help Abby take some pride in her work, I instructed her to visualize herself looking at her work, in front of which there was a large sign that read "Architectural Design by Abby Jones, Architect." As she did so, she experienced a feeling of sadness for all of the other people (especially the women) who had worked on this project but who would not get credit for their work if it went under her name. I do not imagine that there are very many men in our society who would feel this way.

In one sense, it could be said that Abby suffered from a deficiency of a masculine style of individualistic independence. She found it difficult to appropriate her own work in a way that a man does: to pronounce it as her own and take pride in *her* accomplishment. But in another sense, Abby's sadness reflected a compassionate desire for all of the co-workers who labored in this project to share in its rewards. She had a strong awareness of her interdependence with others which was a repudiation of the hierarchical male system of individual careers in which the labor of the "underlings" often remains invisible.

Indeed, there is good reason for women today to fear giving up the valuable aspects of our female capacity for dependent connection to others in favor of a male style of rigid ego autonomy. Our society could benefit from Abby's awareness.

5. *Everywoman's Story: Internalized Anger*

SUSAN'S STORY: CINDERELLA STRIKES BACK

I have been invisible,
weird and supernatural.
I want my black dress.
I want my hair
curling wild around me.
I want my broomstick
from the closet where I hid it.
Tonight I meet my sisters
in the graveyard.
Around midnight
if you stop at a red light
in the wet city traffic,
watch for us against the moon.
We are screaming,
we are flying,
laughing, and won't stop.
(from "Witch," by Jean Tepperman)

Throughout this book, we have seen how central the experience of depression is to many women's lives. Chronic and intermittent forms of depression continue to cripple the lives of millions of women in our society every day. More and more, depression is being treated with chemicals: antidepressants, tranquilizers, lithium. The use of electroshock for depressed patients is also on the rise. And in the past few years, the use of psychosurgery is enjoying a resurgence as a "cure" for depression as well as other psychiatric and behavioral "disorders."

One reason why none of these methods works very well is that they all fail to get at the underlying cause of most women's chronic depression: an abiding, unconscious rage at our oppression which has found no legitimate outlet. We have seen this repressed rage in the stories of Amy, Linda, Nora, and Laura, among others. One of the cardinal assumptions of this book has been that within many female psychological symptoms lies the seed of unconscious rage at male domination. This is nowhere more obvious than in the case of women who suffer from depression. What kind of help do such women require?

Looking back at my own journeys through the mire of depression and self-hatred, the first answer that comes to me has nothing to do with therapy—at least as it is conventionally defined. It has to do with anger, power, and other women. What helped me, more than anything else, to overcome my own depression was the terrifying and exhilarating process of finally, with the help of many other women, letting myself get good and angry.

Becoming undepressed meant learning to love myself as a woman. It meant recognizing that a poisonous arrow perpetually pointed at my own heart could be redirected to its appropriate targets. It meant allowing myself to rage at a society (and at all the particular men in my life) that had perpetuated my own worst ideas of who I was. For much of my life until the women's movement arrived, I had believed (consciously or unconsciously), that since women were only supposed to exist for others, my own needs were "selfish"; that since men were the measure of all value, I would never be worth as much as a man; that my value lay mainly in how I looked; that, no matter how much I might fool people into thinking otherwise, I was, at bottom, stupid and weak. These were just some of the externally imposed messages that I had internalized and with which I was depressing myself.

It was with the advent of the women's movement that I first let myself get angry about all this. When I did, I hated every man I'd ever known. When I passed men on the street, I deliberately moved as far away from them as I could, as though even the nearness of their bodies could somehow harm me. No man was to be trusted. Inside every man was a Rapist. The deep, masculine sound of a man's voice could whip me into a frenzy of fear and loathing. TV commercials I'd seen all my life, displaying sexy women draped over elegant men selling cars or simple housewives cosmically worrying about their wash, were more than I could bear. I dumped my bewildered boy-

friend of the time and became celibate. Every particle of reality
burned with the oppression of women by men. It was as though
I felt, really felt, for the first time, and with no "reasonable,"
conscious censors to stop me, the abiding menace that men
were to women in patriarchal society.

It was not a neat, rational "appropriate" anger that I could
put in a little bag and tie up with a little pink feminine ribbon.
It was not a nice anger. It was not an anger that could be confined to the therapy room with my male therapist. It was not an
anger I could ever have let myself feel unless I had the backing
of thousands of women across the country who were raging
along with me, the immediate support of a few close women
friends who knew exactly what I was feeling and why, and the
encouragement of a consciousness-raising group in which we
could all sort out and understand what this fury was all about,
without judging it out of hand.

The courage to rage, for me, had come from the increasing
knowledge that being this angry did not mean I was crazy—
because for the first time, *women were doing it together.* And,
doing it together, we learned to look at ourselves and each
other in a new way: to see our beauty where male culture saw
only blemishes. To see our strength where the male world saw
feminine weakness. To appreciate the feminine in us that mi-
sogynist culture feared, hated, and envied: our emotionality,
our softness, our capacity to nurture, our ability to be receptive
and "passive." We even learned (and this was the hardest lesson of all) to love our bodies: the bodies we had learned to see
through male eyes as perpetual reminders of our inadequacy,
the bodies whose dark odors and discharges and monthly fertil-
ity we felt we had to hide.

Through the process of allowing my "man-hating," I found
a new way to love men that did not entail my subordination. In
the process of feeling and letting go of my anger, I learned to
love myself and other women.

These lessons in anger and self-love are not something
women ordinarily learn in therapy. (My rage at male society
had been, not surprisingly, both bewildering and off-putting to

my male psychiatrist, who tried his best to put a stop to it. When I trusted my anger enough, I quit the therapy.) In most therapy situations, women merely learn to suppress their rage even further; or to see it as a strictly personal matter, wholly irrational in nature; or to channel it into a kind of male-identified contempt for other women while learning to see oneself as the "exceptional woman," somehow above the rest. Therapy is not known for creating or encouraging people to fight back.

But fighting depression in my (and many other women's) experience grew out of fighting back. It was part of a process of seeing the power women had, potentially and actually, to change ourselves and the way things were for women. In using our power together, to alter the institutionalized ways in which we were kept down, we emerged from our isolated cocoons of self-hate and depression. Self-love was not simply something that I found, like buried treasure in the backyard. It was something that we *won* by acting together as women.

Internalization of oppression is the crux of women's depression and self-hate. It is as though every impulse of a depressed woman's consciousness is finely tuned to a view of herself that is in accord with that of the dominant culture's view of women as inferior. (In a society that has not yet accepted even the minimal principle of equal pay for equal work, the cultural allegiance to the continued supremacy of men over women is clear.) Getting past this pattern of internalization often feels like a defiance too large to undertake. It means getting fighting angry at an entire social universe predicated on institutionalized woman hatred. This is not something that any woman can do easily or alone. There is a tremendous resistance to the enterprise. It is not, as traditional psychologists think, simply a resistance to uncovering unconscious feelings. It is equally, and more important, a resistance to seeing the social basis for one's feelings—and thereby ending the depression, once and for all.

Validating one's feelings in this way entails a kind of cultural/political revolt against the status quo which is often too frightening for anyone to take on alone, in or out of therapy.

Here is a kind of therapeutic cul-de-sac which points to the inherent limits of what any therapy can accomplish, in and of itself.

Nevertheless, therapy *can* help women overcome depression—without drugs. The fundamental lesson to be learned from female depression is that *in anger there is power.* Just as the indirect anger of depression exerts indirect forms of power, so the direct anger of women can help us find more authentic forms of power.

The more severely depressed you are, the more you are likely to give people the message that you are incapable of taking any responsibility for yourself. There is an indirect plea for nurturance here which sometimes works to manipulate others into giving, but can also alienate them from you altogether. All too many people (including many therapists) will agree with you in your belief that you are not responsible for yourself and will paternalize you, thus reinforcing your profound sense of powerlessness. People respond this way, in part, because challenging your helplessness often tends to provoke the profound rage that is there just below the surface. People who are frightened of your anger (and who think of it as irrational) prefer to pacify you, rather than to set you off. It is as though you are a time bomb set to explode; no one wants to be the fuse. But without being set off, you will never be released from your depression. The therapist's job is to help you understand the explosions that result. For there is no way to regain your sense of power without engaging in this process of allowing your anger.

Letting yourself do this may appear to be impossible, not only because it is frightening, but also because, the more depressed you are, the more depleted you feel. That is, the more you feel empty of any inner resources at all, as though there is really nothing in you to come out. To counter this profound sense of inner poverty and powerlessness, the therapist's job is to gratify your needs for nurturance and validation while encouraging you to work responsibly with your anger on your own behalf.

In my own practice with depressed and suicidal women, I replace medications with large doses of respect and support. The more depressed a woman is, the more frequently I see her and the more I tend to give the nurturance and validation she needs. This is not a matter of dispensing chicken soup; rather it means getting to and validating the source of anger behind the depression. It means asking hard questions such as "What do you get out of being depressed?" I also tend to give even more "homework" to the depressed client so that she can feel her independent power to help herself without me. Writing about one's depression or anger, for instance, can be a useful tool for women who feel otherwise unable to express themselves. It is a more controlled medium than speech and doesn't entail the fear that one's anger will overwhelm oneself or others.

Certain active techniques borrowed from the growth therapies can also be valuable in helping women find, name, and express their anger. We have seen how the growth therapist uses these techniques in chapter eight. The difference between the humanist use of these techniques and my own lies in how I understand the process of releasing anger, and how I encourage my clients to understand it. I do not see letting go of anger as a matter of getting it out so that we can forget it. It is a matter of unleashing it from the repressed, indirect, and self-destructive forms that strangle us so that we can use it in more conscious, active, and collective ways. Curing women's depressions is thus neither a matter of finding the right chemical straightjacket nor of finding the right technique of catharsis. It is a matter of helping women *to understand the rage inside our depressions in terms of our oppression,* so that we can use it on our own behalf, even after we have expressed it in therapy. To see how this works, let us look at Susan's story.

Susan was an intelligent woman in her thirties who worked as a physician's assistant. She came to therapy after years of chronic depression, searching for the courage to divorce the man to whom she was still psychically wedded, though they had been separated for several years. She hoped that therapy would help her sort out the confusions she felt in her relationships with other men and that it would help her decide whether or not divorce was the answer to her problems.

Susan's story had all the elements of a modernized Cinderella myth gone awry. When Susan and her husband first met, they had both felt an instantaneous connection so strong that they referred to it as a "mystical" bond. It was as though they were simultaneously struck with Cupid's arrows and knew, at once, that they would never love anyone else the way they loved each other. Within six weeks, they were married.

At first, Susan saw Joe as a kind of Prince Charming. He was handsome, powerful, wise, and he wanted to take care of her. His eyes were filled with love. He told her that their union was fated by God. Susan had high hopes of living happily ever after. But her happiness lasted about two weeks into her marriage. Joe then began to show her another side of himself. Whereas he had once told her how beautiful she was, he now told her that she didn't know how to kiss, that she was fat and stupid. He became maniacally possessive, demanding complete allegiance to his wishes. For instance, she was permitted to read only the books that he recommended. (Because Susan admired his mind so much, she went along.) Her pursuit of even the most traditionally feminine interests, like sewing or potting plants, provoked his rage because it was a sign that she was not paying enough attention to him. She could not visit with her women friends, or even talk with them on the phone, without his consent. If Susan rebelled against these restrictions, Joe would become furious and accuse her of deserting him. He did not hit her—but the threat was always there.

Susan recognized that Joe was irrationally jealous and tried to talk to him about it. But there was no way to get through. In exasperation, because she loved him, she gave up trying to fight him. Slowly, she surrendered her interests and her friends. She hoped that in proving her love for her husband in this way, he would eventually give up his desire to rule her.

But this did not happen. Indeed, the more obedience Susan showed, the more tyrannical her husband became.

Whereas in the first few weeks of their relationship they had both enjoyed making love, Joe now refused to touch her, protesting that their relationship was spiritual in nature and should not be soiled with the cravings of the flesh. At first, Susan had tried to seduce him out of this idea, but this only enraged him all the more. He began to contrast her to a woman he had once known whom he described as "a goddess." This goddess was the epitome of purity and perfection. Susan was the "black witch." Joe blamed Susan's sexuality for the problems in their marriage. Her anger at this accusation only further convinced him of her evil.

Susan found herself a virtual prisoner of her husband, trapped in a dungeon of loneliness, despair, and self-hatred. She began to fear that she was going crazy. She hated her husband's tyrannical hold over her, but she felt, in her own words, "trapped in his spell." The more he told her she was ugly and evil the more mesmerized she became, until she came to believe that he was right. When she brought up the idea of separation or divorce, Joe would declare that Susan's "original sin" of not totally surrendering herself to him without any vestige of withholding or rebellion had destroyed their marriage. At the same time, he did not want to divorce.

For eight years, Susan lived with this man. Her docility and obedience were matched by a fiery rage which emerged in recurrent, irreconcilable fights with her husband. Finally, despite her overwhelming terror of being alone, she moved into her own apartment. She began to date other men. Once she convinced herself that it was all right for her to do so, she had no trouble finding men, for she was very beautiful. To her great surprise and delight, she discovered that there were men who, unlike Joe, appreciated her sexuality and in fact could not get enough of making love to her. At first, this was a great, satisfying revelation. But as the novelty wore off, Susan became more and more aware that the men who appreciated her body did not similarly appreciate her mind. With Joe, she had been able to have serious conversations and there was a feeling of intellectual connection, which was very important to her. In fact, this connection was a strong part of the cement that bonded her to him. But these new, more sexually "liberated" men seemed to have little or no interest in her intellectual capacities. In a different way than with her husband, she still felt profoundly disrespected as a person.

The familiar themes of feminine dependence on men, internalized rage, depression, and the fear of being alone all converge in this story. It might appear that Susan's story is so extreme that it cannot possibly apply to most women in the post–women's liberation era. But one of the core assumptions of my work with women is that the most extreme story of a woman is only the one that most clearly illuminates the commonplace. We may not all share the extent of Susan's dependence on her husband, but I firmly believe that if we look closely enough at ourselves, Susan's story only mirrors the familiar. Susan's depression, as we shall see, was ultimately connected to a terror of her own power as a woman: this is a fear that few of us, however "liberated" we may be trying to be, have totally overcome.

In fact, the most striking thing about Susan, as I got to know her in therapy, was how much her very presence seemed to contradict her story of painful and crippling dependence. In so many ways, Susan appeared to be a strikingly powerful woman: she was remarkably smart, physically vital, and quite willful. She knew how to stand up for herself in many ways. (One time while Susan was traveling in a rush-hour bus, a man ran off with her wallet. She ran after him and demanded to know why he had taken her wallet and how he would feel if someone did that to him. The man was so disconcerted, he returned her wallet. But she didn't let him get away until she let him know, in no uncertain terms, why she thought his petty theft was misguided.) Susan was by no means a "doormat"—she was a feisty woman with a great deal of strength. A good part of her problem was her fear of this strength. It was a fear that started with her fear of her own anger.

The bottom line of Susan's passivity in oppressive relationships with men was her inability to feel, express, or validate her anger. This became the bottom line of our work in therapy. For the most part, in the beginning, Susan did not experience her anger directly. With some work, she began to discover what she did with her anger at men: she would act conciliatory and withholding, taking her anger in and becoming more and more depressed. Or she would pile up the anger until it came out in an altercation in which she felt totally out of control. Gradually, Susan learned to recognize the cues that signaled this process of internalization. But even so, very often she could only talk about her anger without really feeling it. My goal was to help her name her anger *before* she turned it into depression or into an out-of-control fight.

To do this, I sometimes suggested that she have a gestalt conversation between her anger and the represser of her anger; or that she try to punch or kick a symbolic target like a pillow. These suggestions invariably met with great resistance. Susan thought it was silly and worthless to try to get her anger out. The first few times she tried to punch the pillow confirmed her in this belief; she found the experience frustrating and futile. Far from feeling empowered by her anger, she felt defeated by it.

When I asked her to visualize her anger, Susan saw it as "something that came from deep in the ground and would erupt like a volcano" if she let it. She was determined not to let it. The volcano that threatened to bury Susan was the accumulated rage of the Victim. The Victim in Susan experienced her anger as yet another—perhaps the final—indication of her impotence. She could not imagine that her anger could have any effect. This was not incompatible with her view of her anger as an immensely destructive force. She experienced her anger as a force so large that it was utterly incommensurate with her capacity to express it. Consequently, she ended up feeling that her anger was ultimately useless, overwhelming, and self-defeating.

Susan's way of thinking about and experiencing her anger is quite common among depressed women. All of the hurts of being a woman in patriarchal society, accumulating in the unconscious for years, build up to an extraordinarily powerful subterranean rage. To peek into this "Pandora's Box" by examining even the most specific and smallest of angers, often feels very dangerous. The depressed woman who first embarks on the search for her repressed anger inevitably starts out by feeling even more trapped in her consciousness. Anger seems to be the trap. But it is not. It is just that the accumulated sludge of the Victim's rage, which has clogged up the woman's consciousness for years, has to be cleaned out before anything else can happen. Validating and finally letting go of this crippling rage of the past is the necessary precursor to experiencing the genuine sense of freedom and power that comes from using our anger rather than having it use us.

With practice, Susan did learn to feel more empowered by getting her anger out in therapy. As she did so, she found that she was allowing herself to feel and express her anger more directly outside therapy. As she put it, "I find that I just have to feel a good righteous anger sometimes or nothing else works."

The more that Susan learned to accept and free her anger, the more she realized how much of it was there—not only at her husband, but at men in general. Paradoxically, this freeing process then led to a retrenchment of Susan's old patterns of self-hatred and depression. For a period of time, she came to therapy consistently complaining about how hopeless and awful she felt about everything—particularly her relationships with men. When we examined this more closely, it became apparent that Susan felt somehow compelled to denigrate herself precisely because she was beginning to feel more and more powerful! I have referred to this phenomenon before as the "backlash of the feminine."

In many cases, in heterosexual women, the fear of one's own power takes the form of the fear of "man-hating." Increasingly, this became Susan's fear. She was afraid that allowing and validating her anger at specific men in her life would alienate her completely from all men. It was difficult for her to admit that she was already alienated from all men: that her dread of man-hating was a dread of what was already the case. This came through clearly in an autobiographical "Story of My Anger" which she once wrote as "homework":

> When a man first looks at me, my first reaction is to see if he has nice eyes and a pleasant face. That lasts about one second. Then I hate him because I fear that he's like all the rest. Then I want to disarm him—castrate him—render him harmless. Turn them all into eunuchs. Safe for me. No more male arrogance. No more owning the world simply by gender birthright. I'm very jealous that men have the power in the world. They run it all. Own it all. Deal all deals. We (women) are powerless to change the world without major revolutions—war is more like it. How can I be with one of the enemy? Why would my foe want to be with me if he knew how I felt? There's no way out.

The magnitude of Susan's unconscious rage at her oppression comes through vividly in her image of castration and her violent wish to "disarm" men who use their weapons against her in the unequal battle of the sexes. The truth is that women's terror of man-hating belies the fact that most *women in patriarchal society unconsciously hate men*. This hatred is the normal, inevitable consequence of oppression, and it is only furthered in its unconscious forms by being denied. The task for any woman, but particularly for women who are depressed, is to get past the unconscious, indirect forms of this man-hating; to allow it to surface; and to let go of it. Only then is it possible to find more authentic ways to love men that do not entail our subordination, or to find authentic forms of anger that do not entail our self-destruction.

In short, there is no way out of man-hating but through it. For many women, this journey seems too treacherous to undertake, even with help. Hence Susan's strangled cry at the end of the story of her anger: "There's no way out." This is the trapped cry of the Victim. (The depressed woman's way out of her anger is her depression.) Susan's sense of being trapped lay in her deep-seated conviction that her anger at men would condemn her to a life of utter isolation and loneliness. Either it would so

blind her that she would not be able to recognize a "good man"
even if she stumbled over him; or more likely, none of these
potential good men would want any part of her if she was too
angry. An internal voice in her head repeated over and over
again: "If you are angry at men, you will always be alone."

Like Diane, but in a different way, Susan was scared to be
alone. Her image of her aloneness was being suspended in a
great, dark, endless space in which she floated forever, sur-
rounded only by the stars. In fact, Susan was, in many ways,
already alone: she lived alone, had her own work, made her
own living, and perpetuated an attenuated relationship with a
former husband whom she no longer relied on for anything.
Actually Susan quite enjoyed living alone and making her own
way in life without her husband. But this did not eradicate her
terrifying image of her aloneness. The fact that she was technically still married to her husband gave her the illusion that she
was *not* alone. Susan cherished this illusion because she felt
that it protected her. To give up her husband, or the illusion
that he protected her, was to be unloosed into the dark eternity
of her solitary independence.

One of the hardest parts of Susan's work in therapy was the
slow, painful, but ultimately freeing realization that her fear of
being alone disguised an even deeper wish to be alone. Her
fear of being rejected by men for being too angry was, in part,
a projection of her own angry rejection of men! Underneath the
internal voice that said "men won't love me if I'm angry" was a
deeper voice that said "men are not worth loving." Susan's
unconscious wish to be alone was, in part, a function of this
unconscious man-hating side of her that found men arrogant
and worthless.

On the other hand, Susan's wish to be alone also reflected
her most profound longing: to be independent of men, to feel
whole and free without them, to live in the vastness of space
without the illusion that men buoyed her up. Thus beneath
Susan's oft-pronounced fear of loneliness lurked an even
deeper terror of her own power: the fear that she would actually
relish being alone, that she did not essentially need men, that

she could live without them quite well. In short, what Susan feared most was her own freedom.

In the course of a year's work together, as Susan came increasingly face to face with her own anger, she learned more and more about this fear of her own freedom—as well as her deep yearning for it. Despite her fears that she would alienate everyone, she began to trust her anger, to develop deeper relationships with women, to demand both less and more from men (less of being "saved" by them, more of being respected by them). She began, with great trepidation and courage, to come out as a feminist.

At the time of this writing, Susan has not yet decided whether or not to divorce her husband. But she no longer allows him to run her life. She has become more and more dedicated to her own independence. She has come to appreciate herself for the strengths that she hid for so long: her ability to take care of herself, her intelligence, her power to control her own emotions and to love others without putting herself at their mercy. She is no longer depressed.

The emergence of an authentic, woman-identified identity for any woman, but particularly for the woman who is chronically depressed, is contingent upon the surfacing of what she has always been obliged to keep underground: her anger. We have seen how the repression of anger is essential to the maintenance of the Victim psychology of women demanded in patriarchal society, and how this anger is converted into unconscious, passive/aggressive symptoms. It is not surprising that many, if not most, women never allow themselves to experience anger, or never find a comfortable way to express it. It is "unfeminine" to be angry: we are often seen, and see ourselves, as cold bitch, man-hating dyke, ugly witch, crazy broad, or hysterical female. I have frequently heard women say in therapy that they feel "ugly" when they are angry. I have never observed this feeling in men, no matter how difficult it may be for some men to express their anger. Some psychologists would say that this feeling of ugliness is a "displacement" phenomenon—that is, the woman feels that her anger is ugly (depraved, monstrous, irrational, etc.) and she then displaces her fear of her anger into a concern with how she looks. Though this explanation may be partially true, it ignores the very real and serious threat to traditional femininity that anger poses to women who are trained to be charming and beautiful.*

The facial changes produced in the expression of anger indeed alter a woman's visage. In the distorted carnival glass of woman's self-image, she is nowhere uglier than when she is angry. Given the feminine conditioning to be beautiful or be damned, this internalized distortion often works quite effectively to keep the woman's anger down.

Getting angry is a beginning: a way out of the depressions that keep us immobilized. Male society reinforces the idea that we have no right to it: that we look silly or frightened or cute or ugly; that we are acting like bitches, dykes, or witches. We must take these terms and turn them into epithets of self-love and love of other women so that we can begin to see, not how cute, but how beautiful we are when we are angry. To the extent that we are frightened of our own anger, we choose, whether consciously or not, to be Victims.

On the other hand, though our anger may be healthy, clean, and just, it is also, in our society, still dangerous to be an angry woman alone. For woman as an individual, the problem of anger is twofold: anger is necessary, but anger is not enough. The process of liberation is not simply a matter of feeling anger. It is a matter of making connections between the anger we feel and the material conditions of our lives. Of knowing how and where to channel that anger so that we serve our own interests as women and avoid getting burnt out, fired, violently out of control, psychiatrically hospitalized, beaten up, raped, or any of the other consequences that sometimes lie in wait for women who experience and act on their anger without support. Wom-

---

* Think of the all-too-common incidence of women on the street who are admonished by male strangers to smile. A woman's smile is one of the many nonverbal indicators of her submissiveness, a way of assuring these strangers that the woman is not angry.

en's problem with anger is not simply a problem of denial that we feel angry. It is also a problem of knowing how to name our anger properly, understand its origins in our lives, and act on it effectively.

There are some therapists (including some feminists) who would tell us that our anger is sufficient unto itself; that in getting angry we are empowering ourselves. But this is at best a half-truth and at worst a dangerous falsification. We need to know more than how to feel angry. We need to know how to mobilize and organize our anger collectively; to use it to fight for control over our bodies and reproductive lives, our family and sex lives, our paid-work lives, our psychic/emotional lives. For it is the institutionalized lack of control over these conditions that feeds our anger, no matter how personal it may appear. Without beginning to experience our anger as justified rage at certain specific conditions of subordination, we will never undertake the project of changing those conditions; and without undertaking that project, the anger of women as a group (no matter how in touch we are with it) will never be assuaged.

Anger, like love, takes many forms. There are the hidden and self-destructive forms of powerlessness with which we are so familiar: depressions, wrist slashings, overdoses, and other suicidal gestures. There is also a kind of stubborn bitterness and helplessness which poisons our minds and bodies and deadens us to living; or there is unconsciously held resentment at men without an awareness of its meaning. All of these forms of anger keep us immobile: either locked up in the prisons of our selves or antagonistically pitted against one another.

But there is another form of anger, the other side of which is love. Not only a growing love for ourselves and each other as women, but also a growing realization that we are all of us—men and women alike—mutually interdependent. This is not a rigid closing off of our energies but an opening up to a respectful compassion for ourselves as women, and a loving struggle with the men in our lives. Anger is the fuel we need to burn in the struggle to create a society without Victims.

11

The Feminist Model:
Polly Patient Becomes a Person

Polly is nervous as she comes to therapy today. She knows that she will be talking about her boss's sexual harassment. The very word makes her anxious. She has preferred to say her boss's "flirtations," but her therapist thinks Polly's use of this term is her way of pretending that her boss's actions are more harmless than they actually are. She has learned in therapy that sexual harassment is an abuse of her boss's power over her: he is trying to coerce her sexually by implying that she will be rewarded on the job for sexual compliance and punished, perhaps even fired, for sexual "disobedience." After last night's dinner fiasco, Polly is certain that "sexual harassment" accurately describes her situation. Yet somehow she still feels that the term sounds harsh. Her boss seems like a nice man—if he's been playing sexual games with her, perhaps she has been setting herself up for them. Maybe she should give him the benefit of the doubt and quit worrying about all of this. But how?

I wonder if I'll ever get rid of these headaches, she thinks as she rings the doorbell. Suddenly, she remembers that in the last therapy session, her therapist gave her the telephone number of a local organization of women against sexual harassment. She should have called this week—but it completely slipped her mind! *Just like me to blow it,* she thinks, biting her lip.

As I hear the doorbell ring and press the buzzer to let Polly in, I think about where we are in the therapy. My job recently has been to help Polly understand her compliance in her boss's sexual harassment without concluding that her boss's behavior is her fault. This has been tricky work. It has involved more than helping Polly get in touch with her feelings toward her boss. It has meant helping her understand the *meaning* of her feelings: that they are not simply irrational or neurotic, even if they *do* tap into older feelings she has about other people in her life—particularly her father. It has also been my job to help Polly realize the range of real choices in her situation so that she can decide how to act.

Traveling the road to this end has meant meeting the dangerous snares along the way, placed there by Polly herself. One is Polly's inordinate sense of Victim shame, thick as molasses and running through all the sessions. Another is what I have named her chronic Patient Routine, which has been polished up in response to her boss's sexual harassment. Through the many practiced and artful devices of this Patient Routine, Polly has tried to convince herself (and me) that (1) her boss's sexual harassment is only a personal problem she, as a woman, is having with a man and not *also* a political problem she, as a female employee, is having with her boss; and (2) that all of her feelings and behaviors in reponse to this problem are evidence that she is "fucked up."

Polly's Patient Routine is hard to get around. If I ask her why she is always protecting her boss from her anger, even when (as in therapy) it can't possibly hurt him, she tells me that she lacks "assertiveness." If, on the other hand, she sometimes acknowledges that she is furious with him, she then says that this is because of her "problem with anger." If I assure Polly that her anger and fear are natural and to some extent justified, under the circumstances, she looks at me with a raised eyebrow, wondering if I am doing my job properly. She doubts my support as much as she craves it.

At no time in our therapy work together is it clearer that my task is to help educate Polly to the real dimensions of her power as a woman in an oppressive situation. She needs to see that, as an individual, she is neither all-powerful in relation to her boss, nor completely powerless; that though she is being victimized by him, she is more than the Victim. And she needs to understand that, by acting alone on her anger, she might risk further sexual harassment or firing. She can use the help of other women in order to act most powerfully: both women who share her predicament in the workplace, and women who work for organizations that are dedicated specifically to helping women confront sexual harassment without endangering their jobs.

To work with Polly in therapy lately has been to work against the grain of her mammoth resistance to seeing her problem in sexual-political terms. The Victim in Polly hangs on like an ancient reptilian beast at the dawn of a new era. But a newer consciousness is there too, one that I can help her cultivate.

Polly enters and takes a seat without looking at me, so I know something is brewing today—something she's probably feeling scared or guilty about. As I sit down, I try to catch her eye.

"How are you doing, Polly?"

Polly makes a face—one of her more expressive ones—mimicking a combination of exasperation, desperation, and disgust. The face of someone throwing up her hands and giving up. The face of the Victim. She groans.

"That bad, huh? What's happening?"

Polly sobers up at the question, dropping the self-mockery and expelling a long sigh.

"I guess I'm depressed again . . . I'm not sure where to start. I have one of my headaches. I don't know . . . I'm confused."

I gaze at her, sensing her hesitation. She needs encouragement not to run away from herself.

"You know I never let you get away with saying you're confused," I say with a smile. "What are the feelings behind the confusion?"

Polly grins. "I should know your favorite questions by now." There is a pause while she turns her attention inward.

"I'm feeling . . . scared and guilty and angry," she says, and then rushes headlong into her story. "I had a rough time with my boss last night. He kept me late again and then asked me out to dinner. I'm not sure why . . . but I accepted the invitation. It was late and I felt sorry for him because he'd been telling me all about his problems with his wife, you know? Anyway, I think I really set myself up for what happened. . . ." Polly averts her eyes and looks embarrassed.

"So what happened, Polly? You look embarrassed."

"How'd you guess? I *am* embarrassed . . . for being such a jerk!" She giggles nervously and looks a little relieved, then continues. "Well, to make a long story short, during dinner he kept telling me how special I was and subtly promising me things if I put out. It got so late that he ended up driving me home and when we parked in front of my house he tried to . . . he kissed me and I tried to stop him but he just ignored me when I said no. He just kept it up until I had to really yell at him. Then he became furious. He practically shoved me out of the car!" At this point in her story Polly is starting to sound agitated. She is madly fidgeting with her hands and her eyes are glued to a spot on the floor.

"Well, he's been mad at me all day," she continues. "After I made a silly mistake in a letter, he called me lazy and inefficient and threatened to fire me if I didn't shape up. I know it's not really the mistake—he's just angry that I didn't screw him last night. And now I'm terrified that I'll lose my job! I think I set myself up to be sexually harassed by going out with him at all."

When Polly raises her eyes, they are filled with a dumb appeal for a mercy that she doesn't expect. As I look at her and think of her boss, my anger rises in me like steam.

"It sounds to me like he tried to coerce you sexually and you refused him. Yet you seem to blame yourself for what happened. Why is that?"

"I went out to dinner with him, didn't I? I should have *known* that he would try something! And then I even let him drive me home! Granted, it was late and I'm scared of riding the train myself at night. But still . . . I can't believe how stupid I was." Polly is beginning to look like she wants to cry. But she is holding back. Her eyes glass over. She has the look of a defeated woman.

"Polly, your going out to dinner with him doesn't mean he has the right to fuck you on demand, or to threaten to fire you if you don't."

"I know that." *(I can't stand it when she gets so down on him. Sometimes I think she hates men.)* "But why did I do it? When, somewhere, unconsciously, I must have known that I was in for trouble if I did? I think I'm somewhat attracted to him. Not only did I go out with him, I let him pay for dinner. I sort of liked *getting* something from him, you know? I think I really acted-out in a self-destructive way."

This last line is delivered with a slight suggestion of satisfaction, the way a bright student might answer a difficult exam question. At the same time, there is a rehearsed quality, as though the answer has been learned by rote.

"Why did you do it, Polly?"

"I . . . I'm not sure. He asked me to and I felt sorry for him. He really *is* upset about his wife running around on him. He looked depressed and I always soften up when he tells me about his pain. Part of me wanted to take care of him, like I always do. So when he asked me out for dinner, I thought, 'Why not? Secretaries sometimes go out to dinner with their bosses. No harm in that.' I had no intention of anything more than that. But still, unconsciously, I think I must have been leading him on in some way. You know what I mean?"

Polly seems to want some confirmation from me about the neurotic intentions of her unconscious. I can feel the powerful tug of her Patient Routine—the self-hate and shame masquerading as deep psychological insight. She *is* on to something, of course: her attraction to her boss increases her vulnerability to his continued victimization of her and she does comply with him. But she is also way off, like someone so intent on watching the inner landscape that she neglects to see that there is a man in front of her with a weapon pointed at her. The combination of Polly's acute vision and her terrible nearsightedness is often frustrating. Her awareness of her attraction to her boss and the way in which she feeds into his sexual power games is definitely something for me to go after. But to do so now, in this way, is simply to supply her Victim with more nourishment to fatten on. Her insight-mongering is her way of avoiding how angry she is at her boss and blaming the victim instead. I decide that it would be better now to stick close to Polly's feelings.

"Okay. Your boss came on to you about how unhappy he is and turned to you for emotional comfort and, later, for sex. And it sounds like part of you felt compassion for him and felt that it was your duty to oblige him, while the other part of you felt that you ought to be ashamed of yourself for wanting to."

Polly nods her head with relief. "Right! It's been like that the whole time: wanting to play along with him and also wanting to tell him to fuck off. I think going out with him was part of my self-destructive pattern with men—of being drawn to men who aren't good for me, or who are already involved, or somehow getting off on dead-end relationships. I know that what he did last night was harassment, but I think that the problem is that, when he tried to have sex with me, part of me really *wanted* him to, even though I knew it would be a mistake. I'm *attracted* to him, actually, so of course he's going to pick that up and go after me. I've got to stop feeling the way I do about him."

I look at Polly and feel a mixture of empathy and impatience. Part of me wants to take her by the shoulders and shake her, shouting, "It's not all your fault, goddamn it! Stop taking all of this in on yourself! You don't control the universe with your emotions!" My impulse is to argue with her; to remind her that her boss has been harassing her for weeks, though she hasn't gone out with him in all that time; to persuade her that the finer motivations of her unconscious do not really determine his behavior. But I know that this will not work. I sense that my desire to get past the deep murky waters of Polly's self-victimization to some more solid ground stems from the part of me that identifies with her. Her educated compulsion to blame herself, her insightful self-condemnation, is too disquietingly like my own tendencies in that direction. My impatience with her is probably related to my impatience with myself! I decide to take another tack—to go *with* Polly's line of thinking, rather than against it.

"I guess you have a pretty sick unconscious, don't you, Polly! You can't really blame your boss for trying to get you into bed and threatening to fire you. After all, you asked for it, didn't you?" I deliver these lines deadpan.

Polly looks at me blankly, stunned into silence. She is not sure whether I am kidding or not. I continue.

"Is that what you want me to say, Polly? That you ought to be ashamed of yourself? That because of your terrible attraction to him and because of your sick, acting-out behavior, you have single-handedly provoked your boss into harassing you? That you deserve anything you get, including getting fired, because basically you're to blame?"

Polly's eyes redden with the shame she has been feeling all along. She looks pained by what I've said.

"I *do* feel that it's all my fault! And I *am* ashamed of myself. And it's hard for me to talk about this to you because I feel like you're ashamed of me, too." Polly's eyes are watery and her voice quavers. She is still trying her best not to cry.

"I'm not ashamed of you, Polly. But what are *you* feeling toward me right now?" (*If I can only get a little closer to her, maybe we can get past her shame.*)

"Scared of what you must think of me. And a little . . . angry, I guess, because I think you're mad at me."

"Why should I be mad at you?"

"Because I really fucked up with my boss. And because I'm not doing a very good job of dealing with my feelings in here either." Polly turns away from me, feeling sorry for herself.

"Polly," I say gently, "do you want to check out with me what I *really* feel toward you, instead of what you *imagine* I feel?"

"Yes. I guess so." Polly hesitates here. She is usually frightened to find out about my thoughts and feelings, preferring her own imagination.

"Well, why don't you ask me then?"

"Okay. What do you feel about my going out with my boss last night? Do you think I was an asshole?" Polly smiles weakly. For the moment, she looks very young—no more than ten years old. I smile back and think about what I want to say to her, how to tell her that I'm on her side.

"Since you came in here today, you've looked scared and guilty, Polly. I've been trying to find a way to reach out to you. But your Patient Routine seems to keep me at a distance from you. It's hard for me to break through it. Mostly, I feel sorry that your boss got to you, that he found a way to manipulate your softer feelings of compassion for him—and sorry that you've been blaming yourself so thoroughly for that. I'm not mad at you—I'm mad at him! But you may have been picking up some impatience I feel when you blame yourself so much. That may be because, in some ways, I empathize with your way of doing so. I do it to myself often enough. Self-blame seems to come easy to women. I'd like to help you get past it."

Polly looks at me shyly, as she always does when I reveal something of myself to her. The shadow of anxiety that has been in her face from the start of the session is gone. Her face is softer and, for the first time since the session began, she looks as though she is here in the room with me.

"I guess it *is* easy for me to blame myself for everything." The harshness in her voice is gone and she is speaking more slowly. "I can't help feeling that I should know how to handle this whole thing better. That if I were more together, none of this would be happening to me."

"It's not true, Polly," I say gently. "Thousands of women are sexually harassed by their employers every day, whether or not they are attracted to their bosses or go out to dinner with them. Most of them put up with it because they don't know what else to do. They know their jobs are on the line and they're scared. Let's say you *did* set yourself up for some trou-

ble with your boss last night, Polly. It seems that there are ways
you do feed into what he's doing and we need to understand
why. You seem, for instance, to feel compelled to respond to
him when he says he needs you—as though you have no choice
in the matter. It's the old 'compassion trap' that women fall into,
isn't it? Feeling obligated to take care of his needs and losing
sight of what you need to take care of yourself. Certainly we
need to understand your attraction to your boss too. What draws
you to him when you feel you'd be better off, for instance, not
going to dinner with him? But none of these feelings means
that his actions are your responsibility or your fault, Polly. Until
you can see your feelings with a little more compassion for
yourself, all your insight becomes just another excuse for you
to hate yourself—and that's just a dead end, isn't it?"

Polly's eyes are brimming over with tears now. She has
been able to hear my support.

"You know I really don't know *what* to do—besides blame
myself! And that certainly doesn't seem to work too well," she
says through her tears. "I've tried pretending to be sick so I
don't have to work overtime. I've tried being nice to him and
being cold to him and even getting angry with him. And now
I've tried going out with him—and none of it's worked. Nothing seems to help. It all feels so hopeless sometimes!" Polly
cries openly now. Weeks of anxiety, self-loathing, and fear find
their release in her wracking sobs. But then she stops abruptly,
looking up at me with the vulnerable eyes of a child.

"What are you feeling, Polly?"

"Relieved that you're not mad at me, and glad that you told
me about how you blame yourself too. It makes me feel less
crazy, though it's also kind of scary to know that you're not
perfect! I feel better now than when I came in. But I still feel
kind of hopeless about how to deal with him."

"Last week, I suggested you might try asking around at the
office to see if there are other women who are being harassed
so that you could get some emotional and practical support.
And I also gave you the phone number of Women Against Sexual Coercion. Did you try to contact them?"

"I . . . I wanted to," Polly says, averting her eyes, "but every time I went to call, I found something else to do."

"How come, Polly? What got in the way?"

"All my guilt, I guess. It's the same with asking around the office to see if he's been bothering other women. I know I should do it, but I feel like they'd just look at me and say, 'Oh, so you've been leading him on, have you? Well, that's your problem, not ours!' I get to feeling so hopeless that I just feel paralyzed."

"So all the shame and hopelessness gets in the way of your standing up for yourself—and then you only feel more hopeless and helpless than ever! Sounds like the old Victim in you getting the upper hand, doesn't it?"

Polly smiles. "Yes—she has a way of screwing me up every time!"

"Well, what are you going to do about her?"

"I don't know! I can't stand her! It seems like she's always running my life and I hate her!" Polly is back to playing with her hands, clenching and unclenching her fists.

There is a silence. Polly has the look she often gets when she is "stuck." Watching her hands I think that if she could mobilize even half the energy I see in her nervous fidgeting, she would be able to get past her paralysis.

"Polly, why don't you try being your hands for a moment. If they had a voice, what would they be saying right now?"

Immediately Polly stops playing with her hands. She groans: "No way you're going to get me to do this role-playing crap—I don't want to be my hands!"

"Okay. But why not? What are you feeling?"

"Angry. I'm feeling angry."

"Angry at who?"

"Oh, I don't know—angry at myself, mostly."

"Who else? Who else are you angry at?"

"You want me to say my boss, don't you?" Polly breaks into a grin again. "But I don't *feel* angry at him!"

"Who *do* you feel angry at?"

"Well, I feel a little angry at you, just because I hate that role-playing stuff and you're always going after my anger like a shark after blood. Even when I don't *feel* it!"

"You want to yell at me?"

"No!" Polly yells. "I'm not *that* angry!" And then, more quietly, "It's mostly gone, now that I've told you about it."

"At the start of the session, you said that you were feeling angry at your boss. Where is that anger now?" I know Polly would like me to let up, but I resist the temptation to do so. Letting up on her anger now would only mean returning to her hopelessness.

"I know there *is* some anger at him somewhere, because I've had a splitting headache since yesterday and that's always a clue. But like I say, I don't really *feel* it. I guess I end up taking it in, getting depressed and feeling ashamed instead."

"What do you need to get past the anger at *you* to the anger at *him*, Polly?"

"I don't know. Getting angry at him scares me."

"How come?"

"Because I'm scared I'll lose my job if I get angry at him."

"Well, if you let him know about it directly, you just might! That's why I suggested you call WASC—they'd be able to help you strategize about how best to put your anger to work for you. But for right now, it's not a matter of showing *him* your anger. We're one step before that: it's a matter of showing yourself that you're angry. Perhaps if you let yourself feel your anger you wouldn't end up feeling so depressed and hopeless. And your boss is not here in the room." I lower my voice and whisper, "He'll never know."

Polly laughs. "Okay, okay. You win. I'll try getting some anger out at him!" She turns her head in the direction of the tennis racket, standing in the corner of the room.

Polly has been schooled in the use of the tennis racket on a floor pillow: how to hold the racket behind her as she kneels and then, using both hands, to come down hard on the pillow, over and over again. To shout all the angry words and thoughts in her head, or just to let herself grunt or cry or yell. It is a technique I use to help women feel and validate their anger—

to hear the loud, resounding *thwack!* of the tennis racket as it hits the pillow and know that we are capable of making noise and taking up space in the world. It is not a matter of releasing the anger and being done with it. But once the anger is out we can work with it.

It is not Polly's favorite therapy game. She clutches at the tennis racket like a child and her eyes dart around the room, as though looking for a means of escape.

"Give it a try, Polly. And remember that you can always stop whenever you want to."

Polly seats herself with her legs beneath her and arranges the pillow in front of her.

"Okay." She laughs nervously. "But I don't know what to say."

"Just tell your boss what you'd like to say but wouldn't dare."

There is a long silence before Polly starts, while she is getting up her courage. Then she starts to pound, wincing a little with every thumping sound she makes. At first, there are no words, but with some urging from me, her voice emerges with a strangled cry.

"You creep! Get lost! I hate you! I'm sick and tired of all this crap! It gives me headaches. I wish you'd just leave me alone! Leave me alone!" Then, abruptly, she stops, looking up at me accusingly, as though to say "See! I told you this wouldn't work!"

"What are you feeling, Polly? You sound like a child yelling at a parent, knowing it will get you nothing but trouble."

"I feel silly and embarrassed. I keep thinking, what's the point? It's not the pillow I should be hitting, it's my boss. I just feel frustrated."

"It's hard to let yourself get angry. I know. It's not something we're supposed to do as women. So it's bound to feel really alien and uncomfortable when you start. Do you want to continue?"

"I'll try." (*I hate this. But I know I always feel better after I do it.*)

"Okay. Maybe it will help if I provoke you a little. I'll play your self-blaming Victim voice—the one that tries to stop you from being angry. And you just try to stick with your anger and don't give up on it, okay?"

Polly nods and we proceed. This time, I bait her with the words I've heard her use against herself: "It's all your fault! You never should have gone out with him in the first place! You can't blame him—you set yourself up for this! You deserve what you get! You deserve to get fired!" And so forth.

In the face of these onslaughts, Polly musters up her anger and pounds away at the pillow. Occasionally, something I am saying stops her in her tracks, and she starts to listen to and believe the voice that tells her that she has no right to be angry. At these points, I interrupt myself-as-Polly and gently urge her to pay no attention to this Victim voice, to stay with her anger. This continues for a few minutes, until Polly drops the tennis racket, exhausted from the effort. Her eyes glaze over and she stares out the window. I know it is not at the outside that she is looking, but at the inside. I have seen this process again and again: this drifting off into another time and place. I wait and watch Polly's eyes which are staring at the pictures unwinding in her head.

"How old do you feel right now, Polly?"

"Oh, I don't know . . . maybe ten or eleven." Another silence.

"Where are you?"

"I'm with my father." Polly speaks without the usual self-consciousness, almost dreamily. "Getting angry at my boss feels so useless, just like it did with my father. I mean, the one time I got *directly* angry with my boss—I told you about it, remember?—it didn't make the slightest difference! He'd been bothering me and I told him that I thought we should have a more professional relationship or something like that. I couldn't even look at him when I said it. Anyway, he just smiled and told me that I was sweet! My anger meant nothing to him! And that's the same way it always was with my dad. Actually, I very rarely got angry at him because it just never did any good. He was always so cool and unruffled. Nothing seemed to have an impact on him. He was that way toward my mother too. Sometimes she'd get angry at him and she'd cry. And he'd always say something like, 'Okay, Flora, there's nothing to get hysterical about.'" Polly mimics the assured voice of masculine authority. "He'd just treat her like a silly child, you know? He was always the high-school principal, even at home. If you got angry at him, he would somehow make you feel like a student who'd disobeyed some rule of his at school. It wasn't that he was harsh or anything. He never yelled. He didn't have to. Just one of his looks and you would back off, feeling like you were wrong for being mad at him for anything."

"When you were ten or eleven, what made you feel angry at him then?"

"I think it was always his distance that made me mad. The feeling that I could never get through to him. But being the youngest child and the only girl in the family with two older brothers, I had a sort of special relationship with him, you know? I was the one who could get around him. He was sterner with my brothers, but he'd soften up with me. He used to put me on his lap and kiss me and call me "pretty Polly" and I would just feel great—you know, loved. But then, when I was ten or eleven, things changed. My brothers were in high school and one of them was into drugs and my father was always angry at them. He'd fly into rages at the drop of a hat, which he'd never done before. And we'd all be scared of him, of what he might do. When you asked me how old I felt before, I guess I was thinking of that time. I was so angry with him because he was always preoccupied with my brothers and he and my mother would fight all the time about how to handle them. I guess I just sort of felt abandoned. He hardly looked at me anymore. So about that time, I started having temper tantrums, to try and get his attention."

"What do you mean by 'temper tantrums'?"

"I would just scream and cry and sometimes I would throw something. But he would be as unaffected as always. He'd say something like, 'If you're going to act like a baby, then you'll have to get treated like one.' Which meant I would have to go to bed early. But I remember feeling awful, just screaming and crying and knowing that it wouldn't make the slightest difference. Except for this one time, I started taunting and cursing him and I told him that he was a bad father and stuff like that. And that time, he hit me hard—which he'd never done before. And when he did that, even though I was crying and scared, I also . . . well, there was this part of me that almost *liked* his hitting me because at least that was a sign that I'd really gotten to him, you know? I remember that he was all red in the face and furious. And that's the way I felt today when my boss got angry at me about the mistakes I made in the letter. I was scared—but part of me was glad too. Because my boss is always so in control—just like my dad. And today he wasn't. Today I got to him."

Polly stops here, surprised at having so much to say, and then continues.

"You know, most of what I feel so guilty about with my boss is that feeling of somehow *liking* his sexual attention, even though it makes me angry. When he comes on to me, even though I know it's all bullshit, I still want to hear it. I'm almost . . . hungry for it. And when he tried to . . . have sex with me last night, partly, it made me feel good. Getting that kind of, you know, physical attention from him made me feel *special*— the way I felt with my father."

"There's something satisfying about being 'pretty Polly' with him, like being Daddy's girl?"

"Exactly! A lot of the attraction to him is that he's the tall, dark, and distant type, like my father. His strength and control turn me on in some way, because I always feel so weak and out of control myself. I admire in him what also drives me crazy. And then I feel guilty for being attracted to him."

"Why?"

"Because he's such a prick!" Polly blushes momentarily. "He's been toying with me for weeks. Sometimes I'd like to strangle him, I hate him so much. How can I be attracted to someone who's driving me crazy?"

"Well, from everything you've said, it makes sense that you would be. Getting physical attention is one of the ways you felt cared for with your father. Being 'Pretty Polly' was the source of your specialness and power with him. So when your boss appeals to the 'Pretty Polly' side of you, that's going to attract you to him, naturally. Plus, you say that his kind of male self-assurance turns you on. Of course! Isn't that what masculinity is all about? We're all taught as women that powerful men are attractive—that *power* in men is attractive. Well, perhaps you need to find a way to keep that attraction from influencing your behavior with him. But why feel guilty about feeling what a woman is *supposed* to feel toward a man like your boss?"

Polly has the startled look she gets when something obvious hits her for the first time. "Yes," she says, "but I guess I feel I should be above these feelings."

"Oh, right! I forgot—you're supposed to be perfect!"

"Right!" Polly laughs. There is a pause, and then she continues. "I guess when my boss comes on to me sexually, I get confused. Some part of me wants him to do what's making me angry. So I end up thinking that it's all my fault—for wanting it. If I didn't want it, then it wouldn't happen. I can see that's not really true. But my attraction to him makes me feel I have no right to be angry."

I nod at Polly and we both sit in silence while she absorbs what she has just said. Then I decide to push a little further.

"Not only do you feel you don't have a right to your anger, but from what you've told me, your experience of getting angry at your father only made you feel more powerless. As a result, when you get angry now, you seem to feel 'Why bother?' At the same time, at least when you were eleven years old and having what you called temper tantrums, you seemed to use your own anger as a way of provoking your father—a way of connecting to him through all that distance."

"Yes. And that's just how it is with my boss. Most of the time I feel getting angry is just . . . silly, a ridiculous waste of time—like pounding a pillow in here. It doesn't do any good, so why bother? But also, sometimes I *do* want to provoke my boss to get angry with me, that's true. Like making that dumb mistake in the letter—which I knew would irritate him. Or by sexually teasing him and then not coming through—like I did last night." Polly is heating up now, her face animated with the excitement of seeing her feelings fall into place in a new way: making sense of them without blaming herself!

"What do you know about the part of you that wants to tease him sexually?" I think we can get into these issues now without Polly using her insights against herself.

"Well, I sort of knew at the restaurant that he would probably try to seduce me later on and I made a decision to let him drive me home. I think part of me almost looked forward to his finally, actually *openly* trying to have sex with me, after all those weeks of subtle seduction scenes. Part of that is the attraction to him. But I was also enjoying being attractive to him —having him salivating over me." Polly giggles with nervous embarrassment.

"There's something in particular isn't there, about being able to *refuse* him sexually, knowing how much he wants it?"

Polly looks relieved that I can see this part of her without hating her for it, as she does.

"Yes. I did get some pleasure out of seeing him all angry about not being able to sleep with me."

"What was that about?"

"Being able to make him squirm, after all these weeks of him making me squirm. For once, I felt in control in a way. It was *he* who needed me, instead of the other way around. I could say yes or no. I could give or withhold something he wanted. I guess after feeling so much like he could take my job away from me, it felt good. It was like getting even. Revenge is sweet!" Polly giggles again.

"So it sounds like a lot of that anger at him that you haven't shown him directly has come out in this way: using your sexual power, so to speak, to encourage him to think that he might be able to 'win' you, and then denying him. And in that way, feeling like you have him at your mercy. It's a way to reverse your feeling that you're at his mercy. Let's call it 'Pretty Polly's Revenge.' "

Polly smiles and her eyes twinkle. "Yes. That's what I meant at the start of the session when I said that I feel like I was teasing him, setting him up to harass me. It doesn't seem like a very good way to act with him, does it?"

"No, it doesn't. But what you've just put together is important. There's built-up anger in the teasing, anger that you haven't felt you could express directly. And you *do* have a right to be angry with him, Polly, though I agree there are better ways of dealing with it than 'Pretty Polly's Revenge.' The problem is that any other channel for your anger has felt dangerous to you. You've been scared that it would jeopardize your job. And you've also felt at times that you *had* to take part in all these sexual games with him because a flat-out refusal to do so might also lose you your job. Plus, it makes sense that you would tend to rely on the strategy of 'Pretty Polly's Revenge' at moments like this. As women, we've all been taught to think of ourselves as primarily pretty objects, so naturally, we're going to develop the powers that go along with that. And we're all taught not to get angry at men. My hunch is that 'Pretty Polly's Revenge' has felt like the only option available to you. But it isn't. There are other ways to get angry."

Polly is gazing at me intently, as though she's been listening with every fiber of her being.

"Where are you, Polly?"

Polly takes a deep breath and expels it. Pent-up feelings sometimes make her forget to breathe.

"I'm just thinking about what you're saying. And feeling angry! I was angry last night, too, when he lunged at me in the car and wouldn't stop until I yelled at him. Part of me really wanted to kill him. For all his talk about how special I was as a woman and all that baloney, it was like all he wanted was to fuck me, that he didn't really care what I wanted at all."

Polly's anger is apparent now. Her voice is raised, her face is flushed, and she is talking very quickly.

I glance at the clock. It is the end of the hour, time to wind down. But how can we stop here? Instinctively, I decide to go ahead for another five or ten minutes. Every session has a shape and that shape can't be neatly tucked into sixty minutes. With those clients that I know can stay, I sometimes end up stretching the hour. At this point in the session, it is clear to me that the next few minutes could save a few weeks of work. Before Polly has a chance to retrench during the week, it is best to seize the time.

"What do you want to do with your anger, Polly?"

The gleam in Polly's eyes wanes a bit when she hears this question and she stammers her reply: "I guess . . . well, I'm not sure. Don't you think a lot of my anger at my boss is really anger at my father?"

I look at Polly and can't suppress a laugh. The return of the Patient Routine! How many shrinks wouldn't give their leather-bound copies of the *Complete Works of Sigmund Freud* for a patient like Polly?

"Spare me your Patient Routine, will you, Polly? When you were pounding away at the pillow before, you stopped yourself, saying it was really your boss you were angry at—so why pound a pillow? Now that you've let yourself feel your anger at your boss, you've decided it's really your father you're angry at—so why deal with your anger at your boss? Seems like anger is something you always put somewhere else, isn't it?"

We are both grinning. There is mischief in Polly's eyes. She looks like a kid who's been caught at some secret game, embarrassed but relieved at having been found out. We laugh together at the shared secret.

"So what are you going to do with your anger, Polly?"

Polly growls in response. "Goddamn it, you never let up!"

Then swiftly, with no further bidding from me, Polly grabs the tennis racket and begins pounding away again. Like a coach with an athlete in training, I urge her along with goading and encouraging words. The sound of the tennis racket against the pillow gets louder and louder as Polly builds up the force and speed. Her words are belted out, no longer from a constricted throat but from some point further down in her guts. Her voice is not only louder, it *sounds* different than before: deeper, weightier. Her face is reddened and distorted with effort and rage. The whimpering, frustrated child has given way to the angry adult woman.

Then, abruptly, it is over. Polly drops the tennis racket and rests. She is breathless. Her cheeks are red, her eyes clear. When she speaks again, it is with amazement.

"I didn't think I had that in me!"

"Are you surprised?"

"Well, yes. I guess I've never let myself feel this angry before. The other times I tried to hit the pillow, I didn't get anywhere. But this time I felt strong."

"Great! But you know, Polly, the pillow is just a technique. It's not how well you perform at it that matters. What matters is, now that you feel the strength of your anger, how are you going to use it to help yourself?"

"You know," she says, "I think I could probably get in touch with WASC now. I feel like maybe I can handle this after all."

"I'm sure you can, Polly."

Polly and I smile at each other. Looking in her eyes, I can see her affection for me. I hope that she can see mine for her.

She glances at the clock and, in a second, she is sitting up and back to her normal consciousness. As she gathers her belongings, preparing to leave, I ask her to appreciate herself for something she did in the session. She groans a little with displeasure. Self-appreciations are a chore for her, as they are for most of my clients.

"Okay. Let's see . . . I was able to really feel my anger and get most of it out . . . and I talked to you about being a cocktease even though it embarrassed the shit out of me!" She throws back her head and laughs.

As we are standing up together, I ask her, on a scale of one to ten, how much does she really *feel* her self-appreciations? Polly answers seven. I remind her that last time it was only four.

"Terrific! You're coming up in the world!" I say, as we give each other a parting hug and say our good-bys.

A Final Word to Therapists and Clients

It has been observed that some of the most theoretically knowledgeable and expertly trained therapists are singularly unimpressive in helping others change; while some people with little or no training seem to have an innate gift for being therapeutically beneficial to others. Why should this be so? While I make no claims to a complete answer to this question, I would suggest that a crucial part of the answer has to do with the therapist's capacity for compassion. Without compassion, it is unlikely that therapy of any description can be lastingly helpful to anyone. If you have ever been a therapy patient, you know how much of its benefit derives from the feeling that your therapist is someone who empathizes with what you feel, understands who you are, and still seems to care about you. In experiencing the compassion of the therapist, the client learns to love herself. This is especially important for women who have learned, through internalizing this society's misogyny, to hate themselves. A new approach to therapy—for men and women—must replace traditional therapy's emphasis on the therapist's distance, with an unwavering appreciation of the crucial importance of the therapist's compassion.

What do I mean by compassion? Like so many words in our culture, compassion is a degraded word. It has come to mean "pity" or "sympathy." But strictly speaking, compassion and pity are opposite emotions. Pity is something one feels for someone "pathetic," not worthy of respect. It is a distancing emotion. To pity someone is to say to oneself: "I am not like you. I feel sorry for you, because you are in such bad shape, whereas I am not."

Compassion, by contrast, grows out of a deep experience of *connection* to others, an experience of what binds us together as persons in a similar social—and human—condition. It is the opposite of a distancing emotion. It is an embracing emotion. Compassion includes sympathy, but is more than sympathy. It is a respectful opening to the other person. It includes also a knowledge about the sources of suffering. It is not simply a feeling; it is a manner of making contact with a person in a way that dissolves the ordinary illusions of separateness.

Compassion is essentially a form of nonconditional love. Yet "love" itself has become a four-letter word in our society, a word referring to a kind of romantic sadomasochism, or infantile greediness; or used as a synonym for sex.

The traditional approach to therapy is not exempt from this cultural distortion of the word "love." As we have seen, love is not a word that appears in the psychiatric lexicon. If mentioned at all, it is considered a taboo—a "countertransference" problem of the therapist who "overidentifies with the patient," and who has therefore lost the necessary distance to do therapeutic work. Or it is seen as the countertransference problem of the therapist who wishes to (or does) seduce his patient. Love in psychiatry is what it is in the larger culture: power confused with sexuality. For this reason, traditional therapy correctly shuns the sharing of this kind of love between patient and therapist.

Traditional therapy is rightly suspicious of any emotion on the part of the therapist that is likely to infringe upon or manipulate the patient. But the fact that love is seen as such an emotion grows out of a particularly male conception of identity, love, and relationships. The proper professional distance required of the therapist is thought to be contingent upon the therapist's denial of feeling for the patient. Therapeutic expertise, in this sense, is seen as a kind of control: both self-control and control over the patient. It is supposed that the therapist who loves his patient has lost control of himself and of her. He thus either lays himself open to her manipulations, or else manipulates her with his feelings, or both.*

But the love I am talking about does not compromise one's ability to be of service to another. It is neither a way of manipulating nor of being manipulated. It is actually the opposite: a basic respect for the freedom of the other person. Therapists who do not feel this respect, or who do not like their patients as people, should not be working with them. Many cases of therapy failures are due to the simple, but often ignored, fact that the therapists in these cases have no positive feelings for their patients. Patients invariably pick this up and end up feeling like meal tickets instead of people. No amount of therapeutic technique or expertise will work in these cases: the relationship simply never gets off the ground.

Just as no therapy can be successful without the strength of the therapist's compassion, so no therapy can be successful without the strength of the client's will to change. The importance of nurturing this power in therapy is all the more important in the case of the female client—or any client who is socially oppressed. The power of the client starts with her capacity to choose the therapist that she feels will be most beneficial to her.

In the new model of therapy presented in these pages, I have had a female therapist and a female client in mind. How necessary is it for women clients to find women therapists? Certainly, some women have been helped by some male therapists. And having a female therapist does not guarantee that a woman will get the help she needs. The traditional approach to therapy is destructive to female clients, whether the therapist is a man or a woman. And it is theoretically possible for men to

---

* This way of viewing relationships, if exhibited by a patient, would be diagnosed as symptomatic of an obsessive-compulsive character disorder. The confusion of love, control, and manipulation is striking. It is a confusion actually endemic to a masculine form of identity as it is culturally conditioned. Given the rigid ego boundaries of male individualism, losing one's control is very threatening to a male sense of identity. It appears to be dangerous, to entail the risk of being swallowed up in emotions.

become "feminist" therapists. To do so, they would have to start with an honest exploration of how male society and male-style therapy has oppressed women. They would have to be motivated by a strong desire to learn about this process from women themselves—including women clients. I will not venture to guess how many male therapists are especially interested in this project. But I believe that presently, with rare exceptions, help for women in therapy must come from women therapists who have adopted a feminist approach to women and therapy.

At the same time, I believe that the model of therapy presented here can and does work successfully with male clients. The essential ingredient of this approach—an understanding of the social origins of people's emotional pain—is especially applicable to men in the lower classes, who share some of the features of Victim psychology I have examined. A knowledge of how the system of male domination thwarts, distorts, and cripples the emotional lives of men of all classes is indeed essential to working with male clients. This is not a matter of indoctrination into feminism, but of helping men come to grips with how their own sexism works against them and the women in their lives. In my own experience, male clients are usually greatly relieved to know that they are not expected to keep up a male "front" in therapy and that the therapist does not expect them to exhibit a male standard of mental health. (But this is the subject for another book.)

As a last word to women in therapy or looking for a therapist, I urge you to consider your rights as a client: to have a therapist who shows you the basic respect you deserve and who is accountable for his or her part of the therapeutic relationship. While it is generally thought wise for prospective therapygoers to inquire about the professional credentials of the therapist, it is not common for clients to check out the therapist's orientation toward women and therapy. Many therapists would regard this as a hostile challenge to their expertise. I believe that women in therapy today must challenge their therapists in these and other ways.

Many clients who start out in therapy feel uneasy about

their therapist but decide that this is a sign of their own neurosis or illness. Certainly, it is common to feel somewhat distrustful in the beginning, to be cautious about what you're getting into. Given the state of the art of therapy, I would suggest that this caution is not misplaced. But it is not enough to be cautious: the point is to find out just what you're getting into in as clear a way as you can. If you are investing your psyche and your money in therapy, you have a right and a responsibility to find out what your therapist is up to and why. And this means talking to your therapist and asking how he or she sees you as a woman, and functions in the therapy process. If I were to offer any advice in this matter, it would be to trust your judgment and your intuitions. A small feeling of unease at the start of something new is not the same as an overwhelming message that this person or this approach to therapy is not for you. In many cases, this may not necessarily be a fault of the therapy or therapist, but simply a reflection of the fact that not all therapists and all clients are a good match. Some therapists work very well with some clients and not others. And vice versa.

Do not be afraid to ask a prospective therapist if he or she will give you a free first session in which you can both meet and decide if you want to proceed. Some therapists will be responsive to this idea of an introductory meeting, even if they have never done it before. It is always wise to "shop around" for a therapist. You can also start therapy with a four- to six-week trial run to see how it works—or doesn't. In that time, your initial questions about therapy should be answered and your initial caution should begin to diminish. If it doesn't, you and your therapist should talk about what's wrong. How much of your distrust is something you would have to work out with *any* therapist, and how much of it is related to a profound conviction that this is not the therapy or therapist for you? Trust yourself.

The question of how you intuitively feel about the therapy you're in is also crucial when that therapy does not seem to be working. At such times, just as your therapist may ask what's going on inside you that is causing the impasse, so you both need to examine what about the therapy approach itself or about the therapist's attitudes may be contributing to the problem. A responsible therapist should be open to these questions, and to examining his or her contribution to the relationship called therapy. If he or she is not, that tells you something important about who has the power in the relationship, and should be a clue as to how you're being treated in general.

In many cases, dissatisfactions with therapy are related to unrealistic goals or fantasies about what therapy can do, or to transference feelings from the past. But in many cases, they are *also* related to the limitations of the therapy approach or the therapist or both. At such times, you may have a legitimate gripe which has no legitimate outlet—for, as we have seen, client criticisms of traditional therapy are routinely "interpreted." While the issues involved in therapeutic impasses are usually quite complex, such impasses are often a combined result of the feelings of both the therapist and the client. The therapist who claims no responsibility for the relationship is not likely to be responsive to your needs at this time.*

The final right of any therapy client is the right to walk out of therapy. If you find that therapy is consistently unproductive, then it may be time to quit. This is especially true if you've talked the impasse over with your therapist and still nothing changes after a period of time. Many therapists would no doubt regard this last bit of advice as an invitation to patient "resistance." A healthy resistance to the failures of traditional and humanist therapies is not, as far as I'm concerned, a neurotic problem but a sign of increasing strength. Woman as Patient deserves the best help possible. To get it, you sometimes have to fight for it.

If this book has helped give you the courage to do so, it will have served its purpose.

---

* On the few occasions when I have not been able to quickly resolve a therapeutic impasse with a client, I have sometimes called in a "neutral" third party—that is, another therapist who is there to help the client and myself reach an understanding. This can be very effective if both client and therapist are willing to suspend their roles.

Notes

Introduction to the Second Edition

1. The phrase is from Nelle Morton, "The Rising of Women's Consciousness in a Male Language Structure," *Andover Newton Quarterly* 12, No. 4 (March 1972), pp. 177-190.

2. For an overview of the feminist challenge to Family Therapy, see Betty Carter, "Stonewalling Feminism," in the *Family Therapy Networker* (Jan./Feb., 1992). See also Demaris Wehr, *Jung and Feminism: Liberating Archetypes* (Boston: Beacon Press, 1987) for a feminist critique and re-visioning of Jungian psychology.

3. Phyllis Chesler, *Women and Madness* (New York: Doubleday, 1972), and Jean Baker Miller, *Toward A New Psychology of Women* (Boston: Beacon Press, 1976).

4. Anne Kent Rush and Anica Mander's radical *Feminism as Therapy* (New York: Random House, 1974) and Elizabeth Friar William's liberal approach to feminism in *Notes of a Feminist Therapist* (New York: Praeger Publishers, 1976), were the only two trade books published in the U.S. on the subject of feminist therapy before the publication of *A New Approach to Women and Therapy*. An excellent anthology published in Canada in 1975 by Press Gang Publishers was *Women Look at Psychiatry*, edited by Dorothy E. Smith and Sara J. David. The only textbook was Susan Sturdivant's *Therapy With Women* (New York: Springer, 1980). There were some noteworthy books that had emerged from the anti-psychiatry movement of the 1960s and 70s, including one by Hogie Wyckoff that focused on women, called *Solving Women's Problems* (New York: Grove Press Inc., 1977). In the past decade, the literature on feminist psychology and psychotherapy has become enriched, including: Carol Gilligan's *In a Different Voice: Psychological Theory and Women's Development* (Cambridge: Harvard University Press, 1983); Judith V. Jordan, Alexandra G. Kaplan, Jean Baker Miller, Irene P. Stiver, and Janet L. Surrey, *Women's Growth in Connection: Writings from the Stone Center* (New York: Guilford Press, 1991); Toni Ann Laidlaw, Cheryl Malmo and Associates, *Healing Voices: Feminist Approaches to Therapy With Women* (San Francisco: Jossey-Bass Publishers, 1990); Luise Eichenbaum and Susie Orbach, *What Do Women Want: Exploding the Myth of Dependency* (New York: Coward-McCann, Inc., 1983); Marjorie Braude, editor of *Women, Power and Therapy* (New York: Harrington Park Press, 1988); Harriet Goldhor Lerner, *Women In Therapy* (Northvale, NJ.: Jason Aronson, Inc., 1988); Carol Josephowitz Siegel, ed. *Women Changing Therapy* (New York: Haworth Press, Inc., 1986); Doris Howard, *The Dynamics of Feminist Therapy* (New

York: Haworth Press, Inc., 1987). Journals devoted to this area include: *Women and Therapy, A Feminist Quarterly* published by Haworth Press and *The Journal of Feminist Family Therapy.*

5. See Jordan, et. al., *Women's Growth in Connection: Writings from the Stone Center,* ibid., for a collection of some of these papers.

6. See the special issue on "Diversity and Complexity in Feminist Therapy," Part I in *Women and Therapy: A Feminist Quarterly,* ed. by Laura S. Brown and Maria P. Root (Volume 9, No. 1/2, 1990) and also, Part II (Volume 9, No. 3, 1990).

7. For statistics on woman-battering, see Patricia Nealon's three-part series on battered women in the Boston Globe (May 31, June 1-2, 1992). For rape statistics, see Carolyn Skorneck's "683,000 Women Raped in 1990, New Government Study Finds," reported in the Boston Globe (April 24, 1992). See also, the classic by Susan Brownmiller, *Against Our Will: Men, Women and Rape* (New York: Bantam Books, 1975) and ed. Jill Radford and Diana Russell, *Femicide: The Politics of Woman Killing* (New York: Twayne Publisher, 1992).

8. See Susan Faludi, *Backlash: The Undeclared War Against American Women* (New York: Anchor Books, Doubleday, 1991), for an excellent study of the pervasive backlash in this country.

9. A decade ago there were a few confessional books about childhood sexual abuse such as Katherine Brady's *Father's Days: A True Story of Incest* (New York, Dell: 1979) and Michelle Morris, *If I Should Die Before I Wake* (New York: Dell, 1982); as well as the classics by Sandra Butler, *Conspiracy of Silence: The Trauma of Incest* (San Francisco: Volcano Press, 1982) and Florence Rush, *The Best Kept Secret: Sexual Abuse of Children* (Englewood Cliffs, N.J.: Prentice-Hall, 1980). Judith Herman's *Father-Daughter Incest* (Cambridge: Harvard University Press, 1981) had just come out when this book was in its final stages. The landmark self-help book by Ellen Bass and Laura Davis, *The Courage to Heal* (New York: Harper and Row) did not emerge until 1988.

10. Freud's Oedipal theory, considered the cornerstone of psychoanalysis, was in fact based on his denial of the earlier discovery of sexual violence as the trauma that caused female neurosis. Rather than facing up to the widespread sexual violence of respectable male relatives of his female patients (or to the implications of this fact for Victorian society as a whole—not to mention the possible negative effects for his career of exposing this sexual violence), Freud resorted to the idea that women who claimed to be abused by male relatives were in fact suffering from an unconscious wish to be seduced by them. This "theory"—which is really Freud's own fantasy—then became the blame-the-victim legacy for all women in psychoanalysis and psychoanalytic psychotherapy from then on. For the definitive expose of all this, written by a psychoanalytic insider, see Jeffrey Moussaieff Masson, *The Assault on Truth: Freud's Suppression of the Seduction Theory* (New York: Atheneum, 1984).

11. For the feminist classic about incest, see Judith Lewis Herman, *Father-Daughter Incest,* ibid.

12. Because of feminist protest, the American Psychiatric Association did not succeed in listing Masochistic Personality Disorder and Premenstrual Dysphoric Disorder as bona fide diagnoses. Instead, these appeared, re-named as Self-defeating Personality Disorder, and Late Luteal Phase Dysphoric Disorder (!) in an appendix designed to alert diagnosticians and researchers to "proposed diagnostic categories needing further study." See the *Desk Reference to the Diagnostic Criteria from DSM-III-R* (published by the American Psychiatric Association, 1987), pp. 213-217. See also Susan Faludi, *Backlash* (ibid., p. 356-362) for an account of the psychiatric diagnostic backlash.

13. See the classics by Lenore Walker, *The Battered Woman* (New York: Harper and Row, 1979), and The Battered Woman Syndrome (New York: Springer Publicaitons, 1984).

14. From the *Desk Reference to the Diagnostic Criteria from the DSM-III-R*, ibid., p. 146.

15. On the contrary, the psychoanalytic establishment merely shot the messenger who brought the unwelcome news. The shocker, *The Assault on Truth: Freud's Suppression of the Seduction Theory*, which definitively exposed the foundational flaw of Freudian psychoanalysis by destroying the credibility of Freud's Oedipal Theory, was written by a highly credentialized bona fide psychoanalyst, a member of the International Psychoanalytic Association, and Projects Director of the Sigmund Freud Archives. No radical feminist, he! Nevertheless, he was hardly greeted with the neutral impartiality prized by psychoanalysts. Rather than take him seriously, the psychoanalytic profession did to Jeffrey Moussaieff Masson what my own supervisors did to me in my psychology training whenever I raised any questions about psychoanalytic theory: they analyzed his motives for raising the issues in the first place, cleverly pathologizing him as they would anyone they regard as a "patient." For a provocative critique of therapy in general (which asserts that all therapy implies some kind of emotional authoritarianism) see Masson's *Against Therapy: Emotional Tyranny and the Myth of Psychological Healing* (New York: Atheneum, 1988).

16. From Charles L. Whitfield, *Healing the Child Within* (Deerfield Beach, Florida: Health Communications Inc., 1987). See also Melanie Beattie, *Co-Dependent No More!* (New York: Harper Collins, 1987).

17. Words from a talk on co-dependence given at Interface in Boston.

18. Joanna Macy, *Despair and Personal Power in the Nuclear Age* (Philadelphia, Pa.: New Society Publishers, 1983).

19. Sally Miller Gearhart, "The Future—If There Is One—Is Female," in *Reweaving the Web of Life: Feminism and Nonviolence*, ed. by Pam McAllister (Philadelphia Pa.: New Society Publishers, 1982).

20. See Miriam Greenspan, "A Social-Spiritual Model for Feminist Therapy" in *A New Creation: America's Contemporary Spiritual Voices*, ed. by Roger S. Gottlieb (New York: Crossroad, 1990).

21. See *Desk Reference to the DSM-III-R*, ibid., p. 191.

22. A popular book in this area is Joan Borysenko's *Guilt is the Teacher, Love is the Lesson*. (New York: Warner Books, 1991). An excellent journal for those in the helping professions who are interested in exploring the interface between psychotherapy and spirituality is *Common Boundary: Between Spirituality and Psychotherapy*, published in Bethesda, Maryland.

23. For a more complete discussion of this work, see my forthcoming book, *Healing Through the Dark Emotions: Finding the Gifts in Grief, Fear, Anger and Despair*.

24. I am indebted to the ongoing support, creativity, and encouragement of the Global Psychotherapy Group in Boston, which has shared many of my questions and doubts about psychotherapy, as well as many of my hopes for its best uses, while working together on a new paradigm of psychology and psychotherapy that connects the personal and the global. In May, 1991, we offered a course, "Toward A New Model of Psychotherapy: Connecting the Personal and the Global" at the Massachusetts School of Professional Psychology. The course was also sponsored by the Center for Psychological Studies in the Nuclear Age/Harvard Medical School at the Cambridge Hospital. The papers given at this course are examples of the inspired work going on today in this area: Sarah Conn, "The Self-World Connection: Recontextualizing Personal Pain," Janet Surrey, "Mutuality in Psychotherapy: Towards a Global Paradigm," Mary Watkins, "From Individualism to the Interdependent Self: Changing the Paradigm of Self in Psychotherapy," Anne Yeomans, "In Search of a Dialogue that Heals," and Miriam Greenspan, "Healing Through the Dark Emotions: Self/Society/Spirit." See also Theodore Roszak, *The Voice of the Earth* (New York: Simon and Schuster, 1992).

25. See Joanna Macy, *World As Lover, World As Self* (Berkley: Parallax Press, 1991) for an extraordinary compendium of essays on the theme of connecting personal and global pain for the sake of healing the planet.

26. For a beautiful discussion of this idea, see Patricia Reis, *Through the Goddess: A Woman's Way of Healing* (New York: Continuum, 1991).

27. For some important works on the Dark Goddess, see the fascinating book by Vicki Noble, *Shakti Woman: Feeling Our Fire, Healing Our World/The New Female Shamanism* (Harper San Francisco, 1991); the chapter "Facing Medusa: The Shadow Sister"in Patricia Reis, ibid.; and China Galland, *Longing for Darkness: Tara and the Black Madonna* (New York: Viking, 1990).

28. The literature of women's spirituality today is a wonderful cornucopia to dip into. I include here only some of my favorites: ed. Charlene Spretnak, *The Politics of Women's Spirituality: Essays on the Rise of Spiritual Power Within the Feminist Movement* (New York: Anchor Books, 1982) and *States of Grace: The Recovery of Meaning in the Postmodern Age* (Harper San Francisco, 1991); Starhawk, *The Spiral Dance: The Rebirth of the Ancient Religion of the Greek Goddess* (San Francisco: Harper and Row, 1979) and *Dreaming the Dark: Magic, Sex and Politics* (Boston: Beacon Press, 1982); ed. Judith Plaskow and Carol P. Christ, *Weaving the Visions: New Patterns in Feminist Spirituality* (San Francisco: Harper and Row, 1989); Christine Downing, *The Goddess: Mythological Images of the Feminine* (New York: Crossroad, 1990); Merlin Stone, *When God was a Woman* (New York: Harcourt, Brace, Jovanovich, 1976); Vicki Noble, *Shakti Woman Feeling Our Fire, Healing Our World: The New Female Shamanism* (Harper San Francisco, 1991); Patricia Reis, *Through the Goddess: A Woman's Way of Healing* (New York: Continuum, 1991); Riane Eisler, *The Chalice and the Blade: Our History, Our Future* (San Francisco: Harper and Row, 1987); and Elinor W. Gadon, *The Once and Future Goddess* (Harper San Francisco, 1989). For the relationship between women's spirituality and environmental healing, see ed. Judith Plant, *Healing the Wounds: The Promise of Ecofeminism* (Philadelphia, Pa.: New Society Publishers, 1989); and ed. Irene Diamond and Gloria Feman Orenstein, *Reweaving the World: The Emergence of Ecofeminism* (San Francisco: Sierra Club Books, 1990).

Chapter 1

1. For statistics documenting the utilization of mental health facilities by men and women, see S. B. Sobel and N. F. Russo, "Sex Differences in Utilization of Mental Health Facilities," distributed by the American Psychological Association, Washington. D.C.; and "Characteristics of Admissions to Selected Mental Health Facilities, 1975; An Annotated Book of Charts and Tables" (Washington, D.C.: National Institute of Mental Health).

2. D. M. Broverman, I. K. Broverman, F. Clarkson, P. Rosenkrantz, and S. Vogel, "Sex-role Stereotypes and Clinical Judgments of Mental Health," *Journal of Consulting and Clinical Psychology* 34 (1970), 1-7.

3. *Diagnostic and Statistical Manual of Mental Disorders*, 2nd ed. (Washington, D.C., American Psychiatric Association, 1968), Diagnosis #301.6, p. 43.

4. M. Harvey Brenner, *Mental Illness and the Economy* (Cambridge, Mass.: Harvard University Press, 1973).

5. R. D. Laing, *The Divided Self* (London: Penguin Books, 1965), p. 36.

6. For some studies of the importance of the therapist's empathy and supportiveness as vital ingredients necessary to the success of therapy, see C. B. Truax and R. R. Carkhuff, *Toward Effective Counseling and Psychotherapy: Training and Practice* (Chicago: Aldine, 1967); R. R. Carkhuff and B. G. Berenson, *Beyond Counseling and Psychotherapy* (New York: Holt, Rinehart and Winston, 1967); and C. R. Rogers, "The

Necessary and Sufficient Conditions of Therapeutic Personality Change," *Journal of Consulting Psychology* 21 (1957); 95-103.

7. Sigmund Freud, *Dora: An Analysis of a Case of Hysteria* (New York: Collier Books, 1974), p. 142.

Chapter 2

1. The first of these research studies was conducted by H. J. Eysenck ("The Effects of Psychotherapy; An Evaluation," *Journal of Consulting Psychology 16* (1952): 319-324). Eysenck's study showed that of patients who received psychoanalysis, the improvement rate was 44 percent; of those who received psychotherapy, the improvement rate was 64 percent; and of those who received no treatment at all, the improvement rate was 72 percent. Since Eysenck's classic study, the research has upheld his conclusions that therapy is no better and often worse than no therapy for the cure of neurosis. See F. Barron and T. Leary, "Changes in Psychotherapy Patients with and without Psychotherapy," *Journal of Consulting Psychology 19* (1955): 239-245; A. E. Bregin, "The Effects of Psychotherapy: Negative Results Revisited," *Journal of Consulting Psychology 10* (1963): 244-250; R. D. Cartwright and J. L. Vogel, "A Comparison of Changes in Psychoneurotic Patients during Matched Periods of Therapy and No Therapy," *Journal of Consulting Psychology 24* (1960): 121-127.

2. *A Psychiatric Glossary* (Washington, D.C. American Psychiatric Association, 1967).

3. *Diagnostic and Statistical Manual*, Diagnosis #301.4, p. 43.

4. Ibid., Diagnosis #301.5, p. 43.

5. R. D. Laing, *The Politics of Experience* (New York: Ballantine Books, 1967), p. 53.

Chapter 3

1. Phyllis Chesler, *Women and Madness* (New York: Doubleday, 1972), p. 108.

2. For a feminist critique of Freudian and psychoanalytic theories of women, see Kate Millett, *Sexual Politics* (New York: Doubleday, 1970), pp. 179-210; Shulamith Firestone, *The Dialectic of Sex* (New York: Bantam Books, 1971) pp. 41-71; and Betty Friedan, *The Feminine Mystique* (New York: Dell, 1963) pp. 95-116.

3. J. Robert Wilson, Clayton T. Beecham, Elsie Reid Carrington, eds., *Obstetrics and Gynecology* (St. Louis: C. V. Mosby Co., 1963), pp. 47-48.

Chapter 6

1. For a good overview of Rogers's humanist approach to psychotherapy, see Carl R. Rogers, *On Becoming a Person: A Therapist's View of Psychotherapy* (Boston: Houghton Mifflin Company, 1970).

2. Frederick S. Perls, *Gestalt Therapy Verbatim* (New York: Bantam Books, 1972).

Chapter 7

1. Carl Rogers, "The Necessary and Sufficient Conditions of Therapeutic Personality Change," *Journal of Consulting Psychology* 21 (1957), 95-103.

2. Elizabeth Friar Williams, *Notes of a Feminist Therapist* (New York: Praeger Publishers, 1976), p. 187.

3. Ibid., p. 9.

4. Ibid., p. 60.

5. For an economic analysis of women as a "sex class," see Ann Ferguson, "Women as a New Revolutionary Class," in Pat Walker, ed., *Between Labor and Capital* (Boston: South End Press. 1979), pp. 279-309.

Chapter 9

1. See Andrea Dworkin, *Woman Hating* (New York: E. P. Dutton, 1974).

2. See Susan Brownmiller, *Against Our Will* (New York: Bantam Books, 1976).

3. *Diagnostic and Statistical Manual*, Diagnosis #301.82, p. 44.

4. For a fine, detailed account of the socioeconomic relation between the nuclear family and the capitalist workplace, and between the domination of women by men and that of workers by bosses, see Sheila Rowbotham, *Woman's Consciousness, Man's World* (London: Penguin Books, 1973).

5. Ibid., p. 35.

6. Chesler, *Women and Madness*, pp. 39-40.

7. Thomas S. Szasz, *The Myth of Mental Illness*, quoted in Chesler, *Women and Madness*, pp. 40-41.

8. For a wonderful history of the ideological context of feminine disorders and illnesses, see Barbara Ehrenreich and Deirdre English, *For Her Own Good* (New York: Anchor Press, 1978).

9. For some lucid analyses of women's work in patriarchal capitalism, see Rowbotham, *Woman's Consciousness, Man's World*; Jean Gardiner, "Women's Domestic Labor," in Zillah Eisenstein, ed., *Capitalist Patriarchy and the Case of Socialist Feminism* (New York: Monthly Review Press, 1979); Ann Ferguson and Nancy Folbre, "The Unhappy Marriage of Patriarchy and Capitalism," in Lydia Sargent, ed., *Women and Revolution* (Boston: South End Press, 1981); and Heidi Hartmann, "The Family as the Locus of Gender, Class and Political Struggle: The Example of Housework," in *Signs 6*, No. 3 (Spring 1981).

10. Jean Baker Miller, *Toward a New Psychology of Women* (Boston: Beacon Press, 1976), p. 72.

11. Ibid., p. 83.

12. Dorothy E. Smith and Sara J. David, eds., *Women Look at Psychiatry* (Vancouver: Press Gang Publishers, 1975).

13. See Eli Zaretsky, *Capitalism, the Family and Personal Life* (New York: Harper & Row/Harper Colophon Books, 1976).

14. Rowbotham, *Woman's Consciousness, Man's World*, p. 77.

Chapter 10

1. See Andrea Dworkin, *Pornography: Men Possessing Women* (New York: G. P. Putnam, 1979), p. 103.

2. For an interesting account of these conflicts in working-class identity, see Richard Sennett and Jonathan Cobb, *The Hidden Injuries of Class* (New York: Vintage Books, 1972).

Index

socioeconomic subordination and, 205–209

symptoms of femininity and, 182–205

Victorian ideology, 15

Violence against women, 168

Wageless labor of women, 208–209, 222, 225–226

Wechsler Adult Intelligence Scale, 58

Williams, Elizabeth Friar, 135–138, 141

Witches, persecution of, 165–166

Woman as Body, 161–182

(*See also* Body, woman as)

Woman as Patient, 88–91, 123

(*See also* Patient, woman as)

Woman as Victim, 103–106

(*See also* Victim psychology)

Women: changing, 97–98

domination by men, 34, 94

feminine, 94–96

Freudian definition, 89–90, 92

liberated, 98–102

(*See also* "Liberated Woman")

masculinity complex, 89

normal womanhood, 89–98

rebellion against, 94–95

traditional therapy and, 87–102

wageless labor of, 208–209, 222, 225–226

Women and Madness (Chesler), xxii, 87, 184–185

Women-oriented therapy, 33–38, 232–315

goal of, 36–37

model of, vii–viii, 37, 232–252

(*See also* Feminist therapy)

Women's movement, xxiii

career choices and, 136–138

consciousness-raising and, 232

rage at society and, 301–302

sex role differences and, 34, 141–143

Women's rights, 101

Work: role of men and women, 228–231

women's wageless labor, 208–209, 222, 225–226

Work force, women in, 206–207

Working housewife and mother, 22–23, 222

conflict between mothering and work, 138–141

economic condition of, 206–209